Locking Plates in
Veterinary Orthopedics

Locking Plates in Veterinary Orthopedics

Edited by

Matthew D. Barnhart, DVM, MS
Diplomate American College
of Veterinary Surgeons

Karl C. Maritato, DVM
Diplomate American College
of Veterinary Surgeons

WILEY Blackwell

ACVS®
FOUNDATION

This edition first published 2019

This work is a co-publication between the American College of Veterinary Surgeons Foundation and Wiley-Blackwell.

Registered Office
John Wiley & Sons, Inc., 111 River Street, Hoboken, NJ 07030, USA

Editorial Office
111 River Street, Hoboken, NJ 07030, USA

For details of our global editorial offices, customer services, and more information about Wiley products, visit us at www.wiley.com.

Wiley also publishes its books in a variety of electronic formats and by print-on-demand. Some content that appears in standard print versions of this book may not be available in other formats.

Library of Congress Cataloging-in-Publication Data

Names: Barnhart, Matthew D., 1969– editor. | Maritato, Karl C., 1979– editor.
Title: Locking plates in veterinary orthopedics / edited by Matthew D. Barnhart, Karl C. Maritato.
Description: Hoboken, NJ : Wiley-Blackwell, 2019. | Series: Advances in veterinary surgery | Includes bibliographical references and index. |
Identifiers: LCCN 2018024348 (print) | LCCN 2018025478 (ebook) | ISBN 9781119380160 (Adobe PDF) | ISBN 9781119380115 (ePub) | ISBN 9781119380122 (hardback)
Subjects: LCSH: Veterinary orthopedics. | MESH: Orthopedic Procedures–veterinary | Bone Plates–veterinary | Prostheses and Implants–veterinary
Classification: LCC SF910.5 (ebook) | LCC SF910.5 .L63 2019 (print) | NLM SF 910.5 | DDC 636.089/67–dc23
LC record available at https://lccn.loc.gov/2018024348

Cover Design: Wiley
Cover Image: © Matthew D. Barnhart

Set in 9.5/11.5pt Palatino by SPi Global, Pondicherry, India

MIX
Paper from responsible sources
FSC
www.fsc.org
FSC® C013604

Contents

List of Contributors

Boaz Arzi, DVM, Diplomate AVDC, EVDC
Associate professor of Dentistry and
Oral Surgery
Surgical and Radiological Sciences
School of Veterinary Medicine
University of California, Davis
One Garrod Drive
Davis, CA 95616, USA

Matthew D. Barnhart, DVM, MS, Diplomate ACVS
Surgery specialty leader
MedVet Medical & Cancer Centers for Pets
300 E. Wilson Bridge Rd
Worthington, OH 43085, USA

Kevin P. Benjamino, DVM, Diplomate ACVS
MedVet Medical and Cancer Centers for Pets
300 East Wilson Bridge Road
Worthington, OH 43085, USA

Mary Sarah Bergh, DVM, MS, Diplomate ACVS, ACVSMR
Affiliate associate professor
Department of Veterinary Clinical Sciences
Iowa State University College of Veterinary
Medicine, 1809 S. Riverside Dr.
Ames, IA 50011, USA

Adam H. Biedrzycki, BVSc, PhD, Diplomate ACVS, ECVS, MRCVS
Assistant professor
College of Veterinary Medicine
Department of Large Animal Clinical Sciences
2015 SW 16th Ave
Gainesville, FL 32610, USA

Kenneth A. Bruecker, DVM, MS, Diplomate ACVS, ACVSMR
Founder/director
Continuing Orthopedic Veterinary
Education (COVE)
Ventura County, CA, USA

Jessica A. Dahlberg, DVM, MS, Diplomate ACVS – LA
Staff surgeon
Bend Veterinary Specialists and Emergency
Center, 1245 SE 3rd St C3
Bend, OR 97702, USA

Noel Fitzpatrick, MVB, DUniv CVR, DSAS(Orth), MRCVS, Diplomate ACVSMR
RCVS specialist in small animal surgery
(orthopedics)
Director Fitzpatrick Referrals, Fitzbionics &
FitzRegen;
Professor of Veterinary Orthopaedics
University of Surrey Surrey, UK

Janik C. Gasiorowski, VMD, Diplomate ACVS
Department of Surgery
The Mid-Atlantic Equine Medical Center
P.O. Box 188, 40 Frontage Rd.
Ringoes, NJ 08551, USA

Tomás Guerrero, PD Dr. med. vet., Diplomate ECVS
Professor of small animal surgery
St. George's University, School of Veterinary
Medicine
True Blue, Grenada, West Indies

Reunan P. Guillou, DVM, Diplomate ACVS
Orthopedic surgeon
ACCESS Bone & Joint Center
9599 Washington Blvd.
Culver City, California, 90232, USA

Laurent P. Guiot, DVM, Diplomate ACVS, ECVS
Orthopedic surgeon
ACCESS Bone & Joint Center
ACCESS Specialty Animal Hospitals
9599 Washington Blvd.
Culver City, CA, USA

Kei Hayashi, DVM, PhD, Diplomate ACVS, JCVS
Associate professor
Cornell University
College of Veterinary Medicine
930 Campus Rd
Ithaca, NY 14853, USA

Bianca F. Hettlich, Dr. med. vet., Diplomate ACVS
Senior lecturer
Vetsuisse faculty
Department of Small Animal Surgery
Vetsuisse Faculty
Department of Small Animal Surgery
3012 Bern, Switzerland

Ian Gordon Holsworth, BVSc, Diplomate ACVS
Director of VetSurg
2859 Loma Vista Rd
Ventura, CA 93003, USA

Shawn C. Kennedy, DVM, Diplomate ACVS
MedVet Medical and Cancer Centers for Pets
300 East Wilson Bridge Road
Worthington, OH 43085, USA

Karl C. Maritato, DVM, Diplomate ACVS
Cincinnati & Dayton Surgery Departments Representative
MedVet Medical & Cancer Centers for Pets
3964 Red Bank Rd
Fairfax, OH 45227, USA

David R. Mason, B vet. med. (Hons), MRCVS, Diplomate ACVS, ECVS, ACVSMR
Chief of Staff
Las Vegas Veterinary Specialty Center
8650 W Tropicana Avenue, Suite B 107
Las Vegas, Nevada 89147, USA

Noël M.M. Moens, DVM, MSc, Diplomate ACVS, ECVS
Associate professor
Department of Clinical Studies
Ontario Veterinary College
University of Guelph, Guelph, N1G 2W1
Ontario, Canada

Malcolm G. Ness, B vet. med., CertSAO, Diplomate ECVS, FRCVS
Consultant veterinary orthopaedic surgeon
Longframlington, Morpeth, Northumberland, NE65 8EB, UK

Massimo Petazzoni, DVM
Clinica Veterinaria Milano Sud
Orthopedic and Trauma department director
Via Liberazione 26
20068 Peschiera Borromeo (Milan), Italy

Fred Pike, DVM, Diplomate ACVS
Medical director
Veterinary Specialty Hospital of San Diego
by Ethos Veterinary Health
10435 Sorrento Valley Rd.
San Diego, CA 92121, USA

Antonio Pozzi, DMV, Diplomate ECVS, ACVS, ACVSMR
ACVS founding fellow, Minimally Invasive Surgery
Department for Small Animals
Winterthurerstrasse 258c
8057 Zurich, Switzerland

Philipp Schmierer, med. vet., Diplomate ECVS
Vetsuisse Faculty, University of Zurich
Klinik für Kleintierchirurgie
Winterthurerstrasse 260
CH-8057 Zurich, Switzerland

Frank J.M. Verstraete, Dr. med. vet., Diplomate AVDC, ECVS, EVDC
Professor of dentistry and oral surgery
Surgical and Radiological Sciences
School of Veterinary Medicine
University of California, Davis
One Garrod Drive, Davis, CA 95616, USA

Kirk L. Wendelburg, DVM, Diplomate ACVS
Medical director
VCA Animal Specialty Group
4641 Colorado Blvd.
Los Angeles, CA 90039, USA

Foreword

Within months of arriving at the AO Research Institute, Davos, Switzerland, in the spring of 1983, I learned how important the dynamic compression plate (DCP) was for the systematized teaching of internal fracture fixation, the worldwide dissemination of concepts supported by years of research and clinical observation, and the impressive business growth of AO-affiliated manufacturers. DCP was the most visible symbol of the AO Group's accomplishments throughout a historically unique synergy of research, education and industrial endeavors in the medical device field. Being eager to move research ahead, I decided to stay away from anything even closely related to DCP. It seemed beyond challenge and immune to change.

But, inevitably, changes were on the horizon. The dominance of plating in internal fixation was being challenged by the rapid acceptance of interlocking nailing, invented by Gross and Kamp and introduced by Howmedica. Perhaps even more threatening, patent protection for DCP was soon to expire. Copies were appearing in minor markets, testing AO willingness to protect its patent rights. The need for a next generation plate was clear. A number of ideas were put forward and were tested in the lab, in animals, and in human patients.

That the disturbance of blood perfusion was the dominant, unwanted side effect of plating was teased out of several key experimental animal studies. This work was performed at the AO Institute in the late 1970s and early 1980s by Stephan Perren, Institute director, and his collaborators Berton Rahn, Jacques Cordey, Ulrich Pfister, Emanuel Gautier, Mauro Vattolo, and Kaspar Joerger. Prior to that research project, sometimes-dramatic loss of cortical bone beneath the plates was fully attributed to stress shielding. Yet it turned out to be mostly due to a natural bone response to necrosis, the resorption of dead tissue.

These findings defined the major goal for the development of the next-generation plate: reduce the damage to periosteal bone perfusion. Collaboration on an unrelated project with Franz Sutter and Oscar Tchudin, two resourceful engineers at Straumann Institute, Waldenburg, Switzerland, got me started on what soon became FIXIN, a pilot project at the AO Institute aiming at complete avoidance of periosteal blood perfusion disturbance by eliminating the contact between the plate and the bone. Franz Sutter had also provided engineering talent to the THORP system of locking plates and screws for mandibular reconstruction, primarily after tumor resections. However, THORP lacked the strength and robustness needed for treatment of long bone fractures. The only other precedent known to us at the time was the Polish ZESPOL system, which has seen very limited acceptance due to practical limitations.

The FIXIN project tested a plate application on intact sheep tibia with bicortical screws locked to the plate by means of expandable, slotted inserts. These experiments provided convincing evidence that keeping the plate a millimeter or two above the periosteum can practically eliminate disturbance of periosteal perfusion. But, unexpectedly, the histology also showed bicortical screw damage to the endosteal perfusion. Replacing bicortical with monocortical screws eliminated the need for the troublesome, locking, slotted ball and, more significantly, reduced damage to the endosteal perfusion. When locked, monocortical screws provided fully adequate load transfer from the plate to the bone. The project took on a new name, PC-Fix (for point-contact fixator), and began its decade-long testing in the lab, in experimental animals and in clinical veterinary and human applications. With the privileged support of Stephan Perren, I devoted a significant percentage of my time to carrying the project forward with a long list of collaborators whose work was only partially acknowledged because of my failure to encourage and help them publish the results. They are, in alphabetic order: Stephan Arens, Stephen Bresina, Henk Eijer, Christian Foglar, Edward van Frank-Hasnoot, Mark Frankle, Robert Frigg, Maximilian Lederer, Urban Lidgren, Kurt Lippuner, Ted Micklau, Pierre Montavon, Keizo Morikawa, Miljenko Plavljanic, Marco Predieri, Andreas Remiger, and Alex Zehnder.

In spite of unusually positive outcomes of all the studies, in every respect considered, including a human clinical study with close to 2,000 forearm fractures, the ultimate decision by the AO industrial partners was to ignore the demands of the AO to make PC-Fix available.

In parallel with technical developments aimed at solving the problem of iatrogenic damage to the bone, there was a major revision, if not a revolution, in the surgical approach to internal fixation, which came to be known as biological internal fixation. The leaders of this movement, together with Stephan Perren, were Reinhold Ganz, Jeffrey Mast and Roland Jacob, the authors of the surgical manifesto for biological fixation *Planning and Reduction Technique in Fracture Surgery* published by Springer-Verlag in 1989. Failure of the AO and its affiliated producers to embrace and combine the emerging technical and surgical approaches was a major missed opportunity to provide better care for millions of trauma patients.

If the mechanical function of fracture stabilization is to be accomplished without plate-to-bone contact, the screws have to be locked to the plate. Locking the screws brings certain mechanical advantages, but the real goal is to preserve blood perfusion and thus reduce the risks of bone necrosis; infection being the most consequential. The goal of preserving bone perfusion has been lost in the intervening years as locking plates gained acceptance in both human and veterinary surgery. The message from more than a decade of experimental work on hundreds of animals – "keep the bone perfused" – has morphed into a much weaker one – "lock the screws." As a consequence, most locking systems have not been designed to prevent iatrogenic damage to fractured bones.

As witnessed by the appearance of this book dedicated to a variety of locking plates, the veterinary scene has profited from being unconstrained by ever-tighter regulation imposed on the human side and, perhaps, even more importantly, less affected by consolidation of the industry. The editors and the authors of this book are giving their veterinary colleagues a wonderful opportunity to inform themselves of the choices available, the appropriate indications, the techniques and the fairly extensive clinical experience with locking plates.

Slobodan Tepic
Zurich, June 2018

Preface

The American College of Veterinary Surgeons Foundation is excited to present *Locking Plates in Veterinary Orthopedics* in the book series entitled *Advances in Veterinary Surgery*. I know many of us that have incorporated locking plate technology into our clinical practice are still unsure as to "best practices" when using locking implants in a particular fracture or osteotomy scenario. As one of the key missions of the ACVS Foundation is to promote cutting-edge education for diplomates, this topic is timely and very reflective of the educational mission of the Foundation.

Locking Plates in Veterinary Orthopedics is edited by Drs. Matt D. Barnhart and Karl C. Maritato. They have chosen a group of strong contributing authors to detail the areas of *Principles, Applications, and Clinical Case Examples* when using locking plates. We are sure you will find this reference extremely valuable.

The ACVS Foundation is an independently charted philanthropic organization devoted to advancing the educational, scientific, and charitable goals of the American College of Veterinary Surgeons. The mission of the ACVS Foundation is to support the advancement of surgical care of all animals through funding of educational and research opportunities for veterinary surgical residents and board-certified veterinary surgeons.

The ACVS Foundation's collaboration with Wiley-Blackwell benefits all those who are interested in veterinary surgery by presenting the latest evidence-based information on relevant surgical topics. The ACVS Foundation is proud to partner with Wiley-Blackwell in this important series and is honored to present this newest book in the *Advances in Veterinary Surgery* series.

R. Randy Basinger, DVM, ACVS
Chair, Board of Trustees
ACVS Foundation

Acknowledgments

I kept thinking of Sir Isaac Newton's quote, "If I have seen further than others, it is by *standing* upon the *shoulders of giants,*" as I pleaded with distinguished colleagues, whose depth of knowledge and experience is greater than my own, to contribute to this textbook. Thank you all for sacrificing your precious time and withholding any deservedly snarky replies to my barrage of emails delivered during this process. I hope you feel your dedication is rewarded by this final product and it fills a need within our profession.

Thank you, Erica Judisch and Susan Engelken from Wiley Blackwell, for believing in and supporting this book and shepherding us through the process. The longest email threads I have ever been part of now exist because of this book!

I owe so much to the mentors, colleagues, and residents who have kept me on my toes over the years. It would have been far easier to rest, but you showed me that's not how we grow. Credit to Harry Wotton, who began this locking implant journey with me and kept saying, "Someone needs write a veterinary book about these implants." Special thanks to Eric Schertel, for being a truly exceptional mentor, friend, and business partner. Your unselfish guidance in the OR and, more importantly, in life is precious to me.

Ultimately, this book is dedicated to Ashley, Bobby, Billy, and Ben, without whom I am nothing. For my boys, this book serves as a tangible reminder that dad isn't just playing with puppies when he's not home before bedtime. For Ashley, who has blessed me beyond measure with her partnership, friendship, and love. She makes all things possible and wonderful, and she confided in me early on that she's always liked "nerds." Well, this book should reaffirm she made a good choice.

I am indebted to my parents and sister for their unquestioning indulgence and tolerance of my "critter" interests since the very beginning and their support of my education. None of this would be possible otherwise. Ironically, this may be the one book my mother will not read cover-to-cover.

Finally, few of us veterinarians would do what we do were it not for our animal companions and patients and the unconditional love they provide. They inspire a passionate motivation in us, our clients, and our staff to support their well-being that is unique to our profession.

Animals are God's creatures. He surrounds them with his providential care. By their mere existence they bless him and give him glory. Thus, we humans owe them a great kindness.

–Matthew D. Barnhart

First and foremost, I want to thank and dedicate this book to my wife, Maria. No one has supported my goals and dreams more selflessly than she. From the first day of vet school to the day I received the news I passed ACVS boards, she never wavered in that support. She has shared me and our time together with my studies, as well as countless patients and clients, on endless weekends, nights, and holidays, when she could have been living a more "normal life." For this I will forever be grateful. Without her, I would be nothing.

I'd like to thank my parents and brother for always encouraging me to pursue my dreams, no matter how far away from them that took me. Specifically, my parents, who always put my education above all things and constantly pushed me to give my all and never give up. The work ethic, drive, humility, and sense of responsibility they instilled in me prepared me for the life of great dedication I give to my patients every day.

To all of my teachers, professors, and clinical mentors: I owe every bit of knowledge I have to your time, guidance, and patience (and I'm sure teaching me required much patience).

To Matthew D. Barnhart, not only for being one of those patient mentors but for respecting a former resident's knowledge and abilities enough to invite me on this incredible journey. I will always be grateful for our "big brother/little brother" relationship.

To Eric Schertel, again, not only for being one of those patient mentors, but for entrusting a large part of the success of your first expansion to a young new surgeon. The confidence you had in me that I could handle such a responsibility was the driving force a nervous young surgeon needed to succeed. I owe much of my success to you.

To all of the contributors of this book, your expertise is unparalleled. Each time I edited a chapter, I was amazed and humbled at how much knowledge there was to be gained by such amazing people, and how much I and my patients have benefited from the information in this book already.

To all those at Wiley who have supported and helped us so greatly with this project. This was not an easy task but you certiainly made it a lot less painful.

Lastly, to my patients. As Mahatma Gandhi once said, "The greatness of a nation can be judged by the way its animals are treated." The driving force behind my passion for orthopedics are all the dogs and cats (particularly the cats) that endlessly supply love to their undeserving human counterparts. If we could be half as loyal and loving as these creatures, our world would be a much better place. I will always do my best to relieve their suffering and keep them happy.

–Karl C. Maritato

Disclosures

- Matthew D. Barnhart is a paid lecturer for Securos and Everost and receives royalties from the sales of some of their products.
- Kevin P. Benjamino is a paid lecturer for Intrauma.
- Noel Fitzpatrick is the director of Fitzbionics
- Tomás Guerrero is a paid lecturer for Kyon.
- Karl C. Maritato is a paid lecturer for Everost and receives royalties from the sales of some of their products.
- Malcolm G. Ness is a paid lecturer for Orthomed and receives royalties from the sales of some of their products.
- Massimo Petazzoni is a paid lecturer for Intrauma.
- Kirk L. Wendelburg is a paid lecturer for and holds patents with Kyon.

1 A Brief History of Veterinary Locking Plates Applications

Karl C. Maritato

As with all of medicine, orthopedics is an ever-evolving science. While locking implants are a relatively recent addition to veterinary orthopedics, they have been used for humans for some time. To better understand where we are, and where we are going, with fracture repair and locking implants, we first need to look back on the history of fracture fixation – a fascinating journey through the brilliant minds of our predecessors.

In the mid-1700s, John Hunter was the first surgeon to define the four stages of callus formation during fracture repair. Around the same time, Albrecht von Haller noted that bone healing was dependent on the vascularity around the fractured region of the bone, emphasizing the role of blood supply in fracture healing. Henri Duhamel disagreed, thinking that all bone arose from the periosteum, and coined the term *cambium layer* [1].

In 1736, John Belchier was the first to identify the important role of osteoblasts in fracture healing, and in the 1840s, John Goodsir confirmed that osteoblasts were the true bone-forming cells [1]. This led some, including Sir William Macewen, to focus strongly on the osteoblast and ignore the role of the periosteum [1]. In the late 1800s, Louis Ollier, like Duhamel, felt more than osteoblasts were in play in fracture repair. He believed that in addition to osteoblasts, the periosteum and the bone marrow all contributed to bone repair; he recommended the periosteum be protected during surgery [1].

In 1886, Carl Hansmann invented the first bone plate and screws. Ironically, it was a locking plate that protruded through the skin [1]. By contrast, Halsted in 1893 and Lane in 1894, utilized the first completely implanted plates [1].

In 1912, William Sherman, who was a surgeon for the Pittsburgh Steel Company, designed plates with better metallurgy and engineering due to this connection. Because of his improved production knowledge, his plates did not corrode or break and were the most widely used plates until the Association for Osteosynthesis (AO) plates were introduced 50 years later [1].

Up until this point, the plates in use were not designed with compression in mind; rather, they served only to stabilize and align the bone as a replacement for external splinting, similar to current locking plates. In 1946, Eggers performed experiments on animals with induced fractures to show the effects of fracture site compression on the rate of healing and, in 1949,

Locking Plates in Veterinary Orthopedics, First Edition.
Edited by Matthew D. Barnhart and Karl C. Maritato.

Robert Danis was the first to apply compression plating to human patients [1].

A decade later, George Bagby was the first to use a plate similar in design to the dynamic compression plates (DCP) used today. His plates had oval-shaped holes with beveled edges that allowed the plate to slide into compression as the screw was tightened [1].

On November 6, 1958, a critical moment in orthopedics history occurred: Arbeitsgemeinschaft fur Osteosynthesenfragen (Association for Osteosynthesis) was formed by 13 surgeons in Switzerland [1, 2]. This group's unprecedented collective focus on the study of biomechanics, osteogenesis, implants, and instruments, as well as orthopedic techniques and postoperative care, ushered in a new era. Additionally, they focused on orthopedic continuing education through instructional courses and labs and published the first AO manual in 1963 [2, 3] followed by *Techniques of Internal Fixation of Fractures,* published in 1965 [2]. The critical principles of primary focus in these early editions were that of anatomic reduction and rigid fixation [2]. It was thought that fracture healing with no callus formation was most desired, and that the presence of callus formation was considered a sign of instability and inappropriate repair. Willeneger and Schenk's research on direct bone healing reinforced this theory [2, 3].

On 31 August 1969, AOVET was founded in Waldenburg, Switzerland (Figure 1.1a–d) [3]. In the decade prior to its formation, a beautiful collaboration between veterinary and human surgeons and engineers had blossomed. Transfer of knowledge between disciplines was initiated as never before in veterinary surgery, most notably by Dr. Guggenbuhl, one of the original 13 AO founders, and Dr. von Salis, a large animal veterinarian and first president of AOVET. This relationship and collaboration with von Salis's colleagues led to the AOVET formation [3]. One of the first documented fracture cases in a dog repaired using AO principles and plates was a femur fracture in a Spitz, performed on 3 February 1969 by Dr. Geri Kasa with a four-hole 4.5 mm round hole plate (Figure 1.2) [3].

In 1970, Allgowar and Perren continued research on the Bagby design and developed a sophisticated plate called the dynamic compression unit. Compression could be achieved in any equally spaced hole on either side of the fracture. Consistent fracture healing and early return to function were noted in patients treated with these plates, and the previously common "fracture disease" problem was disappearing [2]. It was also noted that complications such as sepsis, sequestrum formation, union difficulties, and re-fracture were occurring using these rigid techniques. Focus was redirected toward the effect of the plate on the bone surface and its blood supply [2].

At this same time, Dr. Hohn began the first, and soon to become annual, AOVET course held in the United States at The Ohio State University (Figure 1.3). Dr. Hohn had been the first to perform a canine fracture repair using AO principles in the United States at the Animal Medical Center in New York, as a part of a fantastic collaboration with Dr. Rosen, the first AO principled human orthopedic surgeon in the United States [3].

In 1982 and 1984, the first AO manuals on internal fixation in the horse and small animals, respectively, were published [3].

Stephen Perren built on the initial research of Ollier and in 1988 focused on the periosteum once again. He disagreed with the thought that stress protection from the plate led to osteoporosis of the bone under the plate, and, through his research, was able to prove that periosteal blood supply damage led to necrosis of the bone under the plate. This led to the development of the limited-contact dynamic compression plate (LC-DCP) in 1990 [1]. He also felt that strong compression and complete stability led to vascular damage, and instead he promoted relative stability and favored callus formation. He used longer plates with fewer screws, which favored faster healing with a mechanically strong callus [1].

Also in 1990, Reinhold Ganz developed the model of biologic fixation, promoting the "open but do not touch" approach and the use of long plates with fewer screws as well. Less emphasis was placed on complete reduction and absolute fracture site stability, but rather on alignment and relative stability with an expectation of callus formation. It was noted that fast and predictable bone healing occurred in this manner [2].

In 1997, this approach was taken even further by Chistian Krettek and Harald Tscherne, who developed the concepts of minimally invasive

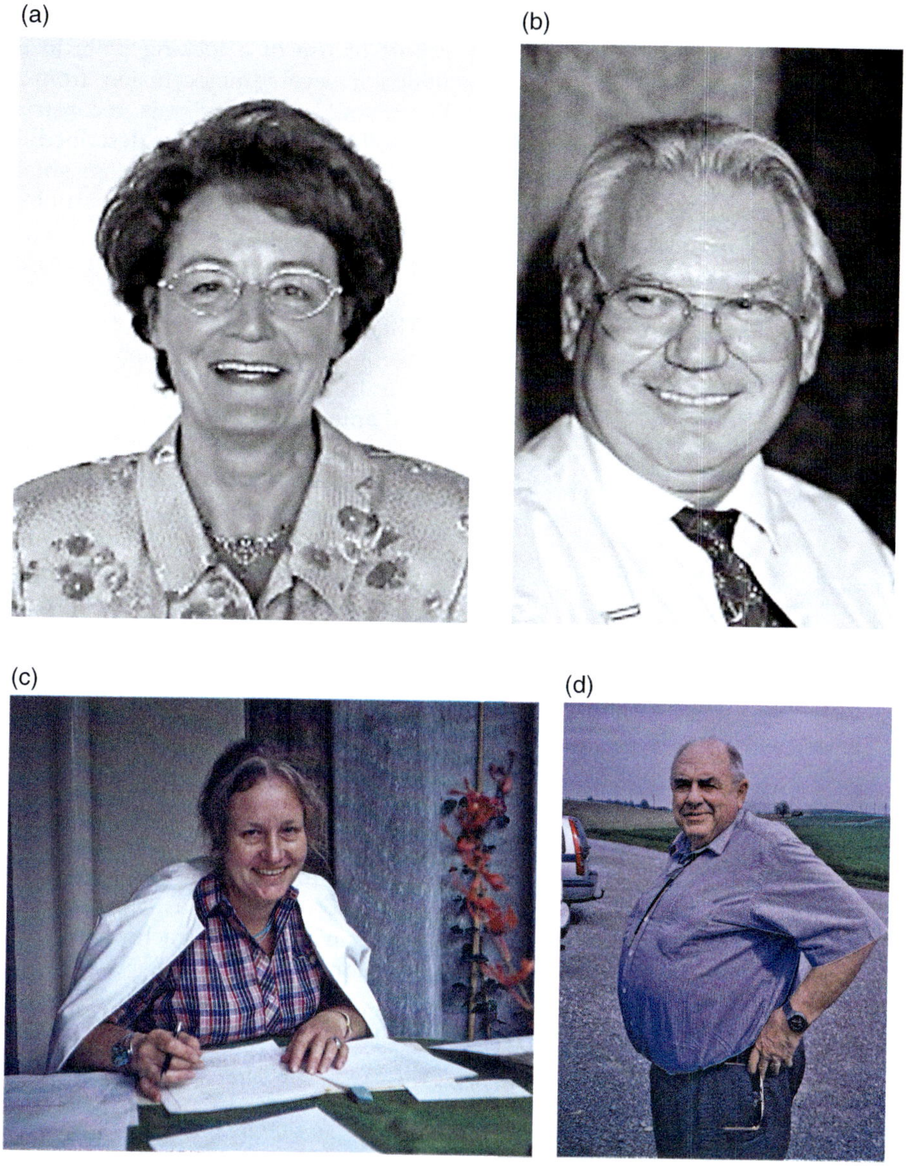

Figure 1.1 (a–d) Four of the primary founders of AOVEET. Geri Kasa, Feri Kasa, Ortun Pohler, Bjorn von Salis. (Source: Courtesy of AO Foundation.)

plate osteosynthesis (MIPO), which produced rapid bone healing with a larger amounts of callus formation [1, 2].

One advantage that external skeletal fixator application historically had over internal fixation was lesser operative injury – that injury caused by the fracture approach, reduction and fixation. This consideration was translated into the creation of internal fixators. Perren and Tepic introduced the concept of locking implants (i.e. internal fixators) in 1993 when they created the Point Contact Fixator using monocortical locking screws and a plate with similar shape and design to the LC-DCP [1]. Next in line was the creation of the less-invasive stabilization system (LISS), which may be considered the first plate particularly designed for MIPO [2].

Seven years later, Wagner and Frigg created the combi-hole plate that allowed both compression screws and locking screws to be used in the same plate. This allowed compression to be used in the portions of a fractured bone where it was desired, such as articular, as well as simultaneous use of the locking mechanism in the diaphyseal portions of the bone fracture [1].

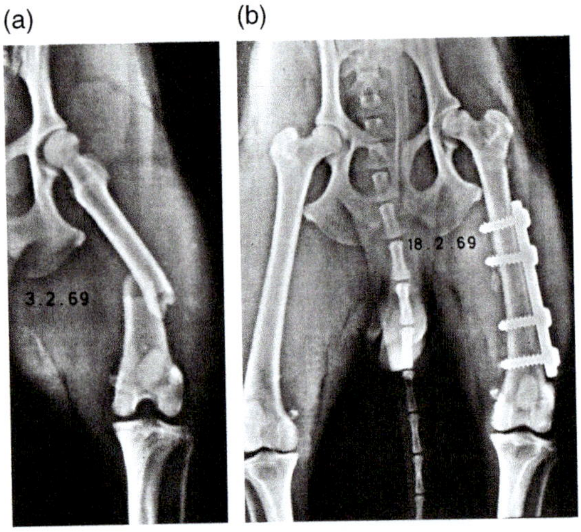

Figure 1.2 (a, b) One of the first documented fracture cases in a dog repaired using AO principles and plates; a femur fracture in a Spitz, performed on February 3, 1969, by Dr. Geri Kasa with a four-hole 4.5 mm round hole plate. (Source: Courtesy of AO Foundation.)

In 2004, Boudrieau published the first case report of use of a locking plate in a dog, in which a severe malocclusion from previous hemimandibulectomy was reconstructed [4]. The following year, Keller described the use of the compact unilock system in small animal orthopedics [5] and Aguila et al. published the first biomechanical study comparing LC-DCP and locking compression plate (LCP) in cadaver canine femurs [6].

The AO research center began testing the concepts of bridging fixation in small animals using 18 different plates commonly used in small animals in 2008 [7]. This laid the groundwork for future research of MIPO. That same year, locking technology moved out of the realm of trauma and was applied to tibial plateau leveling osteotomy [8], and later reports were published on vertebral applications, double pelvic osteotomy and arthrodesis [9, 10, 11]. Since these early reports, research on and the clinical use of locking implant technology has grown exponentially in veterinary medicine.

The founders of orthopedics worked tirelessly to understand bone and biomechanics and their effects on fracture pathology and management, all to better the lives of their patients, both human and animal alike. We must continue to follow their examples and strive for perfection as we pursue the most ideal management of fractures and other orthopedic conditions.

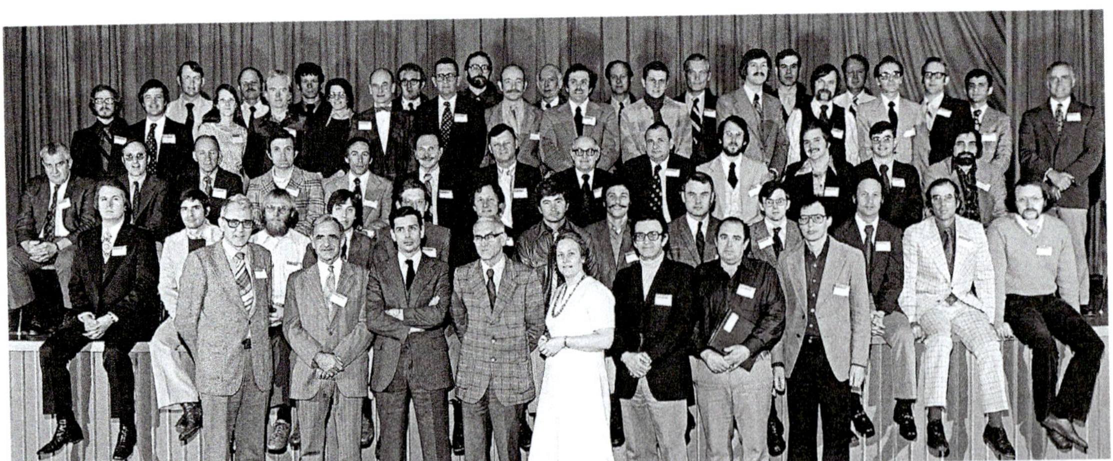

Figure 1.3 The first AOVET course held in the United States at The Ohio State University, 1970. (Source: Courtesy of AO Foundation.)

References

1. Thakur, A.J. (ed.) (2013). Evolution of bone plate … continues. In: *Locking Plates, Concepts and Applications*, 265–281. New Delhi, India: Wolters Kluwer Health.
2. Tong, G.O. and Bavonratanavech, S. (2011). History and evolution of MIPO. In: *Minimally Invasive Plate Osteosynthesis (MIPO): Concepts and Cases Presented by the AO East Asia*, 1e, 3–8. Thieme/AO Publishing.
3. Auer, J.A., Pohler, O., Schlunder, M. et al. (2013). *The History of AOVet, the First 40 Years*. Switzerland: AO foundation.
4. Boudrieau, R.J., Mitchell, S.L., and Seeherman, H. (2004 March-April). Mandibular reconstruction of a partial hemimandibulectomy in a dog with severe malocclusion. *Vet. Surg.* 33 (2): 119–130.
5. Keller, M.A., Voss, K., and Montavon, P.M. (2005). The ComPact UniLock 2.0/2.4 system and its clinical application in small animal orthopedics. *Vet. Comp. Orthop. Traumatol.* 18 (2): 83–93.
6. Aguila, A.Z., Manos, J.M., Orlansky, A.S. et al. (2005). In vitro biomechanical comparison of limited contact dynamic compression plate and locking compression plate. *Vet. Comp. Orthop. Traumatol.* 18 (4): 220–226.
7. Zahn, K., Frei, R., Wunderle, D. et al. (2008). Mechanical properties of 18 different AO bone plates and the clamp-rod internal fixation system tested on a gap model construct. *Vet. Comp. Orthop. Traumatol.* 21 (3): 185–194.
8. Leitner, M., Pearce, S.G., Windolf, M. et al. (2008 June). Comparison of locking and conventional screws for maintenance of tibial plateau positioning and biomechanical stability after locking tibial plateau leveling osteotomy plate fixation. *Vet. Surg.* 37 (4): 357–365.
9. McKee, W.M. and Downes, C.J. (2008 October). Vertebral stabilisation and selective decompression for the management of triple thoracolumbar disc protrusions. *J. Small Anim. Pract.* 49 (10): 536–539.
10. Rose, S.A., Bruecker, K.A., Petersen, S.W. et al. (2012 January). Use of locking plate and screws for triple pelvic osteotomy. *Vet. Surg.* 41 (1): 114–120.
11. Fitzpatrick, N., Yeadon, R., Smith, T.J. et al. (2012 August). Shoulder arthrodesis in 14 dogs. *Vet. Surg.* 41 (6): 745–754.

Section I

Principles of Locking Plate Application

2 Pitfalls of Locking Plate Applications

Matthew D. Barnhart

Locking plates (LP) gradually crept into use in veterinary surgery with little discussion as to the differences between them and the well-established conventional dynamic compression plating (DCP) techniques. The first published clinical application of a LP in a canine fracture case was in 2005 [1]. While thorough reviews on LP theory and its applications existed in the human medical literature, access to these publications required diligent investigation by the interested veterinary surgeon. As such, many of us simply switched an LP for a DCP system in a given trauma application without developing a better understanding of the fundamental differences between the two. This author's own initial misconception, and that most commonly encountered amongst colleagues, was that LP constructs were "stronger" than DCP constructs. We were a bit surprised to learn that LP technology was actually not designed to be stronger or more stable than DCP. Rather, it was created to enhance the principles of biological osteosynthesis in order to promote healing and minimize infection risks that were attributed in part to the periosteal vascular injury caused by the large frictional force generated between DCPs and the bone surface.

Unfortunately, we often learn more from our mistakes than our successes, so this chapter's purpose is to report some of the early pitfalls encountered when using LP systems. It will become clear how basic knowledge and adherence to principles learned later in this book could help minimize or outright avoid complications. Clearly, it is an oversimplification to blame a failure on lack of adherence to a single application principle; however, in some of these cases it is possible that problems could have been avoided had they been followed.

The following fracture repair cases illustrate what can happen if an LP is applied like a DCP without regard for important differences between the two. Fortunately, our contributing authors have done an excellent job reviewing LP principles in detail so these clinical cases will simply act as guides for much more detailed discussions (Figures 2.1–2.5).

Locking Plates in Veterinary Orthopedics, First Edition.
Edited by Matthew D. Barnhart and Karl C. Maritato.

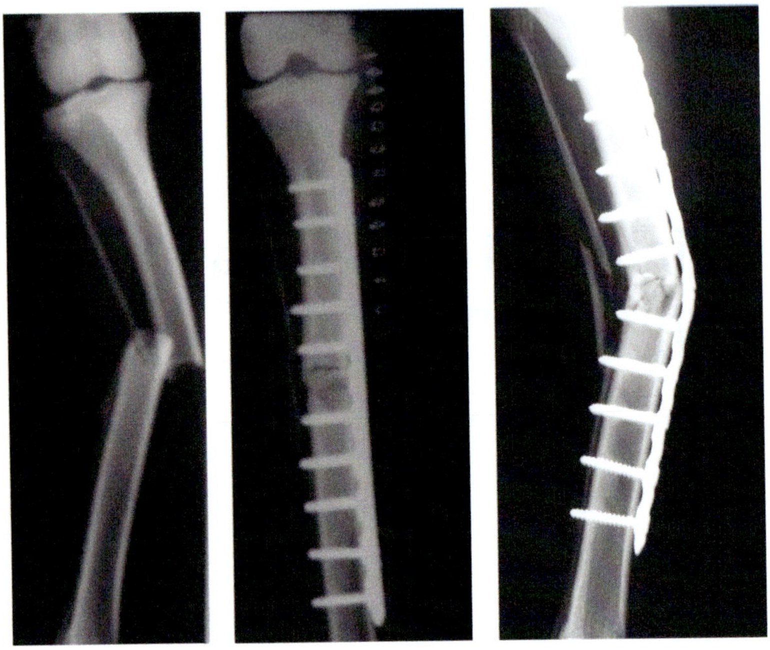

Figure 2.1 The recommended screw density for locking plate (LP) is different than that for dynamic compression plating (DCP). This fracture repair violated this principle, leading to major stress concentration within the implant at the fracture site and its subsequent failure. See pages 34–36 to learn more.

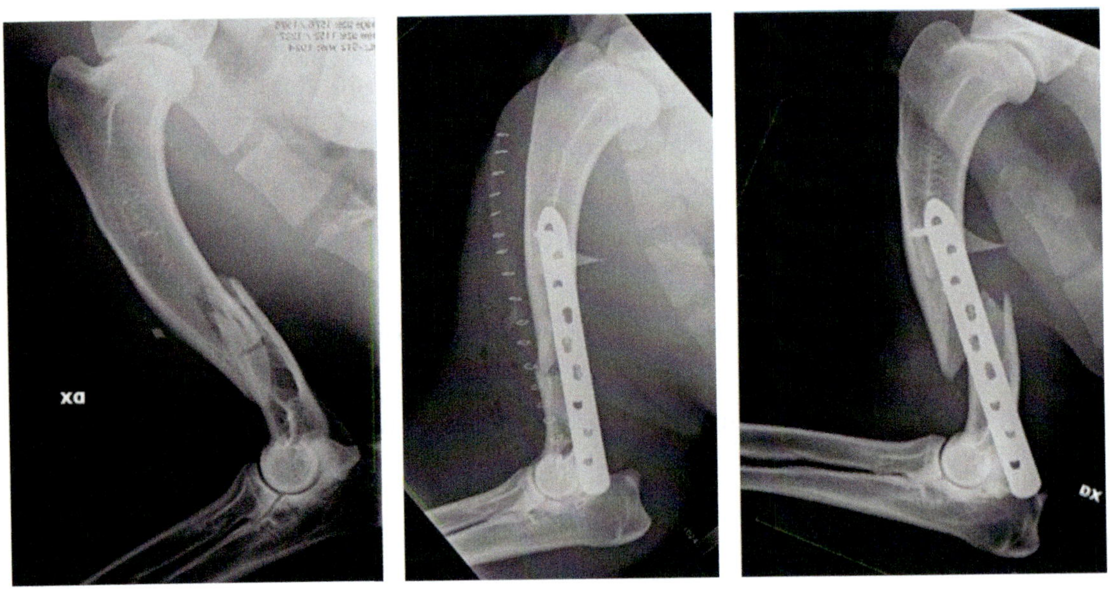

Figure 2.2 Maximizing plate length is particularly important when applying LP. This humerus fracture is a challenging one and may have been best served with bilateral plates. However, at the very least, the LP used was too short, based on the recommended plate length to fracture segment length ratios. See page 43 to learn more.

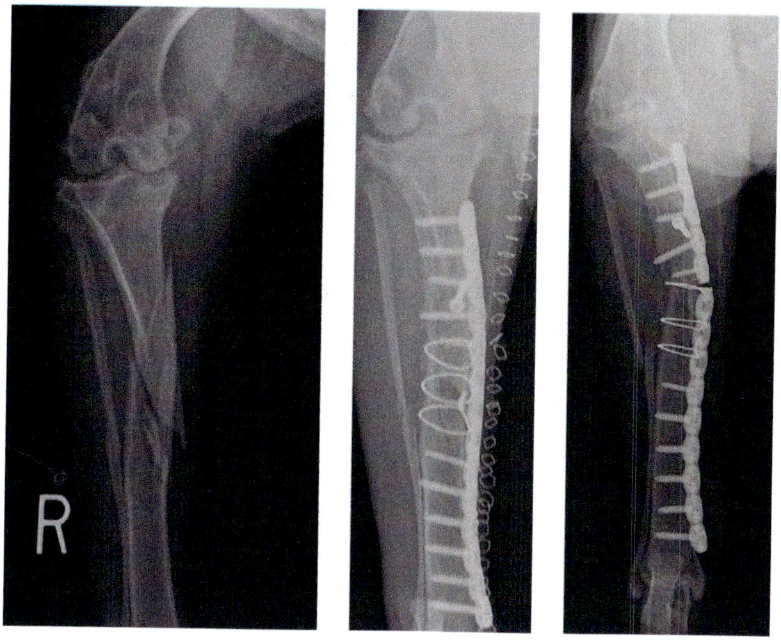

Figure 2.3 As previously stated, LP application provides a very different biological environment for healing compared to the DCP. This means less reconstruction and more elastic plate osteosynthesis principles need be applied. This tibia fracture may have been well reconstructed but was doomed to failure because of the way the LP was utilized. Maximizing the number of screw holes that are filled when using DCPs is typically the norm. By contrast, screw number and position is more critical when using LPs. See pages 34–36 and 130–132 to learn more.

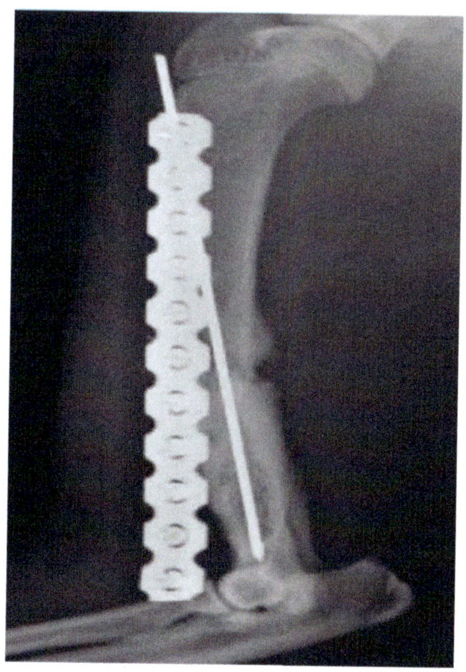

Figure 2.4 One of the things that a surgeon needs to adjust to when using a LP is the difference in "feel" during screw insertion. The physical nuances of the DCP bone-screw interaction that confirm appropriate cortical engagement cannot be relied upon. This was well demonstrated by Voss in a 2009 publication, which warned of the potential dangers of inadequate screw fixation because the surgeon cannot necessarily feel how well the screw engages the bone [2]. Note that the three most distal screws did not engage bone yet; they would have had felt tight because of their locking within the plate. Obviously this would never go unappreciated during a DCP application. See page 27 to learn more.

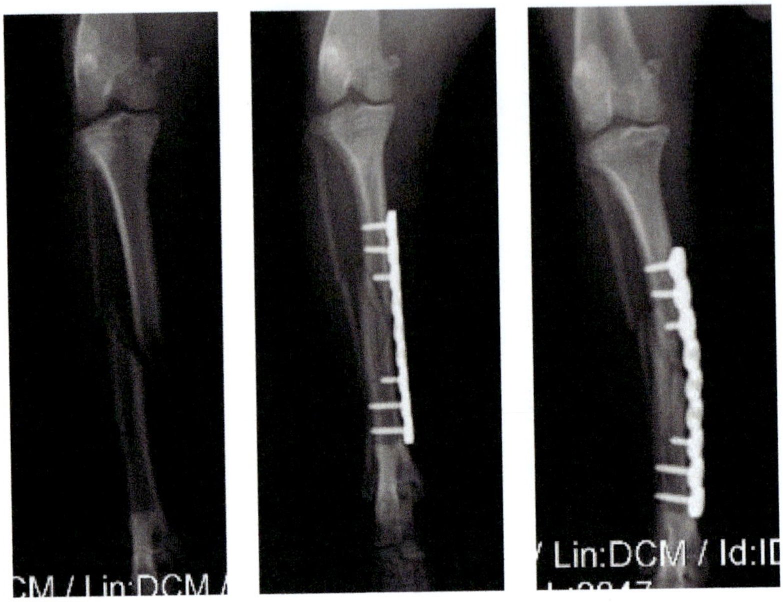

Figure 2.5 The mechanics of the single-beam construct created by a LP are fundamentally different from that of DCP application. Note the progressive bending of this LP without apparent failure at the screw level. Were a DCP to fail in this case, it would likely experience obvious loss of bone-screw stability before any bending took place. Additionally, LPs tend to be less stiff than their similarly sized DCP counterparts, again taking into consideration their different goals relative to elastic bridging and biological osteosynthesis. See pages 31–32 to learn more.

References

1. Scwandt, C.S. and Montavon, P.M. (2005). Locking compression plate fixation of radial and tibial fractures in a young dog. *Vet. Comp. Orthop. Traumatol.* 18 (3): 194–198.
2. Voss, K., Kull, M.A., Haessig, M. et al. (2009). Repair of long-bone fractures in cats and small dogs with the Unilock mandible locking plate system. *Vet. Comp. Orthop. Traumatol.* 22 (5): 398–405.

3 The Biology of Locking Plate Applications

Noël M.M. Moens

Since its introduction in 1969 by AO, the dynamic compression plate (DCP) has arguably become one of the most iconic plates for osteosynthesis and continues to be used successfully around the world. Although the DCP has been the standard bone plate for many decades, research has led to a better understanding of bone biology and the process of bone healing, and has identified shortfalls with the use of the DCP. Extensive zones of bone porosity have been identified underneath the plate following application. The porosis develops within a few weeks but lasts for several months. Although the porotic bone is progressively replaced by normal bone over time, it has been blamed for refracture of long bones after implant removal and may therefore have clinical significance [1–3] (Figure 3.1).

Initially, the development of bone porosis was almost exclusively attributed to stress protection caused by the plate, inducing remodeling of the protected bone according to Wolff's law [4–6]. Although no one can deny the long term effect of the plate on the bone, the pattern of early porosis observed within the first eight weeks of fracture fixation did not appear to match the expected region of stress protection [7]. In an experimental model using dogs, Carter attached plates of different composition and stiffness to the femur of dogs. Despite having a fraction of the rigidity of stainless steel plates, the plastic plates produced a pattern of bone resorption and remodeling similar to that of more rigid steel plates. This suggests that early porosity under the plate occurs even under very low stress shielding, and the remodeling may not be not associated with a change in bone strain but rather be the result of vascular and surgical trauma caused by the plate and its application [8]. Carter also performed a theoretical biomechanical analysis of the bone-plate constructs and suggested that the degree of stress shielding caused by metal plates that had been calculated by others based on theoretical composite beam models might have been overestimated [8]. In dogs, bone resorption following plating of the radius is also frequently observed in miniature breeds but does not appear to be a clinical problem in larger breeds. Stress protection has also often been blamed for the resorption. The fact that the normalized stiffness of the plated radius in miniature breed is similar to that of the large-breed dogs does not support the theory of stress protection and other factors such as damage to the blood supply should be considered [9]. There is

Locking Plates in Veterinary Orthopedics, First Edition.
Edited by Matthew D. Barnhart and Karl C. Maritato.

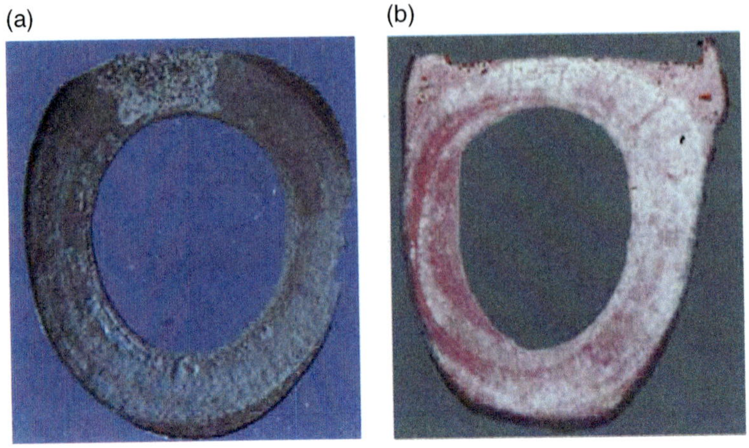

Figure 3.1 (a) Left: Section of a sheep tibia three months after plating with a traditional plate showing extensive osteoporosis corresponding to the width of the plate. (b) Right: Similar section of the tibia, one year after plate application showing the progressive replacement of the porotic bone with new living bone. (Source: Perren [58].)

abundant evidence that implants negatively affect bone blood supply [2, 10–14] (Figure 3.2).

A histological and bone perfusion study in sheep demonstrated a striking correlation between the disturbance of the bone blood supply caused by the plate and the degree and extent of bone necrosis and remodeling observed at 4, 10, and 20 weeks following implantation. In this study, the amount of necrosis observed underneath the plate could be directly related to the amount of contact between the plate and the bone [2]. The correlation between plate contact area and extent of the bone necrosis has also been found in the dog [13]. At the level of the fracture, the bone necrosis and resorption caused delayed healing of the cortex immediately underneath the plate. The focal bone necrosis and the resulting delayed union underneath the plate was suggested to be the cause of refracture of the bone following plate removal [2]. This theory was later supported by a case series of 28 refractures after implant removal. In many, the refracture originated from an area of the cortex underneath the plate that failed to unite despite adequate stabilization [3]. In 1988, Perren made the case that the early porosity observed underneath the plates was more likely the result of bone devascularization and necrosis than the result of stress shielding [10, 15]. The porosity was therefore attributed to an intense bone remodeling following bone necrosis induced by cortical devascularization. The realization of the importance of the bone blood supply and its importance in fracture healing led surgeons to progressively adopt a different approach to bone fixation. Instead of focusing mainly on the preservation of the soft tissue, surgeons realized the importance of also preserving the bone vascular supply and viability [16]. This new approach to fracture fixation was coined "biological plating."

With this changing paradigm, attempts were made to develop bone plates with smaller physical and biological footprints, to decrease the impact on bone biology. The AO group developed the limited-contact DCP (LC-DCP). This plate has a scalloped underside, which reduces the contact surface by more than 50% compared with conventional DCP and should therefore reduce its impact on the bone beneath [16–18] (Figure 3.3). The concept was further developed with the introduction of the point-contact fixator (PC-Fix), which further decreased the contact surface area between the bone and the plate until it became negligible [19–22].

Although the PC-Fix was briefly used in clinical practice, the plate was discontinued for undisclosed reasons and replaced by the locking compression plates (LCP) [23–27]. The radical design of the PC-Fix was abandoned and the LCP reverted to the same overall design and plate undercuts as the LC-DCP but with the addition of the locking screws. Although

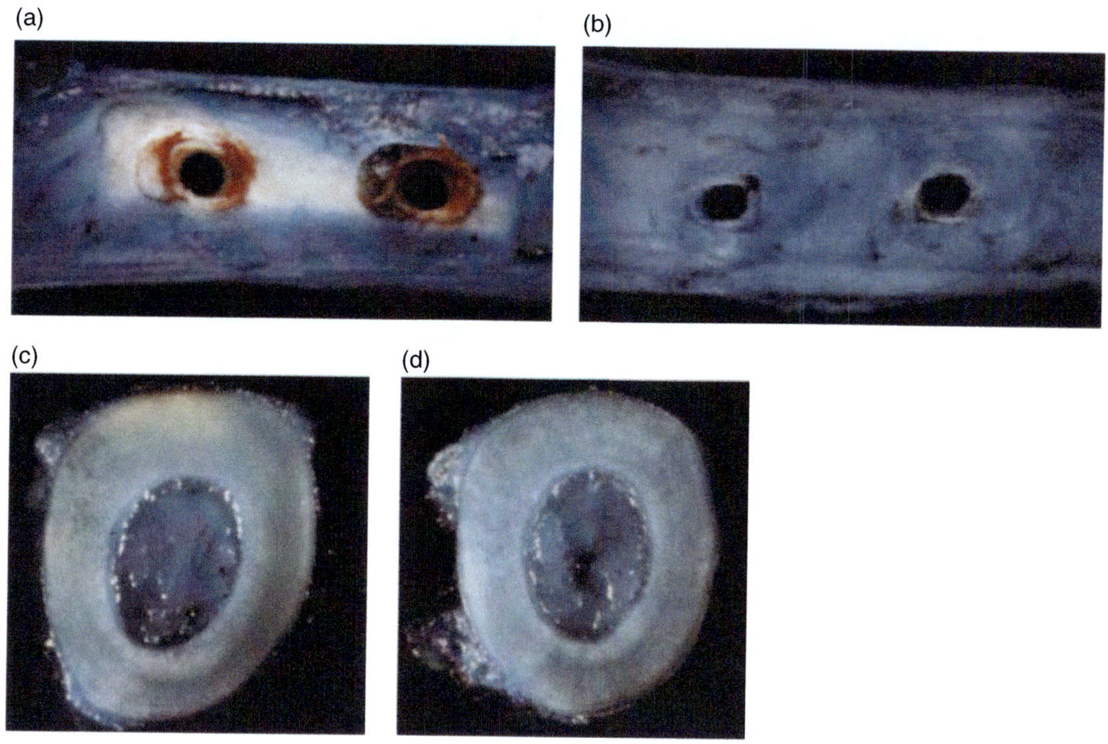

Figure 3.2 Surface appearance of sheep tibia seven hours following plating and injected with disulfin blue immediately prior to euthanasia. Each tibia was plated with either a traditional plate or an experimental plate with the underside designed to lift the plate above the bone surface by 1 mm. (a) Blood flow impairment can be inferred from the large defect in disulfin uptake in the cortex immediately underneath the plate following application of a plate with a solid underside in contact with the bone. (b) Minimal blood flow impairment occurred following plating with the experimental plate that minimize the contact area between the plate and the bone.(c) and (d) Cross section of the tibia after plating with the conventional plate (c) and the limited contact plate (d). (Source: Lippuner et al. [13, p. 80, Figure 1a to 1d]. Springer Verlag.)

the locking screws allow the plate to be placed completely away from the periosteal surface [28, 29], the true extent of plate contact with the bone is likely variable. In clinical cases, the plate is frequently in contact with the bone even if it is not compressed against it. Some locking plates have the option of being used as a hybrid fixation, using a combination of locking and regular screws [30–32]. When used in this fashion, the plate must be properly contoured and the regular screws must be tightened first before the locking screws are added, potentially compressing the bone to the same extent as the LC-DCP. The plate contact surface area and the cortical necrosis induced by locking plates has not been fully investigated and is mostly derived from experience with the LC-DCP and PC-Fix. It is likely variable depending on how the plate is used, but we may reasonably assume that they are less than for nonlocking plates.

Despite the clear trend toward decreasing the plate biological footprint, the causes of the early porosis and the causes for the delayed healing continue to generate debate. Uhthoff studied the pattern of necrosis and bone remodeling after plate fixation in dog and concluded that the pattern of necrosis and the extremely slow bone remodeling of the porotic bone could only be explained by stress protection and not by the compression of the plate onto the bone [4, 5]. Furthermore, in his experiment, the zone of porosity and the zone of bone necrosis did not fully correlate, raising the prospect that they may not be related [4].

Clinically, a decrease in plate footprint and better preservation of bone vascularity should be associated with better healing and a smaller

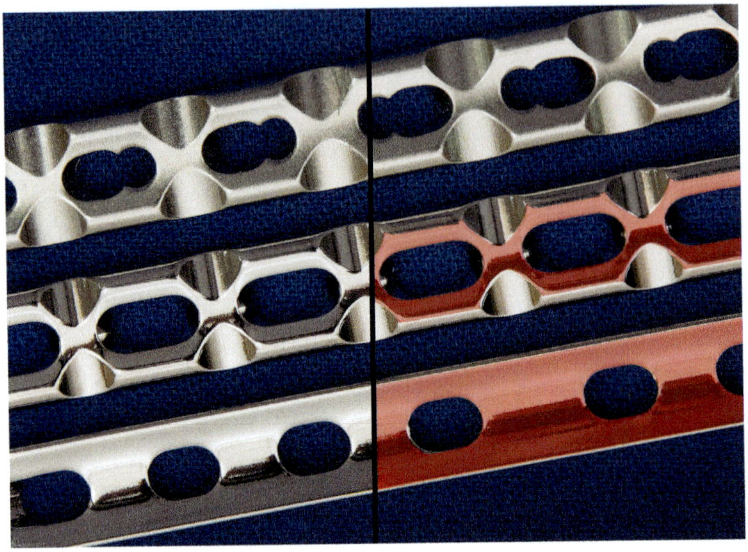

Figure 3.3 View of the underside of the DCP (Bottom), LC-DCP (middle) and LCP (Top). The area colored in red represent the theoretical zones of contact between the plate and the bone. Although the LCP and the LC-DCP have a similar underside, the locking screws in the LCP allow the plate to sit above the periosteum if desired.

risk of refracture following removal. The importance of blood supply to the bone and its effect on bone healing has been well studied [12, 33–35]. Studies in multiple species have shown that disruption of the blood supply, whether from damage to the endosteum, periosteum, cortex or soft tissue envelope, has the potential to delay healing and to increase the risk of fracture complication. Even the fracture hematoma plays a significant role in fracture healing and its removal from the fracture site results in significant healing delays [35, 36]. Fixation methods that minimize damage to the vascular supply to the bone should therefore result in faster bone healing and a decreased rate of delayed unions and nonunions. In a study in sheep, oblique tibial fractures were created and stabilized with a lag screw and neutralized with either a titanium DCP or a PC-Fix plate. Six sheep were euthanized at 12, 24, 48, or 96 weeks and the tibia were subjected to bending until failure. At 12 weeks, in the DCP group, all bones refractured at the level of the original fracture. Two bones refractured at the fracture site at the 24- and 48-week mark and one bone at the 96-week mark. In contrast, in the PC-Fix group all bones (except for one at 96 weeks) refractured in a different location than the original fracture, suggesting that healing was significantly advanced and more complete than in the DCP group. Histology at 12 weeks shows advanced healing and bridging of the bone cortices in the PC-Fix group, while the DCP group displayed extensive bone necrosis and resorption with minimal callus formation [37] (Figure 3.4).

In a radiographic study of tibial fractures in sheep treated with a DCP, LC-DCP, and PC-Fix, bone fusion, a more homogenous bone structure was noted in the PC-Fix group, suggesting better and more advanced bone healing in that group compared to the other two groups [38]. Despite these very encouraging studies showing a clear benefit of the PC-Fix, several others studies failed to demonstrate any benefit of the decreased footprint, under both clinical and experimental conditions. In a comprehensive study in sheep, three types of plates of decreasing contact surface area (DCP, LC-DCP, and partial contact plate) were evaluated for the repair of experimental tibial fractures. Periosteal and bone perfusion, bone density, and porosity, bone remodeling and biomechanical properties of the healing bone, were evaluated at different time points. No significant difference was seen between any of the plate tested for any of the

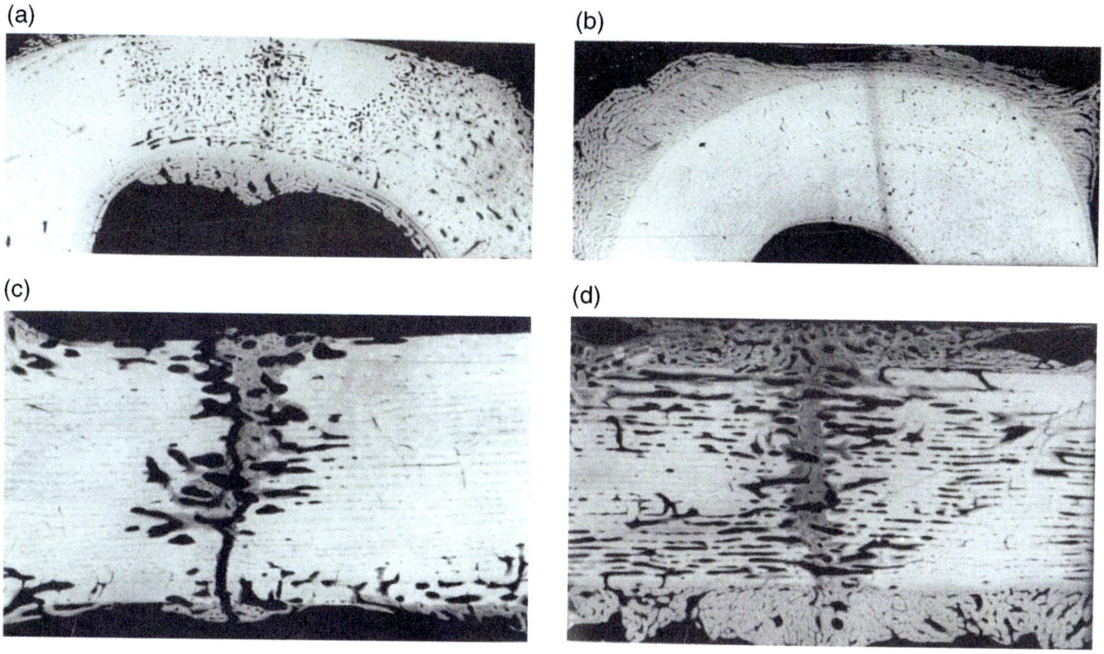

Figure 3.4 (a) Histological section of a sheep tibia 12 weeks following plating with a DCP. Note the extensive area of porosis under the plate. (b) Histological section of a sheep tibia 12 weeks following application of as PC-Fix showing minimal porosis of the cortex underneath the plate. (c) Section of the cortex underneath the plate at the level of the fracture of sheep tibia stabilized with a DCP. Note the lack of bridging at 12 weeks and the minimal callus production. (d) Section of the cortex underneath the plate at the level of the fracture of sheep tibia stabilized with a PC-Fix. The cortex is fully bridged with new callus. Note the presence of periosteal callus immediately underneath the plate (top of the image). (Source: Tepic et al. [37].)

criteria tested, leading the author to conclude that neither of those plates provided any benefit in fracture healing over another [14]. Similarly, in a segmental fracture model in dogs, the DCP and LC-DCP could not be differentiated based on vascularization, remodeling, porosity, or biomechanical properties at 10 weeks postsurgery [39]. It is evident from these contradictory results that plates with smaller footprints may have significant theoretical advantages, but these advantages do not necessarily translate into better and faster healing in all clinical situations. The reasons for the contradictory results remain unclear. One possible explanation could be that differences in design may not translate into clear differences in contact area when applied to the bone. The true difference in plate contact area between the DCP and LC-DCP has been questioned, despite a reported reduction of 50% between the two plates [16]. Using pressure sensitive films on cadaveric bones, Field measured the plate contact area of the DCP and LC-DCP applied to different bones. Despite the lower theoretical footprint of the LC-DCP, no difference in contact area was detected between the two plates when applied to human femora or equine metacarpi. When applied to the caudal surface of the human humerus, a decrease in contact area was observed with the LC-DCP but that difference disappeared when the plate was applied to the medial surface [40]. This suggests that the contact area of the plate is influenced more by the complex surface of the bone and the ability of the surgeon to contour the plate than by the design of the plate itself. The lack of difference in the actual contact surface area could explain the lack of difference in healing observed clinically between the different implants. The more obvious difference in contact area between the traditional plates and the PC-Fix may explain why some better results were obtained with the PC-Fix under strict experimental conditions. As mentioned earlier, the undersurface of the LCP is similar to that of the LC-DCP but with the added benefit of the locking screws. Its impact on bone vascularization has not been fully investigated but can reasonably be expected to be significantly less than traditional plates. Although it has been claimed that locking plates do not induce early temporary porosis [31], in depth and rigorous comparisons between traditional and locking plates have not yet been conducted and much of the information is extrapolated from studies on the LC-DCP, the PC-Fix and other, earlier, plates designs.

In addition to a preservation of the blood biology, physical clearance under the plate at the fracture site, has also been suggested as one the reason for improved strength of the bone following fixation with the PC-Fix [37]. In histological sections of the bone at 12 weeks following fixation with the PC-Fix, callus could be seen immediately underneath the plate, forming almost a 360° ring around the bone. The callus could form because the PC-Fix allowed some clearance under the plate as opposed to the DCP (Figure 3.4c and d). Even though the callus under the plate was smaller than the callus on the opposite cortex, it may have contributed to a stronger healing and prevented the bone from refracturing at the previous fracture site [37]. Greater clearance is expected for locking plates as the plate does not require any contact with the bone and can be placed up to 2 mm away from the periosteal surface without significantly influencing the biomechanical properties of the construct [28, 29, 41]. Interestingly, a lack of callus and delayed healing of the cis-cortex have been observed following locked bridge plating of fractures [42] (Figure 3.5).

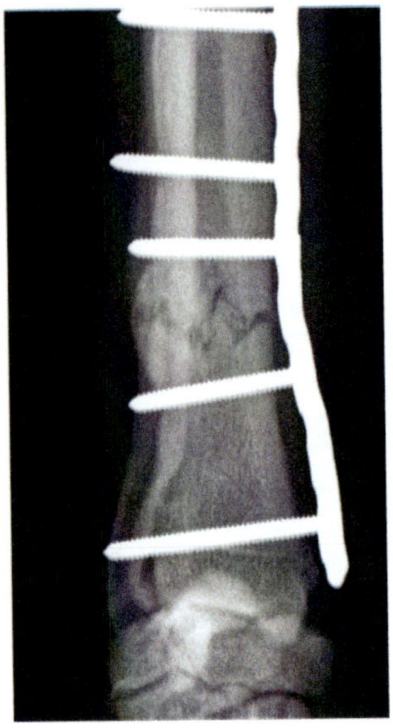

Figure 3.5 One-month postoperative radiographs of a distal radial fracture treated with a locking plate in a bridging fashion. Note the absence of callus at the level of the cortex immediately underneath the plate compared to the well developed callus on the opposite cortex.

The asymmetrical callus formation, however, has not been associated with a lack of blood supply or interference with the plate, but has been linked to the differential strain created by asymmetrical gap closure as the plate flexes during weight bearing [43–45]. Although, the effect of asymmetrical healing has been successfully mitigated by the addition of bone graft to the cis cortex [46], some of the latest developments in locking plate technology have attempted to decrease the strain differential across the fracture gap [45, 47, 48]. Biomechanical reasons have also been suspected for the delayed healing observed in simple transverse fractures of the forearm and tibia treated with locking plates. Simple forearms fractures treated in compression with a DCP healed on average 11 weeks faster than those treated more biologically with a bridging locking plate. However, when the type of fixation was considered, the improvement could be attributed to the compression of the fracture rather than to the plate type [49]. A similar conclusion was drawn from a study comparing open reduction and minimally invasive plate osteosynthesis (MIPO) for the treatment of tibial fractures. Simple tibial fractures treated with a bridging locking plate required twice the time to heal than the fractures treated in compression, regardless of the surgical approach and fixation [50]. These reports highlight the fact that in fracture treatment, biomechanical considerations still play a significant role and may outweigh some of the biological advantages of the implant. Some fractures, particularly the simple ones, may still benefit from anatomical reconstruction and rigid stabilization rather than bridging and relative stability. Although locking plates have been principally designed to be used as bridging implants, some locking plates do allow regular bone screws to be used to create interfragmentary compression if desired. This feature allows the plate to be used as a locking bridging plate, a compression plate, or a hybrid plate [51] (Figure 3.6).

Infection is a frequent but challenging problem following fracture fixation. Implant associated infections are particularly challenging as the bacteria often colonize the implant or necrotic bone and develop a biofilm on their surfaces, rendering them resistant to antibiotics and natural defenses [52]. Healthy bone is naturally resistant to infection but rapidly becomes vulnerable when it becomes devascularized, ischemic, unstable, or in the presence of a foreign body [53–55]. Traditional plates compressed onto the bone surface significantly interfere with cortical and periosteal vascularization. Not only has tissue pressure been shown to increase soft tissues infection rates [56], but the compression also promotes a degree of ischemia in the bone and produces osteonecrosis that is proportional to the footprint of the implant [2, 57]. Although the necrotic bone is progressively remodeled and replaced with living bone overtime, resorption starts at the junction of the healthy and necrotic bone and may result in the formation of a large sequestrum immediately underneath the implant. Necrotic bone provides an ideal substrate for bacteria to adhere and cause infection, and the extent of the sequestrum may allow the infection to propagate along a large, contiguous area underneath the implant [58] (Figure 3.7).

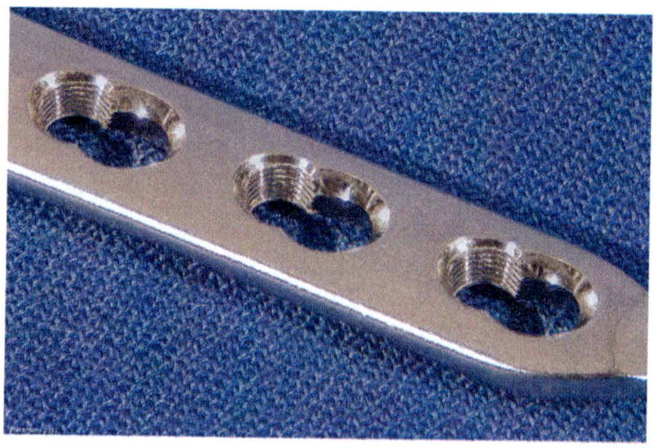

Figure 3.6 Illustration of the "combination hole" of the Synthes LCP™ allowing the plate to be used as a compression plate, a locking bridging plate, or hybrid plate.

Locking plates have several biological and biomechanical advantages over traditional plates that would be beneficial when dealing with contaminated or infected fractures. Because of those characteristics, locking plates have been frequently and successfully used for the treatment of complicated and infected fractures resulting from failed treatment with traditional plates. Despite those excellent results, there is surprisingly a very limited body of evidence demonstrating a decrease in infection rates with locking plates and supporting evidence must be gathered from research on previous versions of the implant.Comparing infections rates between different implants is difficult because many aspects of the implants

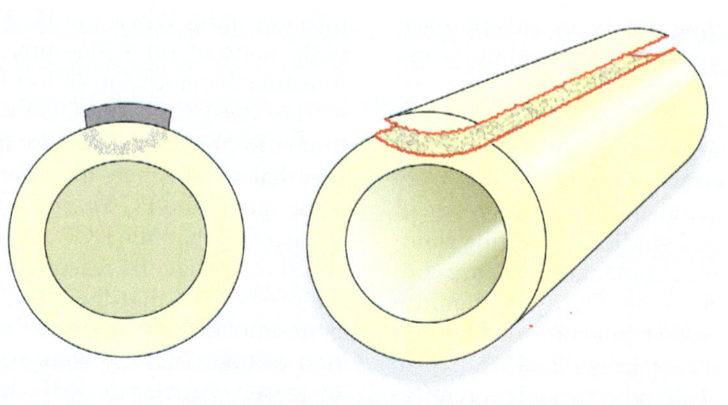

Figure 3.7 Aggressive resorption of the bone at the junction between the live and necrotic bone may lead to the formation of a large, contiguous sequestrum underneath the plate.

can influence infection rates. Design, material composition, biocompatibility, and even surface topography all play a role in the implant resistance to infection and therefore may skew the results. Infections rates associated with the use of the PC-Fix were recorded in a large prospective multicenter study involving 1229 fractures over a six-year period. Of those 1229 fractures, 263 were open. Only 13 PC-Fix became infected, for an overall infection rate of 1.1%. The infection rate was 1.6% when considering only the open fractures and 1% for the closed fractures. Although no concurrent comparison with other implants was made, by comparison with historical data, the author concluded that the infection rates associated with the use of the PC-Fix were low [25]. The infection rates for the LC-DCP were reported in the same study to be around 1.1% [25], while historical Infection rates for fixation of forearm fractures with a DCP were reported to be as high as 5.5% [59]. It is, however, difficult to draw strong conclusions from those numbers, as another contemporary study using DCP for fixation of 134 forearm fractures reports an infection rate of only 0.8% [60]. The authors of this latter study credit their low infection rates on their "biological" approach to fracture fixation by providing relative stability using longer plates with less screws and minimizing disturbance to the periosteum and fracture site. Although the plate design and the limited contact of the implant were credited for the low infection rates in the PC-Fix study, the difference in infection rates from 5.5% to 0.8% between the two DCP studies highlight the fact that surgical technique and biological approach to fracture fixation may be as important as the plate type in determining infection rates.

The material composition of the implants represented another confounding factor in this study because the PC-Fix and LC-DCP were made of titanium, while the DCP were made of stainless steel. Several studies comparing stainless steel and titanium implants have since confirmed the better biocompatibility of titanium and the reduced risk of infection of titanium implants compared to stainless steel [61, 62]. To elucidate the role of all these variables on infection rates, the Association for Osteosynthesis (AO) group conducted a series of experiments isolating each of the variables. Two implants,

Table 3.1 Effect of implant material, implant type and surgical approach on the infection rates and the relative number of colony forming units required to achieve a 50% infection rate in rabbits.

Plate composition	Infection rates			Rel $_{(ID50)}$
Stainless Steel (DCP)	75%	] *	(15/20)	×1
Titanium (DCP)	35%		(7/20)	×10
Plate type				
DCP (Titanium)	63%	] *	(12/19)	×1
PC-Fix (Titanium)	26%		(4/19)	×12
Surgical technique				
Open approach (steel DCP)	38.5%	] NS	(5/13)	×1
Minimally invasive (steel DCP)	25%		(3/12)	×3.1

Source: Data compiled from Schlegel and Perren [63] and Arens et al. [66].
* Denotes statistical difference and NS denotes lack of statistical significance at 0.05%.

only differing by one characteristic, were applied to the tibia of rabbits and infected with increasing concentrations of *Staphylococcus aureus*. Bacterial cultures of bones and soft tissues were performed at 28 days [63]. By determining the infection rates for each bacterial concentration, the bacterial load required to produce 50% infection rates (DI50) was calculated and compared (Table 3.1). As expected, the results confirmed the increased resistance to infection of the titanium implants, which required 10 times more bacteria to cause a 50% infection rate. When the PC-Fix and the DCP, both made of pure titanium, were compared, infection developed in 26% of the PC-Fix, but in 63% of the DCPs. The DI50 was also 10 times higher for the PC-Fix than for the DCP, confirming that even when they are made with the same metal, the PC-Fix has a higher resistance to infection than the DCP. Although the authors could not prove the reason for the difference, it was suggested that the reduced contact at the bone-implant interface and the better preservation of bone biology were responsible for the increased resistance [64]. In a comparison between open reduction and internal fixation (ORIF) and minimally invasive percutaneous osteosynthesis (MIPO), ORIF resulted in a

38.5% infection rate while MIPO resulted in a 25% infection rate. These numbers were, however, not statistically significant. Although this result does not appear to support the benefit of decreasing the biological impact, the plates in the ORIF group were applied in a "biologically friendly" manner with minimal disruption of the soft tissues and periosteum. It is therefore possible that the difference in the biological footprint between these two surgical approaches were not sufficient to influence infection rates. The situation might be different in clinical situations when the tissue covering the fracture is already traumatized. It is important to note that the number of bacteria required to infect an implant cannot be directly translated into risks of infection in a clinical situation, but support the idea that implants with smaller biological footprints offer an increased resistant to bacterial infection. Clearly, other aspects of the surgery, such as minimizing bone and soft tissue damage and preservation of the periosteum also significantly affect infection rates to a degree that may equal or exceed that of the plate type. Massive contamination, on the other hand, is likely to cause infection regardless of the implant type and characteristics [64–66]. Although experimental data suggest an increased resistance to infection for implants with small biological footprints, the difference has not been clearly demonstrated in the clinical setting and infections with locking plates are still observed [67, 68]. In addition to their biological advantages, locking plates have biomechanical advantages that makes them attractive for use in contaminated or infected situations. There are many reports of malunion and multidrug resistant infections that resulted in fracture union and resolution of infection following the replacement of the conventional plates with locking plates suggesting that they have a definite role to play in the treatment of complicated and infected fractures [67, 69–71]. In veterinary medicine, only one retrospective study specifically compared the infection rate of locking and nonlocking tibial plateau leveling osteotomy (TPLO) plates in dogs larger than 50 kg. Although the overall infection rate was high, TPLO stabilized with a locking plate were less likely to become infected than those stabilized with a nonlocking plate (odd ratio: 0.34). Although the reasons for the decreased infection rate remains speculative, the improved stability of the osteotomy provided by the locking plate was the proposed reason for the decreased susceptibility to infection rate [72].

Clinically, locking plates have been very successful and have been widely accepted in both human and animal surgery. Although there is surprisingly little evidence supporting the biological advantages of the locking plate itself, there is a good trail of evidence supporting each step of the plate evolution, from the DCP all the way to the locking plate. It is important to recognize that at the same time as the bone plate evolved, there has been a significant change in the way surgeons approach fracture treatment. From rigid stabilization and anatomical reduction, surgeons have moved toward a more biologically friendly approach by providing bridging fixation and relative stability, while preserving as much of the bone blood supply as possible. The evolution of biological fixation and locking plates are intricately combined, making it difficult to separate the benefit of one versus the other. For this reason, accurate comparison between implants is difficult. It is abundantly evident that the surgical technique and the biomechanical environment are at least as important as the plate itself in guaranteeing a successful outcome. In many cases, despite all the potential biological advantages of the locking plates over traditional plates, a clear clinical advantage is not always observed. Many reports, both in humans and animals, demonstrate good to excellent results with the use of the locking plate. However, for the most part, the results in terms of healing times, infection rates, nonunion, and refracture rates are not different from other plate types or external fixation [68, 71, 73–79]. In some instances, locking plates have been associated with an increased rate of complications compared to traditional plates, making it evident that not every fracture should be treated with a locking plate [49, 51, 80, 81]. There are, however, situations in which the fracture environment is suboptimal and, in which the combined biological and biomechanical advantages of the locking plates offer substantive advantage over traditional plates, making them highly valuable and allowing treatment of difficult fractures that would have been very difficult to treat with other traditional methods of fixation [67, 71, 82, 83].

References

1. Rosson, J., Egan, J., Shearer, J. et al. (1991). Bone weakness after the removal of plates and screws. Cortical atrophy or screw holes? *J. Bone Joint Surg. Br.* 73 (2): 283–286.
2. Gautier, E., Rahn, B.A., and Perren, S.M. (1995). Vascular remodelling. *Injury* 26 (2): B11–B19.
3. Kessler, S.B., Deiler, S., Schiffl-Deiler, M. et al. (1992). Refractures: a consequence of impaired local bone viability. *Arch. Orthop. Trauma Surg.* 111 (2): 96–101.
4. Uhthoff, H.K., Boisvert, D., and Finnegan, M. (1994). Cortical porosis under plates. Reaction to unloading or to necrosis? *J. Bone Joint Surg. Am.* 76 (10): 1507–1512.
5. Uhthoff, H.K. and Finnegan, M. (1983). The effects of metal plates on post-traumatic remodelling and bone mass. *J. Bone Joint Surg. Br.* 65: 66–71.
6. Tonino, A.J., Davidson, C.L., Klopper, P.J. et al. (1976). Protection from stress in bone and its effects. Experiments with stainless steel and plastic plates in dogs. *J. Bone Joint Surg. Br.* 58: 107–113.
7. Cheal, E.J., Hayes, W.C., White, A.A. et al. (1985). Stress analysis of compression plate fixation and its effects on long bone remodeling. *J. Biomech.* 18: 141–150.
8. Carter, D.R., Shimaoka, E.E., Harris, W.H. et al. (1984). Changes in long-bone structural properties during the first 8 weeks of plate implantation. *J. Orthop. Res.* 2: 80–89.
9. Gauthier, C.M., Conrad, B.P., Lewis, D.D. et al. (2011). In vitro comparison of stiffness of plate fixation of radii from large-and small-breed dogs. *Am. J. Vet. Res.* 72: 1112–1117.
10. Perren, S.M., Cordey, J., Rahn, B.A. et al. (1988). Early temporary porosis of bone induced by internal fixation implants. A reaction to necrosis, not to stress protection? *Clin. Orthop. Relat. Res.* (232): 139–151.
11. Jacobs, R.R., Rahn, B.A., and Perren, S.M. (1981). Effects of plates on cortical bone perfusion. *J. Trauma.* 21: 91–95.
12. Smith, S.R., Bronk, J.T., and Kelly, P.J. (1990). Effect of fracture fixation on cortical bone blood flow. *J. Orthop. Res.* 8: 471–478.
13. Lippuner, K., Vogel, R., Tepic, S. et al. (1992). Effect of animal species and age on plate-induced vascular damage in cortical bone. *Arch. Orthop. Trauma Surg.* 111: 78–84.
14. Kregor, P.J., Senft, D., Parvin, D. et al. (1995). Cortical bone perfusion in plated fractured sheep tibiae. *J. Orthop. Res.* 13: 715–724.
15. Cordey, J., Perren, S.M., and Steinemann, S.G. (2000). Stress protection due to plates: myth or reality? A parametric analysis made using the composite beam theory. *Injury* 31 (Suppl 3): C1–C13.
16. Perren, S.M., Allgower, M., Brunner, H. et al. (1991). The concept of biological plating using the limited contact-dynamic compression plate (LC-DCP): Scientific background, design and application. *Injury* 22: 1–41.
17. Schütz, M., and Südkamp, N.P. (2003). Revolution in plate osteosynthesis: new internal fixator systems. *J. Orthop. Sci.* 8: 252–258.
18. Perren, S.M., Klaue, K., Pohler, O. et al. (1990). The limited contact dynamic compression plate (LC-DCP). *Arch. Orthop. Trauma. Surg.* 109: 304–310.
19. Borgeaud, M., Cordey, J., Leyvraz, P.E. et al. (2000). Mechanical analysis of the bone to plate interface of the LC-DCP and of the PC-FIX on human femora. *Injury* 31 (Suppl 3): C29–C36.
20. Miclau, T., Remiger, A., Tepic, S. et al. (1995). A mechanical comparison of the dynamic compression plate, limited contact-dynamic compression plate, and point contact fixator. *J. Orthop. Trauma.* 9: 17–22.
21. Hauke, C., Meisser, A., and Perren, S.M. (2001). Methodology of clinical trials focusing on the PC-Fix clinical trials. *Injury* 32 (Suppl 2): B26–B37.
22. Tepic, S. and Perren, S.M. (1995). The biomechanics of the PC-Fix internal fixator. *Injury* 26 (Suppl 2): B5–B10.
23. Savoldelli, D. and Montavon, P.M. (1995). Clinical handling: small animals. *Injury* 26 (Suppl 2): B47–B50.
24. Auer, J.A., Lischer, C., Kaegi, B. et al. Application of the point contact fixator in large animals. *Injury* 26 (Suppl 2): B37–B46.
25. Eijer, H., Hauke, C., Arens, S. et al. PC-Fix and local infection resistance--influence of implant design on postoperative infection development, clinical and experimental results. *Injury* 32 (Suppl 2): B38–B43.
26. Hertel, R., Eijer, H., Meisser, A. et al. (2001). Biomechanical and biological considerations relating to the clinical use of the point contact-fixator–evaluation of the device handling test in the treatment of diaphyseal fractures of the radius and/or ulna. *Injury* 32 (Suppl 2): B10–B14.
27. Haas, N., Hauke, C., Schütz, M. et al. (2001). Treatment of diaphyseal fractures of the forearm using the point contact fixator (PC-Fix): results of 387 fractures of a prospective multicentric study (PC-Fix II). *Injury* 32 (Suppl 2): B51–B62.
28. Ahmad, M., Nanda, R., Bajwa, A.S. et al. (2007). Biomechanical testing of the locking compression plate: when does the distance between bone and implant significantly reduce construct stability? *Injury* 38: 358–364.
29. Miller, D.L. and Goswami, T. (2007). A review of locking compression plate biomechanics and

their advantages as internal fixators in fracture healing. *Clin. Biomech.* 22: 1049–1062.
30. Roberts, J.W., Grindel, S.I., Rebholz, B. et al. (2007). Biomechanical evaluation of locking plate radial shaft fixation: Unicortical locking fixation versus mixed Bicortical and Unicortical fixation in a Sawbone model. *J. Hand. Surg. Am.* 32: 971–975.
31. Greiwe, R.M. and Archdeacon, M.T. (2007). Locking plate technology: current concepts. *J. Knee Surg.* 20: 50–55.
32. Rowe-Guthrie, K.M., Markel, M.D., and Bleedorn, J.A. (2015). Mechanical evaluation of locking, nonlocking, and hybrid plating constructs using a locking compression plate in a canine synthetic bone model. *Vet. Surg.* 44: 838–842.
33. Whiteside, L.A. and Lesker, P.A. (1978). The effects of extraperiosteal and subperiosteal dissection. II. On fracture healing. *J. Bone Joint Surg. Am.* 60: 26–30.
34. Grundnes, O. and Reikerås, O. (1992). Blood flow and mechanical properties of healing bone. Femoral osteotomies studied in rats. *Acta Orthop. Scand.* 63: 487–491.
35. Ozaki, A., Tsunoda, M., Kinoshita, S. et al. (2000). Role of fracture hematoma and periosteum during fracture healing in rats: interaction of fracture hematoma and the periosteum in the initial step of the healing process. *J. Orthop. Sci.* 5: 64–70.
36. Mizuno, K., Mineo, K., Tachibana, T. et al. (1990). The osteogenetic potential of fracture haematoma. Subperiosteal and intramuscular transplantation of the haematoma. *J. Bone Joint Surg. Br.* 72: 822–829.
37. Tepic, S., Remiger, A.R., Morikawa, K. et al. (1997). Strength recovery in fractured sheep tibia treated with a plate or an internal fixator: an experimental study with a two-year follow-up. *J. Orthop. Trauma* 11: 14–23.
38. Frank Haasnoot, E.v., Münch, T.W.H., Matter, P. et al. (1995). Radiological sequences of healing in internal plates and splints of different contact surface to bone. (DCP, LC-DCP and PC-Fix). *Injury* 26: 28–36.
39. Jain, R., Podworny, N., Hearn, T. et al. (1998). A biomechanical evaluation of different plates for fixation of canine radial osteotomies. *J. Trauma Acute Care Surg.* 44: 193–197.
40. Field, J.R., Hearn, T.C., and Caldwell, C.B. (1997). Bone plate fixation: an evaluation of interface contact area and force of the dynamic compression plate (DCP) and the limited contact-dynamic compression plate (LC-DCP) applied to cadaveric bone. *J. Orthop. Trauma* 11: 368–373.
41. Haug, R.H., Street, C.C., and Goltz, M. (2002). Does plate adaptation affect stability? A biomechanical comparison of locking and nonlocking plates. *J. Oral Maxillofac. Surg.* 60: 1319–1326.
42. Lujan, T.J., Henderson, C.E., Madey, S.M. et al. (2010). Locked plating of distal femur fractures leads to inconsistent and asymmetric callus formation. *J. Orthop. Trauma* 24: 156–162.
43. Bottlang, M., Lesser, M., Koerber, J. et al. (2010). Far cortical locking can improve healing of fractures stabilized with locking plates. *J. Bone Joint Surg. Am.* 92: 1652–1660.
44. Plecko, M., Lagerpusch, N., Andermatt, D. et al. (2013). The dynamisation of locking plate osteosynthesis by means of dynamic locking screws (DLS)–an experimental study in sheep. *Injury* 44: 1346–1357.
45. Tsai, S., Fitzpatrick, D.C., Madey, S.M. et al. (2015). Dynamic locking plates provide symmetric axial dynamization to stimulate fracture healing. *J. Orthop. Res.* 33: 1218–1225.
46. Rizk, A.S. and Al-Ashhab, M.E. (2015). Primary bone grafting with locked plating for comminuted distal femoral fractures: can it improve the results? *Egypt Orthop. J.* 50: 77–83.
47. Gardner, M.J., Nork, S.E., Huber, P. et al. (2010). Less rigid stable fracture fixation in osteoporotic bone using locked plates with near cortical slots. *Injury* 41 (6): 652–656.
48. Bottlang, M., Lesser, M., Koerber, J. et al. (2010). Far cortical locking can improve healing of fractures stabilized with locking plates. *J. Bone Joint Surg. Am.* 92: 1652–1660.
49. Stevens, C.T. and Duis, H.J. (2008). Plate osteosynthesis of simple forearm fractures: LCP versus DC plates. *Acta Orthop. Belg.* 74: 180–183.
50. Hasenboehler, E., Rikli, D., and Babst, R. (2007). Locking compression plate with minimally invasive plate Osteosynthesis in diaphyseal and distal tibial fracture: a retrospective study of 32 patients. *Injury* 38: 365–370.
51. Tan, S.L.E. and Balogh, Z.J. (2009). Indications and limitations of locked plating. *Injury* 40: 683–691.
52. Donlan, R.M. (2002). Biofilms: microbial life on surfaces. *Emerg. Infect. Dis.* 8: 881–890.
53. Ciampolini, J. and Harding, K.G. (2000). Pathophysiology of chronic bacterial osteomyelitis. Why do antibiotics fail so often? *Postgrad. Med. J.* 76: 479–483.
54. Montanaro, L., Testoni, F., Poggi, A. et al. (2011). Emerging pathogenetic mechanisms of the implant-related osteomyelitis by Staphylococcus aureus. *Int. J. Artif. Organs.* 34: 781–788.
55. Norden, C.W. (1970). Experimental osteomyelitis. I. A description of the model. *J. Infect. Dis.* 122: 410–418.
56. Andriole, V.T. and Lytton, B. (1965). The effect and critical duration of increased tissue pressure on susceptibility to bacterial infection. *Br. J. Exp. Pathol.* 46: 308–317.

57. Perren, S.M., Cordey, J., Rahn, B.A. et al. (1988). Early temporary porosis of bone induced by internal fixation implants. A reaction to necrosis, not to stress protection? *Clin. Orthop. Relat. Res.* 232: 139–151.
58. Perren, S.M. (2002). Evolution of the internal fixation of long bone fractures. The scientific basis of biological internal fixation: choosing a new balance between stability and biology. *J. Bone Joint Surg. Br.* 84: 1093–1110.
59. Langkamer, V.G. and Ackroyd, C.E. (1991). Internal fixation of forearm fractures in the 1980s: lessons to be learnt. *Injury* 22: 97–102.
60. Hertel, R., Pisan, M., Lambert, S. et al. (1996). Plate osteosynthesis radius and ulna of diaphyseal fractures of the radius and ulna. *Injury* 27: 545–548.
61. Cordero, J., Munuera, L., and Folgueira, M.D. (1994). Influence of metal implants on infection. An experimental study in rabbits. *J. Bone Joint Surg. Br.* 76: 717–720.
62. Cordero, J., Munuera, L., and Folgueira, M.D. ((1996). The influence of the chemical composition and surface of the implant on infection. *Injury* 27 (Suppl 3): SC34–SC37.
63. Schlegel, U. and Perren, S.M. (2006). Surgical aspects of infection involving osteosynthesis implants: implant design and resistance to local infection. *Injury* 37: 67–73.
64. Arens, S., Eijer, H., Schlegel, U. et al. (1999). Influence of the Design for Fixation Implants on local infection: experimental study of dynamic compression plates versus point contact fixators in rabbits. *J. Orthop. Trauma* 13: 470–476.
65. Arens, S., Hansis, M., Schlegel, U. et al. (1996). Infection after open reduction and internal fixation with dynamic compression plates–clinical and experimental data. *Injury* 27 (Suppl 3): SC27–SC33.
66. Arens, S., Kraft, C., Schlegel, U. et al. (1999). Susceptibility to local infection in biological internal fixation. Experimental study of open vs minimally invasive plate osteosynthesis in rabbits. *Arch. Orthop. Trauma Surg.* 119: 82–85.
67. Kirkpatrick, D., Gandhi, R., and Van, J.E. (2003). Infections associated with locking reconstruction plates: a retrospective review. *J. Oral Maxillofac. Surg.* 61: 462–466.
68. Schepers, T., EMM, V.L., De Vries, M.R. et al. (2011). Increased rates of wound complications with locking plates in distal fibular fractures. *Injury* 42: 1125–1129.
69. Borg, T., Larsson, S., and Lindsjö, U. (2004). Percutaneous plating of distal tibial fractures. Preliminary results in 21 patients. *Injury* 35: 608–614.
70. Hazarika, S., Chakravarthy, J., and Cooper, J. (2006). Minimally invasive locking plate osteosynthesis for fractures of the distal tibia-results in 20 patients. *Injury* 37: 877–887.
71. Sommer, C., Gautier, E., Müller, M. et al. First clinical results of the locking compression plate (LCP). *Injury* 34 (Suppl 2): B43–B54.
72. Solano, M.A., Danielski, A., Kovach, K. et al. (2015)). Locking plate and screw fixation after tibial plateau leveling osteotomy reduces post-operative infection rate in dogs over 50 kg. *Vet. Surg.* 44: 59–64.
73. Uhthoff, H.K., Poitras, P., and Backman, D.S. (2006). Internal plate fixation of fractures: short history and recent developments. *J. Orthop. Sci.* 11: 118–126.
74. Wilcke, M.K.T., Abbaszadegan, H., and Adolphson, P.Y. (2011). Wrist function recovers more rapidly after volar locked plating than after external fixation but the outcomes are similar after 1 year. *Acta Orthop.* 82: 76–81.
75. Egol, K., Walsh, M., Tejwani, N. et al. (2008). Bridging external fixation and supplementary Kirschner-wire fixation versus volar locked plating for unstable fractures of the distal radius: a randomised, prospective trial. *J. Bone Joint Surg. Br.* 90: 1214–1221.
76. Collins, C.P., Pirinjian-Leonard, G., Tolas, A. et al. (2004). A prospective randomized clinical trial comparing 2.0-mm locking plates to 2.0-mm standard plates in treatment of mandible fractures. *J. Oral Maxillofac. Surg.* 62: 1392–1395.
77. Lapcin, O., Arıkan, Y., Yavuz, U. et al. (2016). Evaluation of outcomes in aseptic non-unions of the forearm bones in adults treated with LCP and autograft. *Ulus. Travma Acil Cerrahi Derg.* 22: 283–289.
78. Singh, A.K., Narsaria, N., Seth, R.R. et al. (2014). Plate osteosynthesis of fractures of the shaft of the humerus: comparison of limited contact dynamic compression plates and locking compression plates. *J. Orthop. Traumatol.* 15: 117–122.
79. Gill, S.P.S., Mittal, A., Raj, M. et al. (2017). Stabilisation of diaphyseal fractures of both bones forearm with limited contact dynamic compression or locked compression plate: comparison of clinical outcomes. *Int. J. Res. Orthop.* 3: 623–631.
80. Sproul, R.C., Iyengar, J.J., Devcic, Z. et al. (2011). A systematic review of locking plate fixation of proximal humerus fractures. *Injury* 42: 408–413.
81. Szypryt, P. and Forward, D. (2009). The use and abuse of locking plates. *J. Orthop. Trauma* 23: 281–290.
82. González, Y.H., Martín, A.D., Sánchez, F.J. et al. (2007). Early results with the new internal fixator systems LCP and LISS: a prospective study. *Acta Orthop. Belg.* 73: 60–69.
83. Cronier, P., Pietu, G., Dujardin, C. et al. (2010). The concept of locking plates. *Orthop. Traumatol. Surg. Res.* 96: S17–S36.

4 Dynamic Compression vs. Locking Plating – Is One "Better"? A Review of Biomechanical Principles and *in vitro* Testing

Adam H. Biedrzycki

4.1 Introduction

4.1.1 Background

Advances in fracture repair for both human and veterinary surgery applications continues to expand into areas evaluating shape memory alloys (SMAs) [1], various thermoplastic composites materials such as carbon fiber/polyetheretherketone (CF/PEEK) [2], bone cements, and biocompatible ceramics. These advances stand on the backbone and extensive clinical experience gained using various plates for fracture repair. The primary device used in orthopedic fracture repair in veterinary surgery has been the limited contact dynamic compression plate (LC-DCP) or more recently, the locking compression plate (LCP). Each device has its advantages and disadvantages. However, given the choice, which plate is considered better? Many factors can affect the ultimate clinical outcome, including fracture configuration, patient size, surgical technique with experience, and implant composition. The aim of this chapter is to eliminate all extraneous variables and discuss, from a biomechanical viewpoint of fracture healing, which is better, the LC-DCP or the LCP?

4.1.2 Historical Perspective

The evolution of fracture repair has progressed greatly since it was first reported in 1886 by Carl Hansmann in conjunction with advances in anesthesia, antisepsis, and radiography [3]. Hansmanns' original device consisted of using nickel coated sheet steel with part of the plate and shanks of screws protruding through the skin to allow for percutaneous removal four to eight weeks later (Figure 4.1). Although revolutionary at the time, the concept was limited as it failed to fully appreciate the engineering challenges associated with orthopedic repair such laws of stress, strain, and leverage. The plate functioned merely as a connector without the ability to allow for approximation or even compression of osseous fragments. The progress of osteosynthesis was further advanced in the 1960s by the Arbeitsgemeinschaft fur Osteosynthesefragen (AO) group and the development of the dynamic compression plate (DCP) in 1969 utilizing the laws of friction to allow for fragmentary compression [4, 5]. However, the extensive underside of the DCP interfered with the underlying periosteum and the blood supply to the cortex, which led to the

Locking Plates in Veterinary Orthopedics, First Edition.
Edited by Matthew D. Barnhart and Karl C. Maritato.

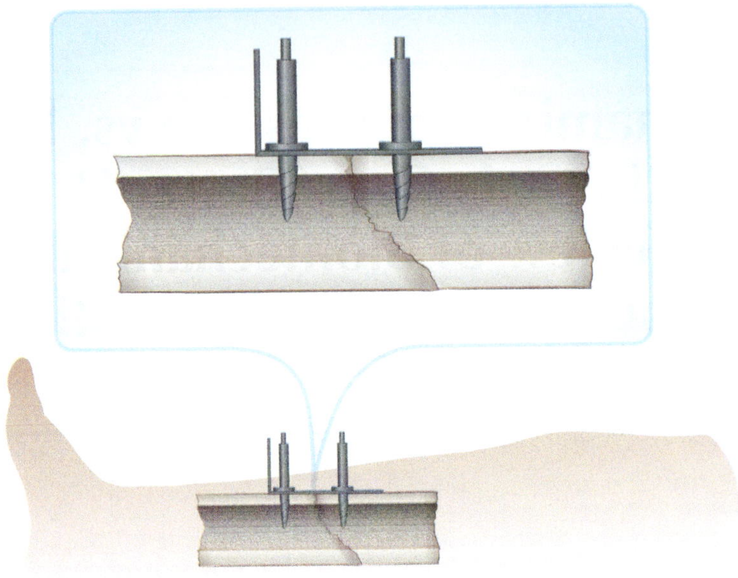

Figure 4.1 The original plate developed by Hansmann [3], providing only basic, monocortical bridging connection across a fracture. (Source: Modified from Hansmann [3].)

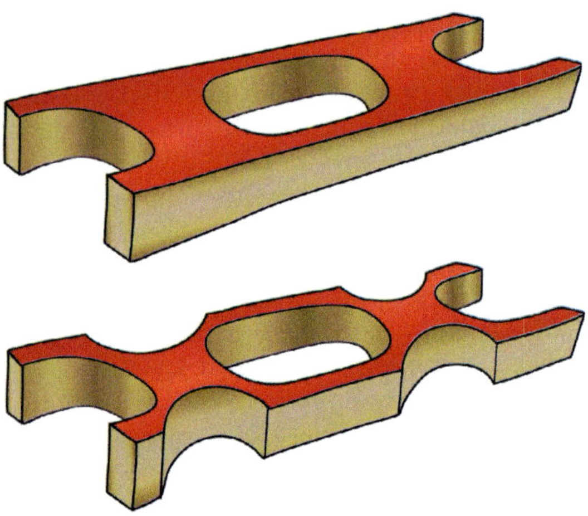

Figure 4.2 Comparison of the footprints of the DCP and the limited contact dynamic compression plate (LC-DCP). The LC-DCP reduces the DCP footprint by 50%. (Source: Modified from Synthes.)

development of the LC-DCP in 1990 (Figure 4.2) [6]. The LC-DCP has an approximately 50% reduced footprint to minimize this interference with biological healing, although the plate is still restricted in that it must be compressed to the bone and thus may cause a disturbance in the vascular supply [4, 7].

The successful use of the LC-DCP is dependent on the frictional forces generated between the remaining, reduced footprint of the plate and the cortex of the bone. This frictional force is essentially limited by the degree of screw torque that can be placed. Using conventional screws, a plate can be compressed to the bone with a force of 2000–3000 N [8]. However, the resulting frictional force this generates in preventing plate sliding is dependent on the coefficient of friction between the two surfaces. To overcome these challenges and increase the coefficient of friction, soft tissue stripping and bone cements have been used. However, both of these have limitations and tissue stripping can further damage the periosteal blood supply. Early attempts to create a device less dependent on the bone-plate frictional force or "internal fixator" included the point-contact fixator (PC-Fix) [9] and less invasive stabilization system (LISS plate) [10] with the resultant development of the LCP in 2001 [11].

4.1.2.1 *What Do We Mean by Better?*

The term *better* can have many connotations. By "better," we are implying we want to achieve optimal fracture healing. This suggest the restoration of the normal functional biomechanics of the bone, i.e. a return to pre-fracture stiffness and strength of the osseous tissues [12]. From a clinical context, there are a plethora of factors that go into determining an optimal outcome. In a biomechanical context, we will assume that the interpretation of "better" is assigned to bone healing and biomechanical superiority of one implant versus the other in conjunction with what each technique may contribute to the overall biomechanical picture. In order to do this, one must understand the biological concepts of bone healing, and fracture repair. A variety of biomechanical concepts, definitions of which are provided in Table 4.1.

4.1.3 Fracture Stability

Stability is a crucial concept in orthopedics in order to permit successful fracture healing. As defined in Table 4.1, stability can be either **relative** or **absolute** depending on the method of repair [14]. Thus, the degree of implant and fragment stability determines the amount of strain at a fracture site; the level of stain present will determine the type of bone healing that occurs. **Absolute stability** occurs where fracture gap strain is less than 2% and results in primary bone healing via osteonal cutting cones if the fracture gap is <200 μm. **Relative stability** occurs where fracture gap strain is 2–10% and healing is via callus formation. At strains in excess of 10%, fracture healing cannot occur, and the site is destined to form a non-union or mal-union.

When fractures are loaded, and the fragments return to their original configuration when unloaded (i.e. elastic deformation), relative stability is present. If after loading, the fracture fragments do not return to their original configuration, plastic deformation has occurred and the fracture is considered unstable. The ability of different tissues to heal in the presence of strain varies. Lamellar bone has the lowest strain tolerance of 2% while granulation tissue can form while undergoing 100% strain [14, 15]. **The advantage of callus and relative stability is that the process occurs much more rapidly than direct primary bone healing with absolute stability** [14].

Compressing a fracture using a DCP can reduce gap lengths between unstable fragment sections to near zero values. As a result, any fracture site motion that occurs in this near zero gap will result in very high gap strains if the motion persists [16]. When presented with high fracture gap strains preventing healing, reduction in strain can occur via (i) increasing gap length, such as occurs with bone resorption at a fracture site, fracture comminution or imperfect reduction, or (ii) decreasing motion present at the fracture gap. Placing the LC-DCP on the tension surface of the bone, where the metallic plate will be the strongest, gap motion and therefore fracture strain, will be limited as long as the LC-DCP can maintain this function.

4.2 The LC-DCP

4.2.1 Construct Basics

Plate-bone-screw constructs can function as either load-sharing or load-bearing devices. The goal of these conventional plating techniques is to provide absolute stability. Occurrences when absolute stability and primary bone healing are essential include articular fractures where joint congruity is crucial; it has been shown that it is important to limit any joint step off to be less than a critical value of 2 mm of incongruity [17–19]. When compression plates are axially loaded in either tension or compression, they serve to convert these forces to shear stress (parallel to the surface) at the bone-plate interface. This shear stress is countered by a frictional force. The normal force, which acts perpendicular to the plate/bone surface, is equal to the axial force generated by the torque applied to the screws fixing the plate to the bone, which is approximately 3–5 Nm for 3.5 mm cortical screws placed into human femora [20]. However, not all screws are tightened with the same degree of torque; therefore, the screw with the greatest insertional torque bears the greatest amount of load in this system. Currently, during screw insertion, surgeons use subjective feel when inserting these screws and stop tightening the screw (stopping torque) when they feel it is "tight," as further torque will strip the threads (stripping torque). It has been demonstrated in several studies that human surgeons achieve a stopping/stripping

Table 4.1 Definition of commonly used biomechanical terms.

Biomechanical Term	Definition
Brittle Material	Material with a low or absent capacity for plastic deformation prior to ultimate failure.
Ductile Material	Material with a high capacity for plastic deformation prior to ultimate failure.
Elasticity	Reversible deformation of a material. When a material is unloaded after loading in the elastic range, it returns to its original shape and dimensions.
Elastic Modulus (E)	Constant of proportionality between stress and strain, also termed Young's modulus., where $E = \delta\sigma / \delta\varepsilon = \tan \phi$.
Friction	The frictional force is directly proportional to the normal force (Amonton's second law). The frictional force F_f is parallel to the surface and is in a directly opposite direction to the net applied external force, F_e the normal force F_n, is force exerted by each surface, directed perpendicular to the surface. F_f and F_n are connection via a proportional constant, μ (frictional coefficient), such that $F_f = \mu F_n$.
Hysteresis	For time-dependent elastic materials, during cyclic loading within the elastic region, hysteresis is the energy dissipated between loading and unloading cycles, usually in the form of heat energy, governed by the coefficient of restitution.
Plasticity	Plasticity describes the irreversible deformation of a material undergoing permanent morphological alterations in response to applied forces.
Stability	Degree of relative movement between structures. Relative stability in orthopedics indicates that motion exists between fracture gaps under loading, but return to the initial position during unloading. Healing is via callus formation (endochondral ossification). Absolute stability is where no motion occurs between fracture fragments during loading, and healing occurs through osteonal cutting cones (endosteal healing).
Stiffness	The resistance of a material to deform under load. Materials with high stiffness (rigid material) deform less under a given load (c.f flexible). The product of the cross-sectional area (A) and the elastic modulus (E) expresses axial stiffness, such that $R_{ax} = A\,E$. Bending stiffness is defined as the product of the axial area moment of inertia and the elastic modulus, such that $R_{be} = I_{ax}\,E$,
Strain, ε	Deformation of a material under a given load. It is expressed as elongation per unit of original length (l) and is dimensionless, although often given as a percentage, where $\varepsilon = \Delta l / l_0$. For a material undergoing deformation, the ratio of transverse strain to axial strain is termed Poisson's ration, or ν.
Strength	Generally, strength indicates how much force a material can support before ultimate failure.
Stress, σ	Force per unit cross-section area. Stress is directly proportional to strain with the elastic modulus as a constant of proportionality. Unit is Newton per m^2 (Pascal, Pa). Can exist as normal stress, acting perpendicular to a surface, or shear stress when the force acts parallel to a surface.
Toughness	The energy absorbed by a structure during the loading process, determined by integrating the stress–strain curve, such that: $\frac{\text{energy}}{\text{volume}} = \int_0^{\epsilon_f} \sigma \, d\epsilon$ where ϵ is strain; ϵf is the strain upon failure; σ is the stress. Generally, toughness indicates how much energy a material can absorb before ultimate failure.
Fatigue	The relationship between stress magnitude and number of loading cycles, described by Wöhler's curve. Fatigue stress is defined as an asymptotic line of Wöhler curve.

Source: Modified from Gautier [13].

torque ratio of 66–92%, resulting in under- and overtightening of screws on a regular basis [21–24]. If screw insertion torque exceeds the shear resistance of the bone, then screws will strip and there may be subsequent loss of fixation. Thus, when an external force, F_e, is applied which exceeds the frictional force, F_f, the plate will slip on the bone (Figure 4.3).

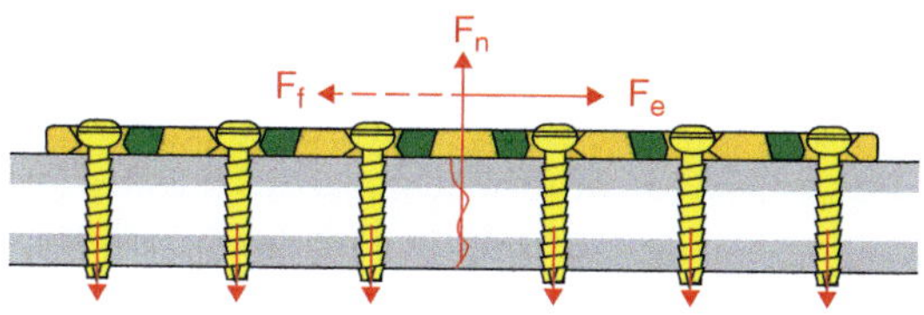

Figure 4.3 The frictional force is directly proportional to the normal force. The frictional force, F_f, is parallel to the surface and is in a directly opposite direction to the net applied external force, F_e. The normal force, F_n, is force exerted by each surface, directed perpendicular to the surface. F_f and F_n are related via a proportional constant, μ (frictional coefficient), such that $F_f = \mu F_n$.

4.2.2 Axial Loads

One of the major benefits of locking screws is that they can be used in bone of poor quality, such as osteoporotic bone. With conventional plating, osteoporotic bone can only withstand a maximum screw insertion torque of approximately 3 Nm, with values often less than this [14]. Experimentally, it has been shown that 3 Nm of screw torque permits motion between the plate and the bone at loads as low as 500 N [9, 20]. This screw torque is insufficient to generate a sufficient normal force, F_n to prevent plate and fracture motion, which can lead to excessive gap strains that exceed the 10% maximum for secondary bone healing. This 3 Nm value is important in veterinary medicine in relation to neonatal surgeries. Although the process of osteoporosis that occurs in humans is less of a concern in animals, it has been shown that a significant number of 4.5 mm cortical screws placed in neonatal calf femora will strip prior to achieving 3 Nm of torque [25].

The success of the LC-DCP is therefore highly dependent on the level of frictional forces that can be generated. As such, increasing the coefficient of friction, μ, or increasing the screw torque to increase the normal force F_n, will lead to increases in the frictional force, F_f, that the plate can generate in order to resist an applied load, F_e. Once the frictional force between the plate and the bone is overcome, the resistance to axial loading is transferred to the single screw furthest from the fracture site in the direction of loading. For a 3.5 mm cortical screw, the maximum load that can be withstood once motion has occurred at the plate–bone interface is 1200 N [20]. As the screwhead is not locked in conventional plating, the cis-cortex for that screw experiences high stresses, which can result in bone resorption and screw loosening if they exceed the strength of the bone. Conventional screws therefore fail by this form of toggling within the bone and, as each screw effectively functions in series, all stresses are concentrated at a single individual screw at any given time [14]. With the resultant screw loosening, there is increased strain at the fracture sites and increased motion, which prevents healing via callus formation once it exceeds 10% strain. It should be noted, therefore, that the LC-DCP construct is strongest immediately after application; with the progress of time, the axial screw forces exerted by the screws is diminished due to remodeling around the screw threads, which leads to a corresponding decrease in normal force F_n and the fictional force F_f at the bone–plate interface.

4.2.3 Bending Loads

For conventional plating methods, resistance to bending loads is equal to the bending stiffness of the plate for gap lengths greater than zero. When bone fragments are compressed and the gap length is equal to zero, the resistance to bending is determined by the resistance of the bone threads of a single screw to shear stress. The location of which screw experiences these stresses is dependent on the biomechanics of the fracture and the plate. When the plate is placed on the tension surface of a bone during bending, the highest shear stresses associated with the screw threads will occur at the screws at the end of the plate. If the plate is placed on the compression side of the fracture, the threads and screws closest to the fracture site will have the highest shear stresses. The most critical screws placed are those in close proximity to the fracture, thus favoring the placement of the LC-DCP on the tension surface of the bone. High screw shear stresses eventually culminate in screw pullout (Figure 4.4c). The required pullout force depends on bone quality, cortical thickness, and outer diameters of the screw.

4.2.4 The Bone–Screw Interface

The importance of the frictional forces generated in axial loading are therefore paramount in

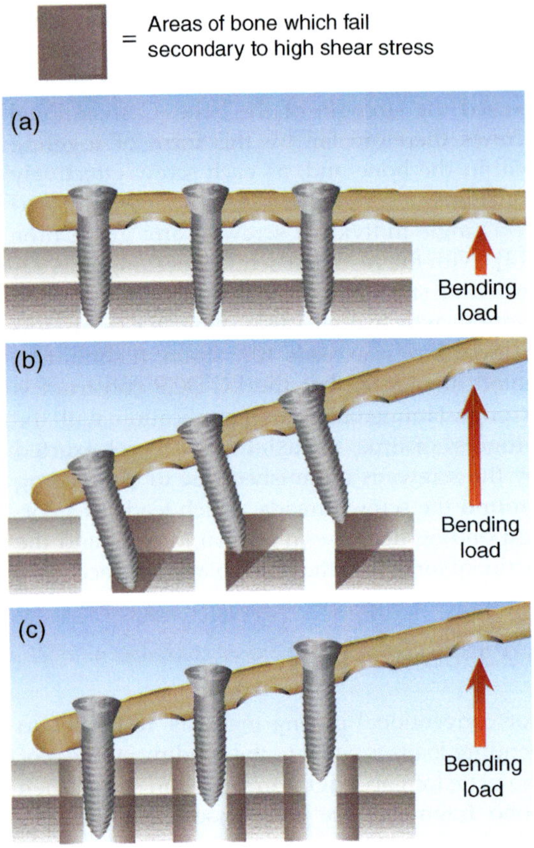

Figure 4.4 (a) Bending load applied to plate–screw–bone constructs. (b) Locking angular stable screws generate compressive forces in the bone resisting pullout. (c) Conventional LC-DCP with nonlocked screws rotate within the plate with the bone in each thread subjected to shear stress. (Source: Modified from Egol et al. [14].)

preventing plate sliding, as are the shear stresses on the bone threads exerted during bending. From both these loading modalities, it can be seen that the weakest point in the plate–bone–screw construct is the bone–screw interface. Therefore, methods that have been attempted to improve this bone–screw interface include (i) increasing the contact area between the screw and bone via bone cement or using larger core diameter screws or cancellous screws, (ii) changing the forces at the bone–screw interface from shear stresses associated with pullout to compressive stress that occurs with the use of locking plates, (iii) increasing the coefficient of friction between the plate and the bone, or (iv) the use of Schuhli nuts, which create angular stability of cortical screws [13]. Schuhli nuts are threaded washers placed underneath the plate and are tapped to receive cortical screws. As the screws are tightened, the nut is pulled toward the plate, which creates an angular stable screw with enhanced holding power. However, the use of Schuhli nuts is technically cumbersome and therefore more elegant forms of angle stable screw fixation are used, such as the LCP.

4.3 The LCP

4.3.1 Construct Basics

The LCP is the successor of the PC-Fix system, which utilized the theory of bridging plate osteosynthesis [14]. In this application, fracture healing occurs via secondary healing, in contrast to the LC-DCP, where it occurs via primary bone healing. The PC-Fix and the LCP systems function much more like a conventional external fixator, even though they are placed internally. Thus, the principles governing the application of external fixators must be applied to locked plates, in which the stiffness of the construct is greatly increased as the connected bars are moved closer to the bone; screw lengths for locked plates being 10–15 times shorter than the pins for external fixators, which greatly enhances construct rigidity [14]. A further benefit to the locking construct is that it is no longer necessary for the plate to be placed on the tension surface of a bone.

The development of the LCP led to angular and axial stability, which eliminated the necessity for exact plate contouring. Thus, when using LCPs as an internal form of an external skeletal fixator, healing will occur via secondary mechanisms with callus formation, progressing more rapidly than the primary healing and absolute stability of an LC-DCP construct.

The need for absolute stability and primary bone healing has been questioned, and the goals of the newer biological fixation techniques are to achieve relative stability and secondary bone healing [14]. The limitations of the conventional plate system included (i) inadequate fixation in pathologic or osteopenic bone, (ii) necrosis-induced bone loss, which can lead to necrosis of bone segments, (iii) stress shielding due to absolute stability, which can predispose to fracture after device removal, and conversely, (iv) due to lack of stability during to motion at the plate–bone–screw interface, can result in increased gap strains resulting in delayed or nonunions.

Biomechanically, the major benefit of the LCP is that it results in a single beam construct, where there is no motion between the plate–bone–screw interfaces. It has been demonstrated that single beam constructs are four times stronger than load sharing beam constructs once motion occurs between the individual components of the beam construct [13, 26]. Thus, conventional plates function as single beam constructs only in ideal circumstances when good-quality bone permits high screw insertion torque and no motion occurs between the plate and the bone. Deviation from the ideal in any one of these three circumstances results in failure of the conventional plate. The benefit of the locking plate is that it will continue to function as a single beam construct even when one or more of these critical components are violated.

Conventional plate screw insertion is reliant on the shear stresses placed at the bone–screw interface, whereas locking plates convert this shear stress into compressive stress. Biomechanically, this is advantageous, as bone has much higher resistance to compressive forces than shear forces. Furthermore, as described in the axial and bending loading models of the conventional plate, the strength of the fixation becomes dependent on an individual screws axial stiffness or pullout strength, respectively. By contrast, locking screws are not individually and sequentially besieged by forces, but rather, the strength of the construct is equal to the sum of all the bone–screw interfaces. This also results in angular stability of the screws, which, in turn, results in a lower incidence of screw loosening and secondary displacement of fracture fragments. While in many instances this is an advantage, it can also be a disadvantage. For a straight LCP, all screws are inserted parallel to each other; thus, all screw loading is identical, as the screws face the same direction. In thin, osteoporotic bone or in neonatal tissue, this can be problematic, as failure in the one direction will result in failure of all screws (Figure 4.5). However, slight wave formation in the plate will result in converging and diverging screws, enhancing their pullout strength, which is also one of the purported advantages of the variable angle-LCP (VA-LCP) over the fixed-angle LCP. Although there is some angulation possible with the standard LCP, the angle is limited to less than 5° [27]. The benefits of the VA-LCP are that it is able to form a fixed-angle-type construct at customizable screw angles. The design of the VA locking hole permits screw

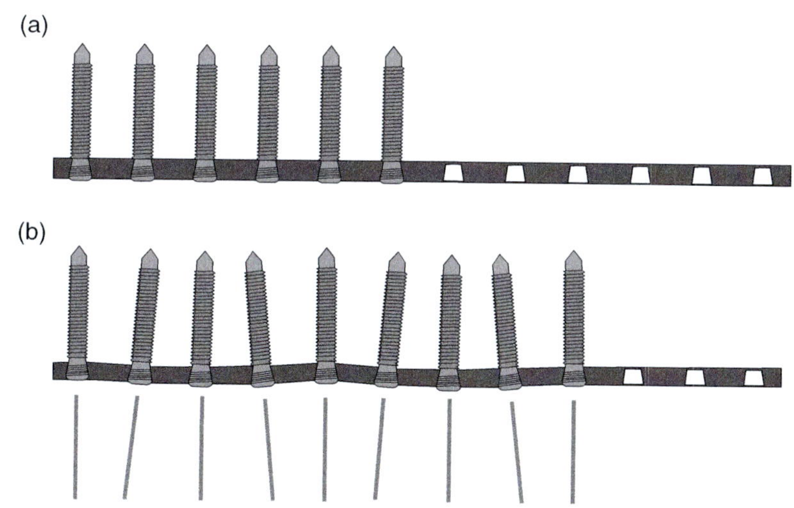

Figure 4.5 Bending the internal fixator to avoid parallel screw insertion. (a) In osteoporotic bone, parallel insertion of all locked screw may be disadvantageous; (b) The pullout resistance of the construct can be improved when the plate slightly is bent forth and back resulting in divergent and convergent locked screw directions. (Source: From Gautier et al. [26].)

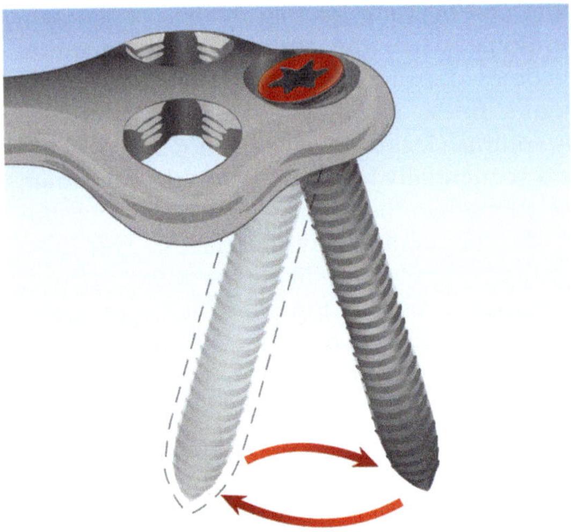

Figure 4.6 Variable angle locking compression plate (VA-LCP) plate combi hole. Four columns of threads in locking hole provide four points of locking between the VA LCP Plate and the specially designed variable angle locking screw. (Source: Modified from Synthes.)

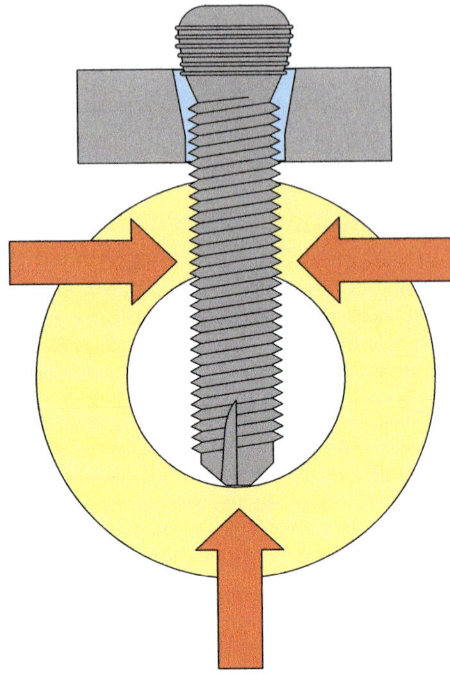

Figure 4.7 In a low diameter bone the tip of the screw can contacts the opposite bone cortex before the screwhead engages in the plate hole thread. This leads to the destruction of the bone thread in the near cortex and complete loss of anchorage of the screw. (Source: From Gautier et al. [26].)

angulation within a 30° cone around the central axis of the plate hole (Figure 4.6). However, VA systems still provide the greatest resistance to rotation when the screws are inserted perpendicular to the plate. As the off-axis angle of insertion increases, the resistance to rotation at the screw-plate interfaces decreases in a near linear fashion; it is unknown if this relationship results in a clinically significant difference in fracture healing [28].

4.3.2 LCP Technical Challenges

One technical challenge associated with the placement of locking screws is that there is a complete loss of the surgical sensation of screw tightening in the bone; the LCP screws feel secure as the threads on the head engage the plate, but the shaft threads in the bone may be stripped or may not even be engaging bone, without the surgeon's awareness. This may be particularly true when placing monocortical screws, especially in narrow bones, in which the screw tip contacts the *trans* cortex while the threads engage in the plate, leading to stripping of the *cis* cortex (Figure 4.7).

As mentioned previously, another disadvantage associated with a fixed-angle locked screwhead position is an inability to angle screws, which, under some circumstances, can have disastrous consequences when plates are placed eccentrically [26, 29] (Figure 4.8). This is of particular concern in the distal aspect of the ulna when repairing olecranon fractures in the equine species, which can lead to catastrophic consequences via radial fracture (Figure 4.9) [30].

Additionally, inappropriately inserted screws can produce failure via cross threading, whereby the head of the screw is offset in the threads of the plate and may disengage from the plate. Cold welding can also occur between the screw and the plate, particularly in softer titanium locking screws [31]. However, several reports indicate that fusion is rarely found, in which case the term *jamming* should be used [32]. The concept of cold welding is a true phenomenon that occurs when reactive metals come into close contact and the rough asperities on their surfaces form junctions under high pressures [33]. Lastly, if locking screws are inserted with insufficient torque, they may not engage adequately within

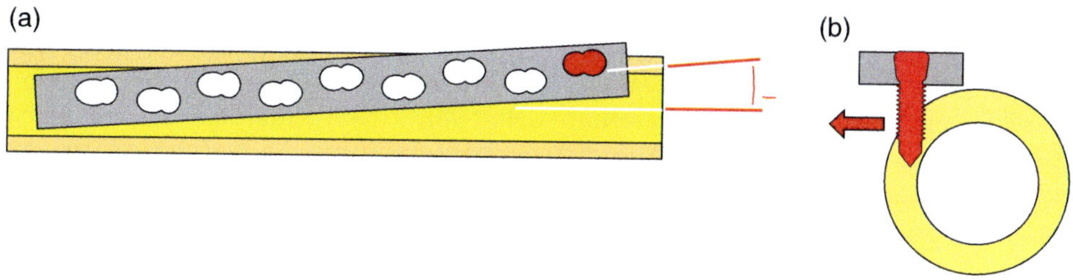

Figure 4.8 Malalignment between bone axis and plate. (a) Malalignment between bone axis and plate leads to an eccentric plate position; (b) At the far end of the plate, a monocortical screw will not anchor in bone in such circumstances. (Source: From Gautier et al. [26].)

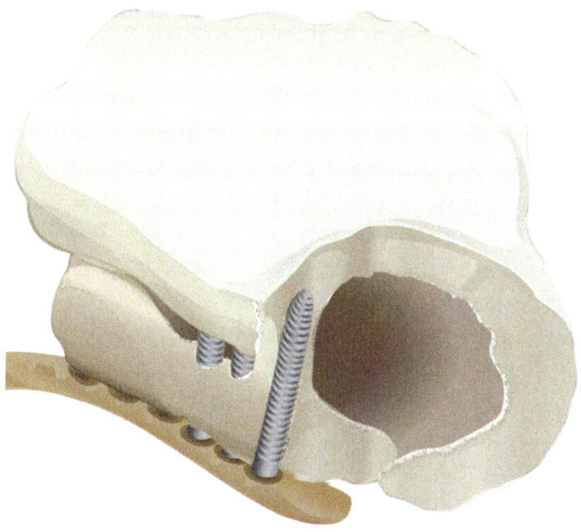

Figure 4.9 Example of an ulnar fracture repair with a locking screw placed entirely within the lateral cortex of the radius, resulting in catastrophic radial fracture. Note also that the inserted screw is shorter than the predrilled screw hole. (Source: Modified from Jackson et al. [30].)

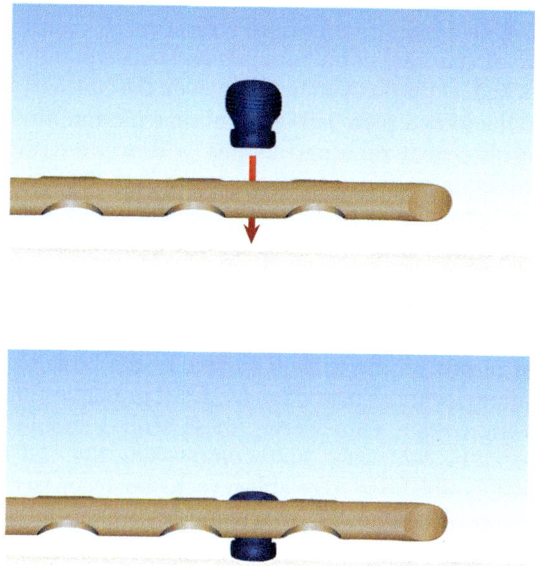

Figure 4.10 Specially designed LCP spaces can be placed in the locking holes to ensure the plate remains at an optimal distance of 2 mm or less away from the bone. Once other locking screws are placed to hold the plate in position, the spacers can be removed and replaced with locking screws. (Source: Modified from Synthes.)

the plate, and ultimately back out. This is especially true when using these systems in large animals; however, this can be avoided with the aid of a torque-limiting driver.

Since locking constructs are not dependent on friction generated between the plate and the bone, the blood supply underneath the periosteum to the cortical bone is preserved [34, 35]. Improved blood supply may accelerate healing, reducing risk of infection and bone resorption. To take full advantage of this principle, specially designed LCP spacers are available that create a 2 mm buffer zone between the plate and the bone when locked screws are placed (Figure 4.10). However, while distance off the bone may have biologic advantages, increasing the distance from 2 to 6 mm decreases torsional and axial stability of the construct by 10–15% [36, 37]. The current recommendation is therefore that the LCP is to be placed no more than 2 mm off the osseous surface.

4.3.3 Composite Locked and Compression Plating

Thorough knowledge of the biomechanics of conventional plates and locking plates is critical in order for a surgeon to be able to successfully blend the two techniques since a number of locking plate systems are specifically designed to accept both locking and nonlocking screws. Failure to understand the principles governing LC-DCP and LCP models can result in a lack of absolute or relative stability of the fracture repair creating an environment with high fracture gap strains which prevent callus formation and healing. If both sides of a fracture are already locked and fixed in position, the use of cortical screws will be suboptimal, as the bone-plate contact is already fixed and the friction required to produce stability will not be generated. Additionally, if a fragment is first compressed with cortical screws, creating a smaller fracture gap and subsequently locked in this position but, however, the elasticity of the locked plate fails to minimize motion, the result is that high gap strains will occur with subsequent failure of osseous union [14]. The recommendation is therefore that when combining techniques, the principles of the more stringent LC-DCP application be followed. Accordingly, while a pure LCP construct can be placed on any surface of a bone, a composite construct should be placed on the tension surface of the bone to follow the more restrictive LC-DCP principles. If using compression screws, these screws should be all be completed first, compressing the LCP plate to the bone to establish plate–bone contact and set up frictional forces in the system, prior to locking screw application. An example of the use of pure LCP constructs is application for minimally invasive surgery for medial condylar fractures in horses. Cortical screws are placed distally to allow for fragment compression and joint congruity, with proximal application of an LCP with locked screws occupying every available plate hole. A hybrid construct, blending locking and cortical technology on the same plate, is often used for the repair of olecranon fractures in horses, where cortical screws can be used to provide fragmentary compression on the tension surface of the bone applied as a tension band principle, or for screw angulation purposes, followed by subsequent locking of the construct through the remaining holes in position using locking screws.

4.3.4 Monocortical vs Bicortical Screws

Consider a simple transverse fracture from a basic biomechanical perspective when two monocortical screws are placed on either side of the fracture. Failure of this construct will occur due to either screw breakage or due to failure of the screw bone interface. Since the bending stiffness of screw (i.e. rod) is proportional to its radius to the fourth power, using a bicortical screw will not change the screw failure load, but it will improve the screw bone interface [13, 26]. The bone–screw interface is therefore an important foundation principle governing the use of monocortical or bicortical screws.

Monocortical screw fixation has several advantages over bicortical fixation: (i) ease of measuring screw lengths percutaneously when performing minimally invasive procedures, (ii) ease of insertion and decreased instrument complexity as there are less stringent requirement for depth measurements, (iii) axial control of the screw is provided by the plate–screw interface, (iv) decreased damage to the endosteal blood supply, (v) no need to generate high axial loads to compress the plate to the bone, and (vi) avoidance of intramedullary implants when using plate/rod combinations. However, two principles regarding the screw's working length need to be adhered to when using monocortical screws (Figure 4.11). The use of monocortical screws should be limited to bone segments loaded in bending or axial load only. Bones loaded in torque create high stresses at the bone–screw interface. Therefore, a longer working length is needed in these cases and a bicortical screw is preferable to resist rotational screw displacement. For a similar reason, the use of monocortical screws is not recommended in bones with a thin bone cortex, which also serves to decrease the working length of the screw. Additionally, the axial pullout of screws is determined by the outer diameter of the screw, a monocortical 5.0 locking screw provides between 60–70% of the holding force of a conventional 4.5 mm bicortical screw [38].

4.3.5 Number of Screws

The optimum screw ratio (number of screw holes filled: number of holes in the plate) has not been sufficiently researched, particularly in large animal models where there's an impetus to fill every available hole to provide a more rigid construct. In respect to the human and

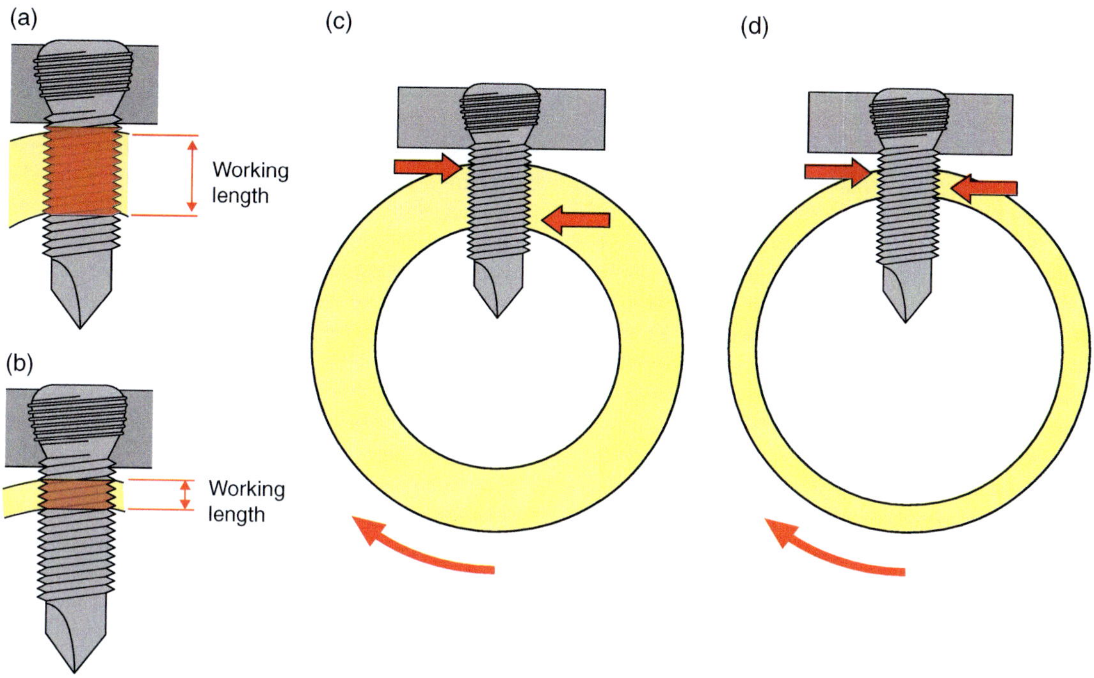

Figure 4.11 Importance of cortical thickness on the working length of monocortical screws. The working length of monocortical screws depends on the thickness of the bone cortex. (a) In normal bone, this working length is sufficient; (b) In osteoporotic bone, the cortex is very thin and thus, the working length of a monocortical screw is insufficient. This difference of the working length is important when osteoporotic bones mainly loaded in torque have to be stabilized. (c) In normal bone, the length of anchorage of the screw thread is sufficient to withstand rotational displacement. (d) In case of osteoporosis, this working length is very short due to the thin cortex, and under torque the bone thread soon will wear out and secondary displacement and instability will occur (d). (Source: From Gautier et al. [26].)

small-animal applications of LCPs, a screw ratio of 0.4–0.5 for bridging fixation with three or four screws either side of the fracture gap is recommended [26, 39]. In these applications, increasing the number of screws in the construct does not necessarily equate to an increased construct stability [26, 36]. As fewer screws are inserted, the leverage on the plate increases, which results in decreasing the load on each screw (Figure 4.12) [26].

The difference between filling every hole with a screw and leaving some holes open also has an impact on the construct stability. By omitting a single hole on either side of a fracture, constructs become more flexible in compression and torsion by 60 and 30% respectively [36]. Noteworthy is that the distance from nearest screw to the fracture site is of most importance, as it has the greatest influence on axial stiffness and torsional rigidity [36]. However, in terms of axial stiffness, more than three screws on either side of the fracture offers little advantage, and no benefit to torsional stiffness occurs after four screws are placed each side of a fracture fragment.

The nearest screw-fracture distance is also critical, as the bending forces exerted on a plate that spans a short distance increase the local strains in the implant; the same bending forces over a longer segment decrease local strain by spreading the strain load throughout an increased span length, thereby improving implant fatigue resistance (Figure 4.12). In human orthopedics, some locking constructs were determined so stiff that they prevented callus formation, which led to the development of the principles of far cortical locking (FCL), whereby screws were locked in the plate and in the far cortex only (no thread purchase in the near cortex) [40]. By contrast, in the horse, this

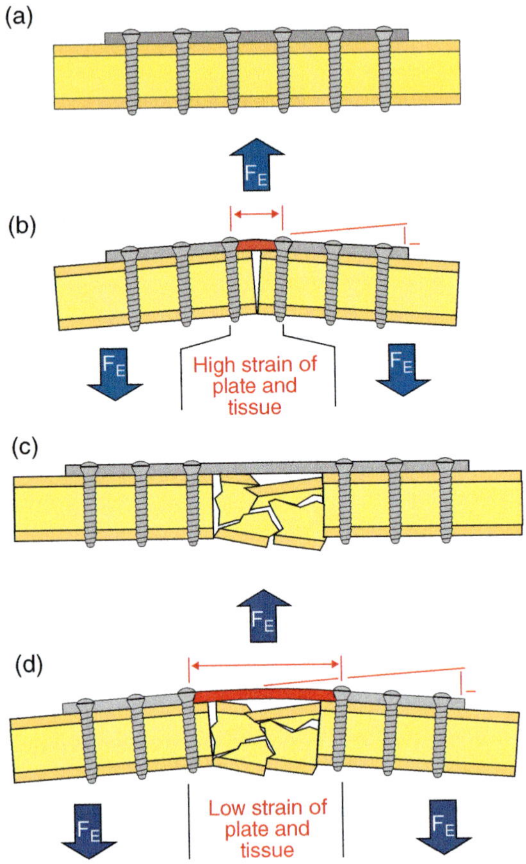

Figure 4.12 Plate strain in three-point bending. When the segment to be bent is short (a, b) the relative deformation (strain) is high and the implant is increasingly likely to undergo fatigue failure. When the plate spans a longer comminuted fracture area (c, d) the same three-point bending leads to an equal absolute deformation (angulation) of the plate. But, the deformation is distributed over a longer distance leading to low implant strain and higher resistance against fatigue. (Source: From Gautier et al. [26].)

degree of overall stiffness preventing fracture healing is unachievable with current implants. In such large animals, the majority of implant failures occur due to loosening (as result of screw–bone interface failure) and bent or broken screws (due to screw failure) [41] and less often due to catastrophic plate failure (Figure 4.12). Therefore, since it is important to decrease the cycling on each screw and maintain the screw–bone interface as much as possible in large animals, the recommendation is to utilize every available hole in a given plate (Figure 4.13).

4.4 DCP vs. LCP

From an economic standpoint, both LCPs and locking screws are more expensive than their nonlocking counterparts and while the cost difference may be small when using a single plate with a few screws, the larger, double-plated constructs sometimes used in equine surgery with a majority of locking screws can rapidly escalate the costs of the hardware involved. Biomechanically, testing of LCPs has been performed *in vitro* on cadaver models [42–45], animal models [46–49], and artificial models [36, 42, 50]. In general, all the tests involve static loading, cyclic loading, or both, in either compression or torsion.

There are a variety of studies where the LCP has been shown to have superior biomechanical properties compared to the LC-DCP, particularly in bone of poor quality [43, 51]. However, there are also several publications that have demonstrated that for specific situations (e.g. pastern arthrodesis in horses), no mechanical advantage is offered by the LCP over the DCP [52, 53].

Where clinically applicable, differences are not only reported for axial, torsion, or bending properties but also for fatigue resistance to cyclic loading [42]. It is important to stress, however, that to the author's knowledge, no studies have revealed any biomechanical disadvantage of the LCP system compared to conventional plating. However, some conventional plating combinations (e.g. the LC-DCP combined with an intramedullary rod system) have been shown to have superior biomechanical properties over an LCP alone [54]. Particularly for the equid species, the use of the LCP in fracture repair has been shown to have superior biomechanical properties in comparison to the LC-DCP, and the use of LCP for the repair of ulnar fractures in horses has been shown to have a high success rate [55, 56].

4.5 Conclusion

Historically, the appearance of callus at an operated fracture site was determined to be a failure of appropriate osteosynthesis, as it implied a lack of stability. As time has progressed, this indirect method of healing is no

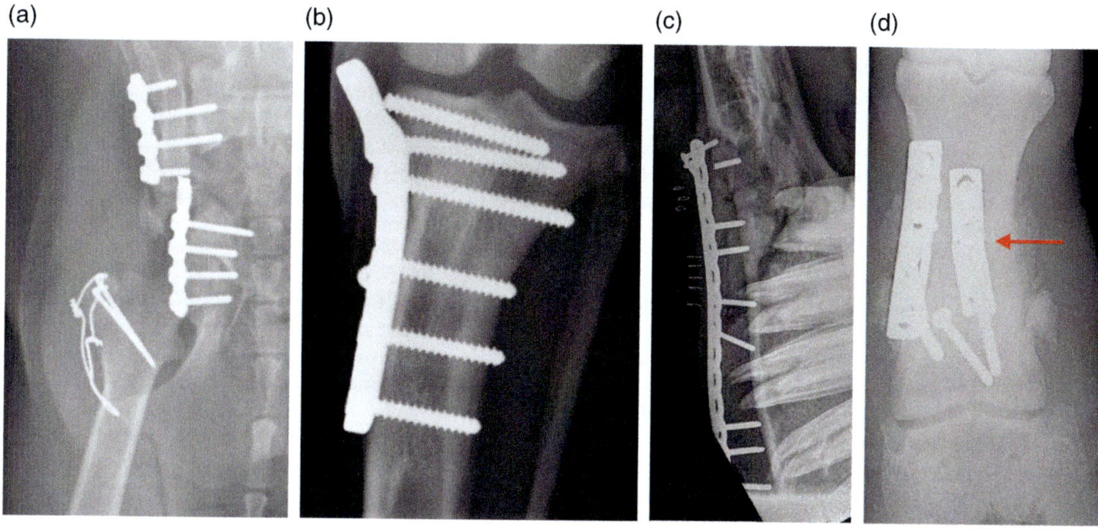

Figure 4.13 (a) Plate failure during repair of a right ilial fracture in a canine; (b) screw fatigue resulting in breakage at the screwhead post TPLO in a canine; (c) screw breakage in a mandibular fracture in an equine; and (d) catastrophic plate failure following a two-plate repair of a pastern fracture necessitating arthrodesis in an equine (red arrow).

longer considered a disadvantage but is now rather a clinical goal. It is clear that the biomechanical principles and function of LC-DCPs and LCP are inherently different and each system can have its advantages and disadvantages. Therefore, clinical judgment must be used when deciding on which is the better method to use. Despite the extensive biomechanical and clinical studies concerning the LC-DCP and LCP implants, the use and most appropriate application of the LCP remains in question. Many parameters (e.g. screw placement, screw size, plate length, bone quality, location, plate placement, anatomy, etc.) complicate the biomechanical behavior of these implants, and differences in testing modalities make direct comparison between biomechanical studies challenging.

It is imperative that the surgeon fully appreciates the concepts and laws of leverage, strain, and stress. The compression plates favor an environment for primary bone healing through absolute stability by reducing fracture gap strains to under 2%. The function of a locking plate is as an internally placed external fixator, favoring an environment for secondary bone healing via callus formation through relative stability by maintaining fracture gap strains under 10%. Compression plates are therefore well-suited and may be advantageous to use for periarticular fractures and situations that demand absolutely stability. Locking plates tend to be more forgiving as a fracture repair technique and may be preferable in applications of indirect fracture reduction with minimally invasive procedures, when bone is of poor quality is present, for bridging comminuted fractures and, where due to fracture configuration or anatomy, a plate cannot be placed on the tension surface of the bone. While there are no absolute contraindications for the use of the LCP, there are clinical situations where their use may be unnecessary.

References

1. Malekani, J., Schmutz, B., Gu, Y. et al. (2012). Orthopedic bone plates: evolution in structure, implementation technique and biomaterial. GSTF. *J. Eng. Technol.* 1: 135–140.
2. Tarallo, L., Mugnai, R., Adani, R. et al. (2014). A new volar plate made of carbon-fiber-reinforced polyetheretherketon for distal radius fracture: analysis of 40 cases. *J. Orthop. Traumatol.* 15: 277–283.
3. Hansmann, C.M. (1886). Eine neue Methode der Fixierung der Fragmente bei complicirten Frakturen. 15. In: *Congress Verhandl Dtsch Gesell Chir.*
4. Perren, S.M., Allgöwer, M., Ehrsam, R. et al. (1969). Clinical experience with a new compression plate 'DCP'. *Acta Orthop. Scand.* (Suppl 125): 31.

5. Allgöwer, M., Ehrsam, R., Ganz, R. et al. (1968). Clinical experience with a new compression plate 'DCP'. *Acta Orthop. Scand.* (Suppl. 125): 45–61.
6. Perren, S.M., Klaue, K., Pohler, O. et al. (1990). The limited contact dynamic compression plate (LC-DCP). *Arch. Orthop. Trauma Surg.* 109: 304–310.
7. Rüedi, T.P., Buckley, R.E., and Moran, C.G. (eds.) (2007). *AO Principles of Fracture Management*. AO Publishing.
8. Miller, D.L., Goswami, T., and Prayson, M.J. (2008). Overview of the locking compression plate and its clinical applications in fracture healing. *J. Surg. Orthop. Adv.* 17: 271–281.
9. Borgeaud, M., Cordey, J., Leyvraz, P.-F. et al. (2000). Mechanical analysis of the bone to plate interface of the LC-DCP and of the PC-FIX on human femora. *Injury* 31: C29–C36.
10. Frigg, R., Appenzeller, A., Christensen, R. et al. (2001). The development of the distal femur less invasive stabilization system (LISS). *Injury* 32: 24–31.
11. Frigg, R. (2001). Locking compression plate (LCP). An osteosynthesis plate based on the dynamic compression plate and the point contact fixator (PC-fix). *Injury* 32: 63–66.
12. Chidgey, L., Chakkalakal, D., Blotcky, A. et al. (1986). Vascular reorganization and return of rigidity in fracture healing. *J. Orthop. Res.* 4: 173–179.
13. Gautier, E. (2016). *Biomechanics and Biomaterials in Orthopedics*, 341–372. Springer.
14. Egol, K.A., Kubiak, E.N., Fulkerson, E. et al. (2004). Biomechanics of locked plates and screws. *J. Orthop. Trauma* 18: 488–493.
15. Wraighte, P.J. and Scammell, B.E. (2006). Principles of fracture healing. *Surg.* 24: 198–207.
16. Hente, R., Cordey, J., and Perren, S.M. (2003). In vivo measurement of bending stiffness in fracture healing. *Biomed. Eng. Online* 2: 8.
17. Bai, B., Kummer, F.J., Sala, D.A. et al. (2001). Effect of articular step-off and meniscectomy on joint alignment and contact pressures for fractures of the lateral tibial plateau. *J. Orthop. Trauma* 15: 101–106.
18. Karnezis, I.A., Panagiotopoulos, E., Tyllianakis, M. et al. (2005). Correlation between radiological parameters and patient-rated wrist dysfunction following fractures of the distal radius. *Injury* 36: 1435–1439.
19. Llinas, A. et al. (1993). Healing and remodeling of articular incongruities in a rabbit fracture model. *J. Bone Joint Surg. Am.* 75: 1508–1523.
20. Cordey, J., Borgeaud, M., Perren, S.M. et al. (2001). Force transfer between the plate and the bone: relative importance of the bending stiffness of the screws and the friction between plate and bone. *Injury* 32: C21–C28.
21. Cordey, J., Rahn, B.A., and Perren, S.M. (1980). Human torque control in the use of bone screws. In: *Current Concepts of Internal. Fixation of Fractures* (ed. H. Uhthoff), 235–243. Berlin: Springer-Verlag.
22. Cleek, T.M., Reynolds, K.J., and Hearn, T.C. (2007). Effect of screw torque level on cortical bone pullout strength. *J. Orthop. Trauma* 21: 117–123.
23. Tsuji, M., Crookshank, M., Olsen, M. et al. (2013). The biomechanical effect of artificial and human bone density on stopping and stripping torque during screw insertion. *J. Mech. Behav. Biomed. Mater.* 22: 146–156.
24. Aziz, M.S.R. et al. (2014). Biomechanical measurements of stopping and stripping torques during screw insertion in five types of human and artificial humeri. *Proc. Inst. Mech. Eng. H* 228: 446–455.
25. Hoerdemann, M., Gédet, P., Ferguson, S.J. et al. (2012). In-vitro comparison of LC-DCP-and LCP-constructs in the femur of newborn calves–a pilot study. *BMC Vet. Res.* 8: 139.
26. Gautier, E. and Sommer, C. (2003). Guidelines for the clinical application of the LCP. *Injury* 34: 63–76.
27. Kääb, M.J., Frenk, A., Schmeling, A. et al. (2004). Locked internal fixator: sensitivity of screw/plate stability to the correct insertion angle of the screw. *J. Orthop. Trauma* 18: 483–487.
28. Tidwell, J.E. et al. (2016). The biomechanical cost of variable angle locking screws. *Injury* 47: 1624–1630.
29. Jackson, M., Kummer, M., Auer, J. et al. (2011). Treatment of type 2 and 4 olecranon fractures with locking compression plate osteosynthesis in horses: a prospective study (2002–2008). *Vet. Comp. Orthop. Traumatol.* 24: 57–61.
30. Kuemmerle, J.M., Kühn, K., Bryner, M. et al. (2013). Equine ulnar fracture repair with locking compression plates can be associated with inadvertent penetration of the lateral cortex of the radius. *Vet. Surg* 42: 790–794.
31. Kumar, G. and Dunlop, C. (2011). Case report: a technique to remove a jammed locking screw from a locking plate. *Clin. Orthop. Relat. Res.* 469: 613–616.
32. Cronier, P., Pietu, G., Dujardin, N. et al. (2010). The concept of locking plates. *Orthop. Traumatol. Surg. Res.* 96: 17–36. doi: 10.1016/j.otsr.2010.03.008.
33. Raja, S., Imbuldeniya, A.M., Garg, S. et al. (2012). Difficulties encountered removing locked plates. *Ann. R. Coll. Surg. Engl.* 94: 502–505.
34. Farouk, O., Krettek, C., Miclau, T. et al. (1998). Effects of percutaneous and conventional plating techniques on the blood supply to the femur. *Arch. Orthop. Trauma Surg* 117: 438–441.
35. Farouk, O., Krettek, C., Miclau, T. et al. (1999). Minimally invasive plate osteosynthesis: does percutaneous plating disrupt femoral blood supply less than the traditional technique? *J. Orthop. Trauma* 13: 401–406.

36. Stoffel, K., Dieter, U., Stachowiak, G. et al. (2003). Biomechanical testing of the LCP–how can stability in locked internal fixators be controlled? *Injury* 34.
37. Ahmad, M., Nanda, R., Bajwa, A.S. et al. (2007). Biomechanical testing of the locking compression plate: when does the distance between bone and implant significantly reduce construct stability? *Injury* 38: 358–364.
38. Niemeyer, P. and Sudkamp, N.P. (2006). Principles and clinical application of the locking compression plate (LCP). *Acta Chir. Orthop. Traumatol. Cech.* 73: 221–228.
39. Hertel, R., Eijer, H., Meisser, A. et al. (2001). Biomechanical and biological considerations relating to the clinical use of the point contact-fixator–evaluation of the device handling test in the treatment of diaphyseal fractures of the radius and/or ulna. *Injury* 32: 10–14.
40. Bottlang, M. and Feist, F. (2011). Biomechanics of far cortical locking. *J. Orthop. Trauma* 25 (Suppl 1): S21–S28.
41. Bischofberger, A.S., Fürst, A., Auer, J. et al. (2009). Surgical management of complete diaphyseal third metacarpal and metatarsal bone fractures: clinical outcome in 10 mature horses and 11 foals. *Equine Vet. J.* 41: 465–473.
42. Gardner, M.J. et al. (2005). The mechanical behavior of locking compression plates compared with dynamic compression plates in a cadaver radius model. *J. Orthop. Trauma* 19: 597–603.
43. Kim, T., Ayturk, U.M., Haskell, A. et al. (2007). Fixation of osteoporotic distal fibula fractures: a biomechanical comparison of locking versus conventional plates. *J. Foot Ankle Surg.* 46: 2–6.
44. Edwards, S.L., Wilson, N.A., Zhang, L.-Q. et al. (2006). Two-part surgical neck fractures of the proximal part of the humerus. A biomechanical evaluation of two fixation techniques. *J. Bone Joint. Surg. Am.* 88: 2258–2264.
45. Lill, H., Hepp, P., Korner, J. et al. (2003). Proximal humeral fractures: how stiff should an implant be? *Arch. Orthop. Trauma Surg.* 123: 74–81.
46. Sod, G.A. et al. (2010). An in vitro biomechanical comparison of a 5.5 mm locking compression plate fixation with a 4.5 mm locking compression plate fixation of Osteotomized equine third metacarpal bones. *Vet. Surg.* 39: 581–587.
47. Sod, G.A., Riggs, L.M., Mitchell, C.F. et al. (2010). In vitro biomechanical comparison of a modified 5.5 mm locking compression plate fixation with a 5.5 mm locking compression plate fixation of osteotomized equine third metacarpal bones. *Vet. Surg.* 39: 833–838.
48. Sod, G.A., Mitchell, C.F., Hubert, J.D. et al. (2008). In vitro biomechanical comparison of locking compression plate fixation and limited-contact dynamic compression plate fixation of osteotomized equine third metacarpal bones. *Vet. Surg.* 37: 283–288.
49. Aguila, A.Z. et al. (2005). In vitro biomechanical comparison of limited contact dynamic compression plate and locking compression plate. *Vet. Comp. Orthop. Traumatol.* 18: 220–226.
50. Fulkerson, E. et al. (2006). Fixation of diaphyseal fractures with a segmental defect: a biomechanical comparison of locked and conventional plating techniques. *J. Trauma* 60: 830–835.
51. Frigg, R., Frenk, A., and Wagner, M. (2007). Biomechanics of plate osteosynthesis. *Tech. Orthop.* 22: 203–208.
52. Nguyentat, A., Camisa, W., Patel, S. et al. (2016). A biomechanical comparison of locking versus conventional plate fixation for distal fibula fractures in trimalleolar ankle injuries. *J. Foot Ankle Surg.* 55: 132–135.
53. Rocconi, R.A., Carmalt, J.L., Sampson, S.N. et al. (2015). Comparison of limited-contact dynamic compression plate and locking compression plate constructs for proximal interphalangeal joint arthrodesis in the horse. *Can. Vet. J.* 56: 615.
54. Matres-Lorenzo, L., Diop, A., Maurel et al. (2016). Biomechanical comparison of locking compression plate and limited contact dynamic compression plate combined with an intramedullary rod in a canine femoral fracture-gap model. *Vet. Surg.* 45 (3): 319–326.
55. Florin, M., Arzdorf, M., Ing, D. et al. (2005). Assessment of stiffness and strength of 4 different implants long-bone fracture model using a bone substitute. *Vet. Surg.* 34 (3): 231–238. doi: 10.1111/j.1532-950X.2005.00035.x.
56. Jacobs, C.C., Levine, D.G., and Richardson, D.W. (2017). Use of locking compression plates in ulnar fractures of 18 horses. *Vet. Surg.* 46: 242–248.

5 Minimally Invasive Plate Osteosynthesis

Philipp Schmierer and Antonio Pozzi

5.1 Introduction

Minimally invasive plate osteosynthesis (MIPO) is defined as reduction and fixation of a fracture with a bone plate without direct surgical exposure of the fracture site. Small skin incisions are used to prepare an epiperiosteal, subcutaneous, or submuscular tunnel that allows one to insert and apply the plate to the fracture fragments [1]. The first descriptions of MIPO in human patients dates back to the early 1990s [2], although the most significant progression has occurred in the last decade, largely thanks to the introduction of new implants such as the locking plate. In the last decade, MIPO was also introduced in veterinary medicine and is nowadays an accepted technique in dogs, cats, and horses [3–5]. Reported benefits of MIPO include reduction in operative time, reduced risk for bacterial infection, decreased soft tissue trauma, and preservation of the fracture hematoma [6]. Furthermore several studies in human, as well as in veterinary, medicine showed that MIPO preserves periosteal blood supply compared to open plating, which may accelerate bone healing [7, 8]. Reported disadvantages of MIPO include the technical difficulty and the inability of direct observation of the fracture fragments leading to an increased risk of malalignment [9, 10].

Clinical results after MIPO in dogs have been promising [11–13]. The initial reports of MIPO for tibial fractures in dogs and cats showed early radiographic union and return to full limb function. These positive results were confirmed in a larger study where the average healing time was 45 days and no major complications were reported [12]. The effect of MIPO on fracture healing was evaluated in a cohort of dogs with radius-ulna fracture using ultrasonography, power Doppler ultrasonography and radiographs. The results of this study showed significantly shorter healing times for dogs that underwent MIPO compared to dogs treated with open reduction and internal fixation (ORIF). [11] However, the effect of MIPO on fracture healing time remains a controversial issue. Baroncelli et al. found no difference in time to clinical union evaluated by radiographs in a retrospective study comparing MIPO and ORIF in 22 dogs with tibial fractures [14]. Other studies concluded that MIPO allowed rapid healing, but the lack of a control make the interpretation of the results difficult [11, 12].

Locking Plates in Veterinary Orthopedics, First Edition.
Edited by Matthew D. Barnhart and Karl C. Maritato.

The evolution of MIPO in human orthopedics was accelerated by the development of locking plates. These angular stable implants serve as ideal implants to implement the principles of biological osteosynthesis for several reasons (Figure 5.1). Locking plates act as internal fixators, which eliminate the need for exact contouring. Additionally, the limited contact between bone and implant further helps to preserve the vascular supply to the bone [15]. This chapter aims to give an overview of MIPO principles and techniques, with special focus on the use of locking implants for fracture reduction and fixation.

5.2 Biology and Biomechanics in MIPO

MIPO preserves an optimal environment for fracture healing by limiting surgical dissection and avoiding disruption of the fracture hematoma. It is clearly understood that careful soft-tissue handling is very important in preserving blood supply to the injured bone. However, it is the combination of not exposing the fracture site and indirectly reducing the fracture that makes MIPO an excellent model for biological osteosynthesis. The fracture hematoma that forms following rupture of endosteal and extraosseal vessels plays an important role in initiating fracture healing [16]. For progressive fracture healing, however, adequate blood supply and oxygen tension at the fractured site is mandatory. The soft tissues surrounding the bone and the periosteum play a critical role in establishing the early blood supply after a fracture [17]. Thus, soft tissue and periosteum preservation using a minimally invasive technique may allow more rapid healing.

The effect of MIPO and ORIF on periosteum preservation and early bone healing was studied in two separate experiments. In a cadaveric study of the canine antebrachium, MIPO caused less disruption of periosteal blood supply of the radius when compared to ORIF [8]. In a separate clinical study, earlier vascularization of the fracture callus compared to open plating was demonstrated using ultrasound, confirming the benefit of MIPO in the initial phase of bone healing [11].

Locking plates are ideal implants for preserving periosteal vessels. The periosteal blood supply beneath locking plates is not compromised because compression between the plate and the bone does not occur (Figure 5.1b); this may improve healing and decrease the risk of cortical bone necrosis and infection [18]. A large multicenter clinical study in people reported an infection rate of 1.1% after using the point-contact fixator (PC-Fix), one of the earliest locking plate designs [19]. Other studies have shown decreased damage to the periosteum and underlying bone and improvements in bone healing with maintenance of a sound bone structure [20]. It is clear that locking plates should be considered as an excellent implant choice for MIPO.

The process of bone healing is dependent on numerous interactions between biologic and mechanical factors. If the local circulation is adequate to support fracture healing, the pattern of bone healing is then dependent on the surrounding biomechanical environment. Most fractures repaired with MIPO techniques heal in conditions of relative stability. Relative stability involves placement of implants that provide somewhat flexible fixation, allowing an acceptable degree of fracture segments displacement. Fixation modalities that are commonly employed in MIPO are plates or plate-rod constructs applied in bridging fashion to span a bone defect, resulting in a relatively stable environment. Understanding the difference between locking and nonlocking plates and the effect of plate type, size, length, position, screw type, and screw placement is important because successful fracture healing depends on appropriate fixation stability.

The principal biomechanical differences between conventional and locking plates is the mode of load transfer through a fractured bone. In conventional compression plate constructs or nonlocking bridging plate constructs, fixation stability is limited by the frictional force generated between the plate and the bone. These frictional forces are the result of axial screw force and the friction coefficient between the bone and the plate [21]. If the force exerted on the bone while the dog is ambulating exceeds the frictional limit, relative shear displacement will occur between the plate and the bone, causing a loss of reduction between the bone fragments, or loosening of the screws, or both. Locking plates differ from nonlocking plates

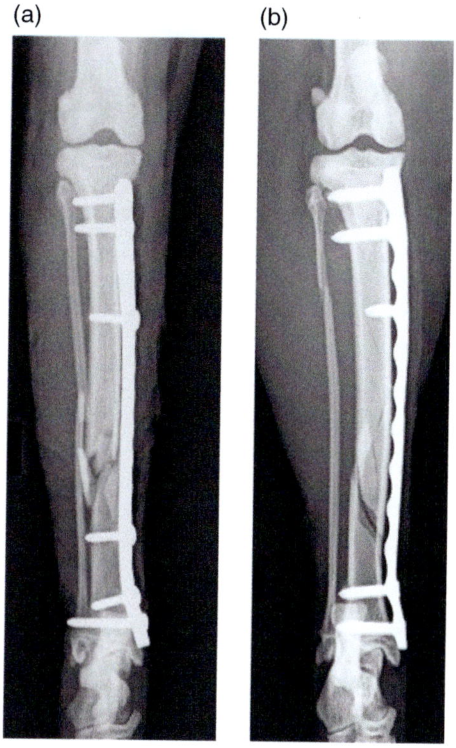

Figure 5.1 Cranio-caudal radiograph of a three year-old Domestic Short-Haired Cat presenting with a comminuted distal diaphyseal tibial fracture. The fracture was reduced manually and a precontoured veterinary cuttable plate (DePuySynthes VET, Oberdorf, BL, Switzerland) was applied to the medial aspect (a). Cranio-caudal radiograph of a five-year-old Domestic Short-Haired Cat presenting with a mildly comminuted distal diaphyseal tibial fracture. Multiple fissures extend from the fracture site into the proximal fragment. The fracture was reduced manually and Advanced Locking Plate System (KYON, Zurich, ZH, Switzerland) was applied (b). Note that exact contouring is necessary with the nonlocking implant (a) while only approximate contouring is adequate in the locking implant because plate standoff is tolerated (b).

because stability is not dependent on the frictional forces generated at the bone–plate interface. These implants consist of a plate and locking head screws, which together act as an internal fixator. Locking the head screw into the plate hole confers axial and angular stability of the screw relative to the plate. Because the stability of the construct does not depend on frictional forces generated between plate and bone, the bone–screw threads are unlikely to strip during insertion. With the screwhead locked in the plate, screw orientation is fixed to the plate resulting in a single beam construct functioning as an internal fixator. With the fixed-angle and the screw locked in the plate, no movement at the plate screw interface is allowed, resulting in a decreased risk of screw pullout and screw loosening [22–25].

When performing bridging osteosynthesis, the selection of an implant of appropriate length is a crucial step. With longer plates, screw-working leverage is improved and bending forces are well distributed along the plate, thereby lowering pullout forces on screws [26]. To determine the adequate length of the plate in the preoperative plan for bridging osteosynthesis in MIPO, two values have been used to determine the plate length to be used. The plate span ratio is the quotient of plate length and segmental length of fractured/comminuted bone. The plate screw density is the quotient of number of screws inserted and number of screw holes. Plate span ratio in comminuted fractures, in which MIPO with bridging osteosynthesis is most commonly performed, should be more than two to three. Values for simple fractures range between eight to ten [26]. Plate screw density should be smaller than 0.5 to 0.4 in comminuted fractures. A value of 0.4 to 0.3 is recommended for simple fractures [26].

Besides plate span ratio and plate screw density, the location of the screws along the plate and in relation to the fracture should be considered. The plate working length is defined as the distance between the distal and the proximal screw nearest to the fracture. Its influence on plate strain, construct stiffness, and cyclic fatigue of the plate construct has been evaluated in human and veterinary studies. Recommendations aim toward increased plate working length in order to reduce axial stiffness of the construct and to allow interfragmentary movements [26, 27]; however, conflicting results have been found in several mechanical studies [28–30]. The plate working length in comminuted fractures might not be equal to the distance between the screws closest to the fracture, but rather to the unsupported area of the plate, which correspond to the length of the fracture gap. Also of interest is the location and number of monocortical and bicortical screws in the construct as they are influential on its biomechanical properties. Less torsional stiffness is reached with monocortical screws compared to bicortical screws. Torsional stiffness of the fixation construct is especially relevant in bones undergoing combined axial and torsional loading such as the tibia [31, 32]. A minimum of one screw placed bicortically in each major bone fragment has been shown to significantly increase torsional stability in a biomechanical study using bone models. Interestingly, when the bicortical screw was placed at the innermost position, closest to the fracture, greatest improvement in torsional stability was observed [34].

5.3 Surgical Technique

5.3.1 Approach and Dissection

Before performing MIPO the surgeon should be familiar with the regional and topographic anatomy to avoid harm to neurovascular structures and to minimize postoperative morbidity [34, 35]. The position of the animal on the table is important for access, but also for the use of fluoroscopy without interference with the table or the other limbs. The skin incisions are centered over the expected proximal and distal ends of the plate and an epiperiosteal soft tissue tunnel connecting the two incisions is created with blunt dissection. Long blunt scissors or periosteal elevators are best suited for tunnel creation (Figure 5.2).

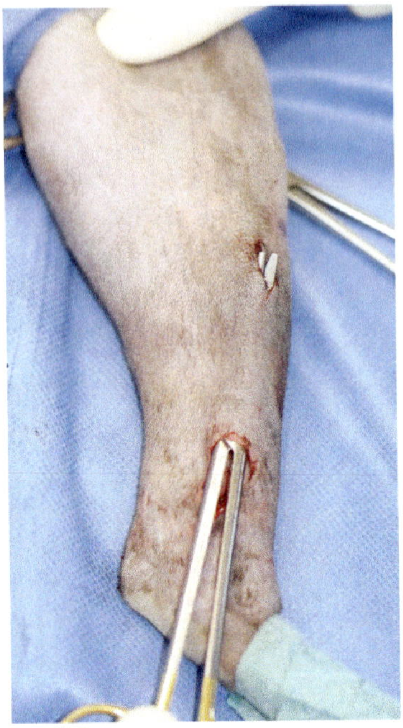

Figure 5.2 Minimally invasive plate osteosynthesis in a tibial fracture of a cat. Metzenbaum scissors are used for creation of the epiperiosteal soft tissue.

5.3.2 Fracture Reduction

Fracture reduction for MIPO is performed using indirect techniques, consisting of repositioning the bone fragments using specific distraction and translation techniques without direct exposure of the fracture site [36–38]. Fracture fragments are manipulated applying forces distant to the fracture [37, 38]. Indirect fracture reduction adapts perfectly to the concept of biological osteosynthesis because the fracture hematoma and the soft tissue envelope around the fracture is preserved [38, 39]. However, it can be challenging to accomplish and maintain reduction compared to conventional direct reduction techniques. In addition, intraoperative imaging is mandatory to assess alignment, reduction, and implant positioning, especially in cases in which the anatomical landmarks are harder to palpate due to a larger soft tissue envelope [40].

Described techniques for indirect reduction include the hanging limb technique, bone-holding forceps, IM pinning, skeletal traction tables, linear and circular external fixation, fracture distractors, and reduction through plate application [6, 36]. In the hanging limb technique the animal's weight is used to assist in distraction of the affected, vertically suspended limb [6, 36]. This technique may offer adequate distraction, especially in fractures of the distal extremity. Final alignment can be achieved by manipulation of the fragments either manually or with bone reduction forceps placed through stab incisions in the distal and proximal segments (Figure 5.3) [6]. In the author's opinion, extreme care must be taken with this technique applied to the radius of cats and small dogs as fissuring can occur.

Intramedullary pinning is an effective way to achieve distraction and in aiding restoration of the original limb length. As some force can be necessary to achieve distraction, the pin should be blunted before it is introduced in the segment to be distracted [6, 36]. To achieve this, the pin is

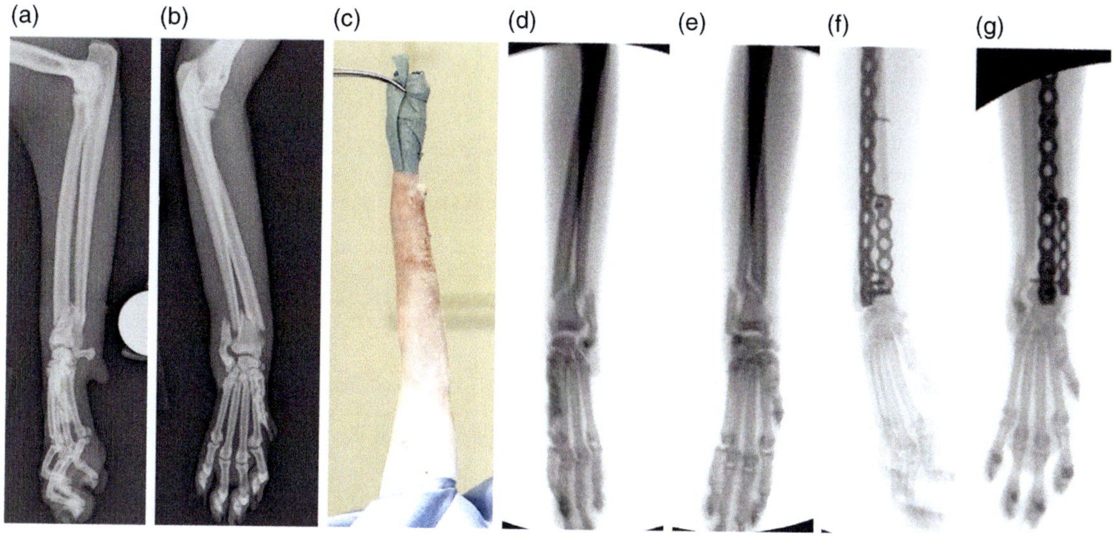

Figure 5.3 Orthogonal radiographs of a two-year-old Domestic Short-Haired Cat presenting with (a) a distal oblique radius and (b) ulna fracture. The hanging limb technique (c) was used for fracture reduction. Intraoperative fluoroscopy was used to assess reduction and implant position (d, e). Double plating in minimally invasive fashion was selected due to the small metaphyseal fragment (f, g).

inserted through the cortex of the proximal fragment in order to open the medullary canal, and is then withdrawn and blunted and consecutively reinserted. Reduction using traction tables is a technique frequently used in people, especially in femur fractures [41–43]. To the authors' knowledge, there is currently only one skeletal traction table available for small animals [5, 43]. Reported benefits are the controlled management of muscle contractions, eventually reaching original limb length and maintenance of reduction throughout the procedure [5, 44]. However their use is not without risk. As described in human medicine, patient positioning and adequate use of traction is crucial to avoid complications such as neurologic injury, malalignment, soft tissue injury, well-leg compartment syndrome, and crush syndrome [44]. External skeletal fixators, either linear or ring constructs, can be used for indirect fracture reduction during MIPO. Fixation wires are introduced in the proximal and distal fragment. One wire per fragment of adequate size is usually sufficient. For the circular construct, two rings or arches/half rings can be used. For linear constructs, full pin frames should be used [5].

Both circular and linear constructs are most commonly used in the antebrachium and tibia. External fixators are less commonly applied to the femur and humerus due to the large muscle mass and the interference with the thoracic and abdominal walls [5]. Fracture distractors consist of two pin housing arms, one of which is fixed at one end. The other end slides along a linear threaded or serrated rod, depending on the device. Large distraction forces can be applied, requiring a cautious use in small animals. They are mostly reserved for femur fractures in large dogs or old, contracted fractures [5].

Indirect fracture reduction is also possible using a precontoured plate. Orthogonal radiographs of the contralateral, unaffected side are obtained. Correct length is determined, and adequate contouring can be achieved using the normal contralateral bone [12]. The craniocaudal view is usually most valuable for plate contouring [4]. The authors prefer to contour the plate preoperatively only on one plane, while the torque is generally applied intraoperatively. Distraction is performed using one of the previously described techniques (i.e. IM pinning). Consecutively, the plate is inserted in the epiperiosteal tunnel and the contour evaluated using fluoroscopy. Care is taken that the plate is centered over the bone. Usually, the proximal end of the plate is fixed first, as it is easier to manipulate the distal part of the limb for axial alignment.

It is important to note that with both conventional and locking plates, cortical screws are inserted first to "pull" the bone fragments to the plate. In locking plates, the first cortical screw is inserted perpendicularly in the proximal end of the plate and is not completely tightened [37]. This allows some movement of the plate distally. The distal end of the plate is centered over the bone and bone forceps are applied to ensure bone-plate contact. The authors prefer point-to-point or lobster claw-type (or clamshell-type) reduction forceps for this step. A second cortical screw is placed perpendicularly and both screws are tightened. Fluoroscopy is used to assess plate positioning and reduction before additional locking screws are inserted. Finally, the cortical screws can be replaced with locking screws. Alternatively, instead of using cortical screws, temporary plate reduction devices such as the push-pull device (De-Puy Synthes) or the pin stopper (Fixin, Intrauma, Rivoli, TO, Italy) can be used (Figure 5.4).

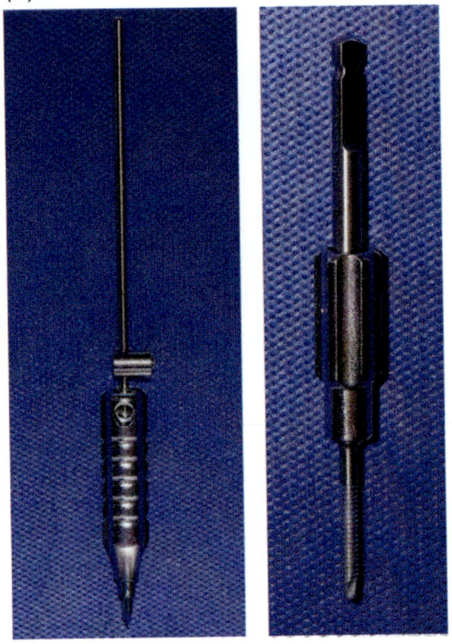

Figure 5.4 Temporary reduction devices. The pin stopper (A) (Fixin, Intrauma, Rivoli, TO, Italy) can be used to secure the plate by using a pin inserted in a sleeve locked with a clamp. The push-pull device (DePuySynthes VET, Oberdorf, BL, Switzerland) allows securing the plate by applying compression to the implant.

Another way to use locking plates for indirect fracture reduction is to use them as a navigation device. In the preoperative planning, the implant is approximately contoured to allow bone contact at the level of the most proximal and distal holes. In surgery, the implant is inserted with the most distal or proximal hole centered over the bone at the level of the anatomical landmark determined in the preoperative planning. With this technique, the most distal or proximal locking screw is inserted first, while maintaining proper alignment of the plate relative to the bone. The fragment can then be manipulated with the plate used as joystick. In case of fixation to the distal fragment first, the plate is pushed distally until the most proximal hole is leveled with the predetermined proximal landmark and centered over the bone. In case of fixation to the proximal fragment first, the distal fragment is pulled distally until the most distal hole is leveled with the predetermined distal landmark. A bone-holding forceps is placed for temporary stabilization of the implant. Fluoroscopy is used to assess implant position and fracture reduction before the most proximal locking screw is placed. Additional screws can be inserted as needed. This technique is especially useful in minimally to moderately displaced fractures of the distal extremities in small dogs and cats. Alternatively, plates offering the option of temporary fixation with pins can be secured before screws are inserted (Figure 5.5).

5.4 MIPO Technique with Locking Plates

5.4.1 Humerus

Comminu ted diaphyseal and metaphyseal fractures that are considered nonreducible are best-suited cases for MIPO in the humerus [45]. A lateral approach for MIPO in the humerus is described in the dog and a lateral and medial approaches have been described in the cat [34, 35]. Locking plates are well-suited for the humerus as precise contouring can be difficult on its cranio-lateral side with the

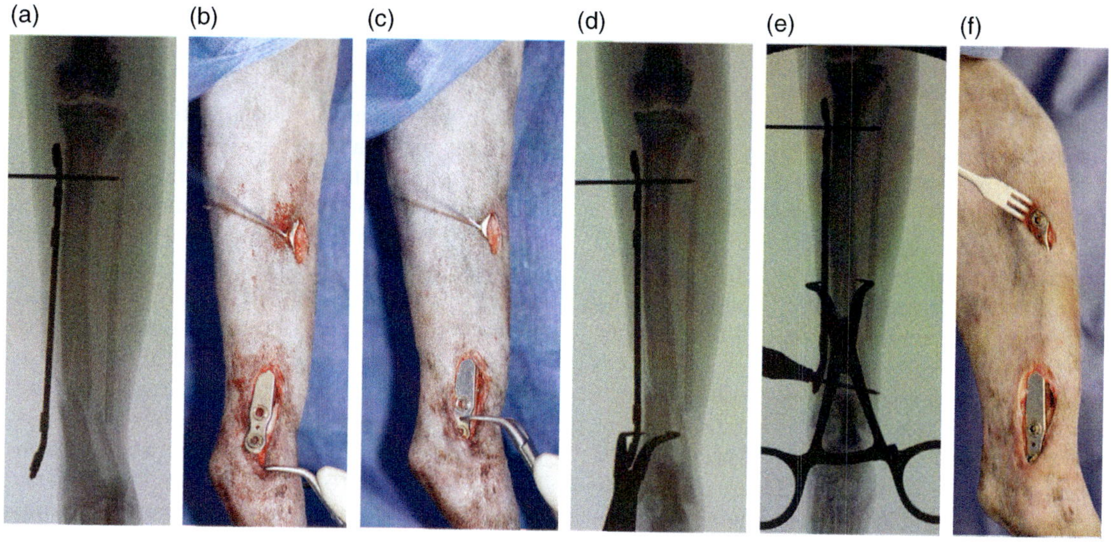

Figure 5.5 Intraoperative images and fluoroscopy of a three-year-old Domestic Long-Haired Cat presenting with a comminuted distal tibial fracture. (a) The implant is approximately contoured to allow bone contact at the level of the most proximal and distal holes in the preoperative planning. In surgery, the implant is inserted with the most proximal hole centered over the bone at the level of the anatomical landmark determined in the preoperative planning; (b) Point-to-point reduction forceps are used to pull the distal fragment distally until the determined distal anatomical landmark is level with the most distal hole; (c, d, e) Point-to-point reduction forceps are used to reduce the distal fragment to the plate and a pin is inserted to secure the bone to the plate; (f) Screws are then inserted for final fixation.

prominent lateral supracondylar crest and the deep brachial groove. In addition, monocortical screw placement, only recommended with locking implants, is valuable to avoid the supratrochlear foramen and intraarticular screw placement. Furthermore, the supracondylar foramen, representing a unique feature to the distal feline humerus should be considered when plating the feline humerus. Bicortical screws placed from the lateral to the medial side of the distal humerus can be associated with the risk of iatrogenic damage to the brachial artery and median nerve as they pass through the foramen [36]. With the available polyaxial locking systems, this risk might be reduced as they offer multidirectional insertion of the screw of up to 10° without cross threading or influence on locking strength [25].

In the proximal humerus of the dog and the cat, the bone cranial and proximal to the tricipital line is usually of cancellous nature with the cortex being relatively thin [46]. In this area, locking implants offer the advantage of decreased risk of screw pullout and screw loosening [22]. In the humerus, intramedullary pinning is a convenient way of indirect fracture reduction. However, when using locking implants, interference between the IM pin and the screws should be considered. This might influence the number of screws placed in bicortical fashion [47]. Use of polyaxial systems can help reduce this difficulty.

5.4.2 Radius and Ulna

Locking implants are an ideal choice for radius and ulna fractures in cats, while in dogs the nonlocking plates adapts well to the flat dorsal surface [48]. The radius of the cat shows a significant change in the orientation of the cranial surface. The cranio-medial orientation in the distal aspect changes to a cranio-lateral orientation in the proximal radius [36]. This change in orientation can make adequate contouring difficult and renders plating with locking implants helpful in cats. Especially in cats and small dogs, the locking implant can be used for fracture reduction without contouring, as described in the fracture reduction section.

5.4.3 Femur

Among the different fixation techniques for MIPO in femoral fractures [49], locking implants are especially valuable in proximal and distal metaphyseal fractures because of limited bone available for screw purchase and the risk for joint violation. In proximal comminuted fractures, as they frequently occur in cats, monocortical screws can be used with limited bone stock. When screws are placed close to the joint, monocortical screws can be useful to avoid joint penetration (Figure 5.6). As in the humerus, IM pinning is a convenient way of indirect fracture reduction in the femur. Interference with the pin when placing locking screws can also occur in the femur. Interference between pin and screws can make pin withdrawing impossible when cutting it to final length [50]. As stated above, polyaxial implants can reduce this difficulty.

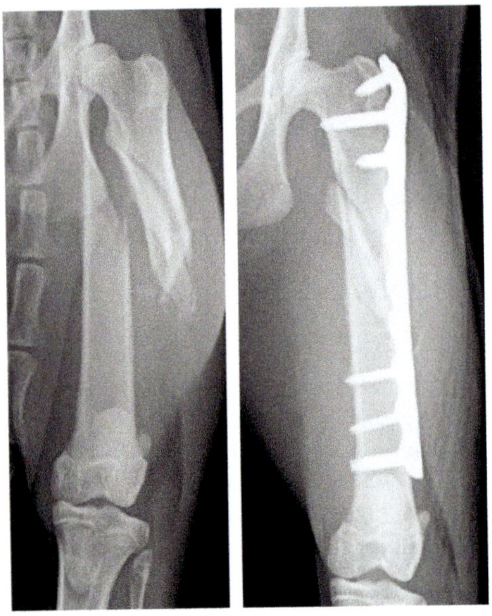

Figure 5.6 Cranio-caudal radiograph of a two-year-old Domestic Short-Haired Cat presenting with a proximal comminuted femoral fracture. The proximal fissures, the deficiency of the medial cortex, and the proximity to the joint obviates the benefits of monocortical screws.

5.4.4 Tibia

Several advantages have to be considered in MIPO with locking implants in tibia and fibula fractures, especially when affecting the metaphiseal regions. In some large and giant breed dogs, the bone of the proximal metaphysis can be of poor density. This, in turn, may increase the risk of screw pullout. With locking implants, this risk can be reduced [22, 50]. Proximal and distal metaphyseal fractures of the tibia often present a challenge to the surgeon, as only limited space for implant positioning can be available. The superior resistance of locking screws to pullout compared to cortical screws is beneficial when only monocortical or a limited number of screws can be placed in a small metaphyseal fragment [22, 50]. However, the reduced torsional stability of monocortical screws should be considered especially in the tibia due to the torsional forces occurring in this specific bone [31–33, 51].

5.4.5 Percutaneous Carpal and Tarsal Arthrodesis

Locking plates have been successfully used to perform minimally invasive percutaneous plate arthrodesis in dogs. The features of locking plates such as lower rate of screw pull-out and the limited need for contouring are also beneficial in percutaneous arthrodesis. However, the fixed angle of screw insertion was reported to be difficult for fixation of the plate to the metatarsal bones [52]. Polyaxial locking systems may help to improve these problems [25].

References

1. Rüedi, T.P., Buckley, R., and Moran, C.G. (2015). AO principles of fracture management. *Ann. R. Coll. Surg. Engl.* 91: 448–449.
2. Brunner, C.F. and Weber, B.G. (1981). *From: Besondere Osteosynthesetechniken*. Berlin: Springer.
3. James, F.M. and Richardson, D.W. (2006). Minimally invasive plate fixation of lower limb injury in horses: 32 cases (1999-2003). *Equine Vet. J.* 38: 246–251.
4. Schmökel, H.G., Stein, S., Radke, H. et al. (2007). Treatment of tibial fractures with plates using minimally invasive percutaneous osteosynthesis in dogs and cats. *J. Small Anim. Pract.* 48: 157–160.

5. Peirone, B., Rovesti, G.L., Baroncelli, A.B. et al. (2012). Minimally invasive plate osteosynthesis fracture reduction techniques in small animals. *Vet. Clin. North Am. Small Anim. Pract.* 42: 873–895.
6. Hudson, C., Pozzi, A., and Lewis, D. (2009). Minimally invasive plate osteosynthesis: applications and techniques in dogs and cats. *Vet. Comp. Orthop. Traumatol.* 22: 175–182.
7. Farouk, O. and Krettek, C. (1998). Miclau, T. et al. effects of percutaneous and conventional plating techniques on the blood supply to the femur. *Arch. Orthop Trauma. Surg.* 117: 438–441.
8. Garofolo, S. and Pozzi, A. (2013). Effect of plating technique on periosteal vasculature of the radius in dogs: a cadaveric study. *Vet. Sur.* 42: 255–261.
9. Kim, J.W., Oh, C.W., Oh, J.K. et al. (2017). Malalignment after minimally invasive plate osteosynthesis in distal femoral fractures. *Injury* 48: 751–757.
10. Choudhari, P. and Baxi, M. (2016). Minimally invasive plate Osteosynthesis: a review. *Indian J. Orthop.* 2: 194–198.
11. Risselada, M., Kramer, M., de Rooster, H. et al. (2005). Ultrasonographic and radiographic assessment of uncomplicated secondary fracture healing of long bones in dogs and cats. *Vet. Surg.* 34: 99–107.
12. Guiot, L.P. and Déjardin, L.M. (2011). Prospective evaluation of minimally invasive plate osteosynthesis in 36 nonarticular tibial fractures in dogs and cats. *Vet. Surg.* 40: 171–182.
13. Pozzi, A., Risselada, M., and Winter, M.D. (2012). Assessment of fracture healing after minimally invasive plate osteosynthesis or open reduction and internal fixation of coexisting radius and ulna fractures in dogs via ultrasonography and radiography. *J. Am. Vet. Med. Assoc.* 241: 744–753.
14. Boero Baroncelli, A., Peirone, B., Winter, M.D. et al. (2012). Retrospective comparison between minimally invasive plate osteosynthesis and open plating for tibial fractures in dogs. *Vet. Comp. Orthop. Traumatol.* 25: 410–417.
15. Frigg, R. (2001). Locking compression plate (LCP). An osteosynthesis plate based on the dynamic compression plate and the point contact fixator (PC-Fix). *Injury* 32: 63–66.
16. Mizuno, T., Kazuo, M., and Tachibana, T. (1990). The osteogenetic potential of fracture hematoma. Subperiosteal and intramuscular transplantation of the hematoma. *J. Bone Joint Surg. Br.* 5: 822–829.
17. Macnab, I. and De Haas, W.G. (1974). The role of periosteal blood supply in the healing of fractures of the tibia. *Clin. Orthop. Relat. Res.* 105: 27–33.
18. Baumgaertel, F., Buhl, M., and Rahn, B.A. (1998). Fracture healing in biological plate osteosynthesis. *Injury* 29: 3–6.
19. Eijer, H., Hauke, C., Arens, S. et al. (2001). PC-Fix and local infection resistance-influence of implant design on postoperative infection development, clinical and experimental results. *Injury* 32 (Suppl 2): B38–B43.
20. Tepic, S., Remiger, A.R., and Morikawa, K. (1997). Strength recovery in fractured sheep tibia treated with a plate or an internal fixator: an experimental study with a two-year follow-up. *J. Orthop. Trauma* 11: 14–23.
21. Miller, D.L. and Goswami, T. (2007). A review of locking compression plate biomechanics and their advantages as internal fixators in fracture healing. *Clin. Biomech.* 22: 1049–1062.
22. Haidukewych, G.J. (2004). Innovations in locking plate technology. *J. Am. Acad. Orthop. Surg.* 4: 205–212.
23. Cabassu, J.B.,.K.,.M.P.,.S.,.J.K. et al. (2011). Single cycle to failure in torsion of three standard and five locking plate constructs. *Vet. Comp. Orthop. Traumatol.* 24: 418–425.
24. Haaland, P.J., Sjöström, L., Devor, M. et al. (2009). Appendicular fracture repair in dogs using the locking compression plate system: 47 cases. *Vet. Comp. Orthop. Traumatol.* 22: 309–315.
25. Barnhart, M.D., Rides, C.F., Kennedy, S.C. et al. (2013). Fracture repair using a polyaxial locking plate system (PAX). *Vet. Surg.* 42: 60–66.
26. Gautier, E. and Sommer, C. (2003). Guidelines for the clinical application of the LCP. *Injury* 34: 63–76.
27. Kubiak, E.N. (2006). The evolution of locked plates. *J. Bone Joint Surg. Am.* 88: 189–113.
28. Hoffmeier, K.L., Hofmann, G.O., and Mückley, T. (2011). Choosing a proper working length can improve the lifespan of locked plates. *Clin. Biomech.* 26: 405–409.
29. Chao, P., Conrad, B.P., Lewis, D.D. et al. (2013). Effect of plate working length on plate stiffness and cyclic fatigue life in a cadaveric femoral fracture gap model stabilized with a 12-hole 2.4mm locking compression plate. *BMC Vet. Res.* 9: 1–1.
30. Maxwell, M., Horstman, C.L., Crawford, R.L. et al. (2009). The effects of screw placement on plate strain in 3.5 mm dynamic compression plates and limited-contact dynamic compression plates. *Vet. Comp. Orthop. Traumatol.* 22: 125–131.
31. Demner, D., Gracia, T.C., Serdy, M.G. et al. (2014). Biomechanical comparison of mono- and bicortical screws in an experimentally induced gap fracture. *Vet. Comp. Orthop. Traumatol.* 27: 422–429.
32. Gautier, E., Perren, S.M., and Cordey, J. (2000). Strain distribution in plated and unplated sheep tibia an in vivo experiment. *Injury* 31 (Suppl 3): C37–C44.

33. Demianiuk, R.M. et al. (2015). Effect of screw type and distribution on the torsional stability of 3.5mm string of pearls locking plate constructs. *Vet. Surg.* 44: 119–125.
34. Pozzi, A. and Lewis, D. (2009). Surgical approaches for minimally invasive plate osteosynthesis in dogs. *Vet. Comp. Orthop. Traumatol.* 22: 316–320.
35. Schmierer, P.A. and Pozzi, A. (2017). Guidelines for surgical approaches for minimally invasive plate osteosynthesis in cats. *Vet. Comp. Orthop. Traumatol.* 30: 272–278.
36. Rüedi, T.P., Sommer, C., and Leutenegger, A. (1998). New techniques in indirect reduction of long bone fractures. *Clin. Orthop. Relat. Res.* 347: 27.
37. Johnson, A.L. (2003). Current concepts in fracture reduction. *Vet. Comp. Orthop. Traumatol.* 16: 59.
38. Palmer, R.H., Hulse, D.A., Hyman, W.A. et al. (1992). Principles of bone healing and biomechanics of external skeletal fixation. *Vet. Clin. North Am. Small Anim. Pract.* 22: 45–68.
39. Guiot, L.P. and Déjardin, L.M. (2012). Perioperative imaging in minimally invasive osteosynthesis in small animals. *Vet. Clin. North Am. Small Anim. Pract.* 42: 897–911.
40. Sonmez, M.M. et al. (2017). Strategies for proximal femoral nailing of unstable intertrochanteric fractures. *J Am Acad Orthop Surg* 25: e37–e44.
41. Wang, P.-C., Ren, D., Song, C.-H. et al. (2016). Surgical technique for subtrochanteric fracture of femur. *Orthop. Surg.* 8: 516–518.
42. de Souza, E.F., Hungria, J.O.S., Rezende, L.R.S. et al. (2017). Comparative study between lateral decubitus and traction table for treatment of pertrochanteric fractures with cephalomedullary nails. *Rev. Bras. Ortop.* 52: 24–28.
43. Rovesti, G.L., Margini, A., Cappellari, F. et al. (2006). Intraoperative skeletal traction in the dog a cadaveric study. *Vet. Comp. Orthop. Traumatol.* 19: 9–13.
44. Flierl, M.A., Stahel, P.F., Hak, D.J. et al. (2010). Traction table-related complications in Orthopaedic surgery. *J. Am. Acad. Orthop. Surg.* 18: 668–675.
45. Hulse, D. (2012). MIPO techniques for the humerus in small animals. *Vet. Clin. North Am. Small Anim. Pract.* 42: 975–82vi.
46. Moses, P.A., Lewis, D.D., Lanz, O.I. et al. (2002). Intramedullary interlocking nail stabilisation of 21 humeral fractures in 19 dogs and one cat. *Aust. Vet. J.* 80: 336–343.
47. Pearson, T., Glyde, M., Hosgood, G. et al. (2015). The effect of intramedullary pin size and monocortical screw configuration on locking compression plate-rod constructs in an in vitro fracture gap model. *Vet. Comp. Orthop. Traumatol.* 28: 95–103.
48. Hudson, C.C., Lewis, D.D., and Pozzi, A. (2012). Minimally invasive plate osteosynthesis in small animals: radius and ulna fractures. *Vet. Clin. North Am. Small Anim. Pract.* 42: 983–96vii.
49. Kowaleski, M.P. (2012). Minimally invasive osteosynthesis techniques of the femur. *Vet Clin North Am Small Anim Pract* 42: 997–1022.
50. Beale, B.S. and McCally, R. (2012). Minimally invasive plate osteosynthesis. *Vet. Clin. North Am. Small Anim. Pract.* 42: 1023–1044.
51. Gautier, E., Perren, S.M., and Cordey, J. (2000). Effect of plate position relative to bending direction on the rigidity of a plate osteosynthesis. A theoretical analysis. *Injury* 31 (Suppl 3): C14–C20.
52. Pozzi, A., Lewis, D.D., Hudson, C.C. et al. (2012). Percutaneous plate arthrodesis in small animals. *Vet. Clin. North Am. Small Anim. Pract.* 42: 1079–1096.

Section II

Principles of Locking Plate Applications in Large Animals

6 Principles of Locking Plate Applications in Large Animals

Janik C. Gasiorowski

6.1 Principles

The basic principles of application of locking plates are the same in large animals as they are in the other species covered in this text. The benefits of locking implants include elimination of the need for plate/bone compression, greater construct stiffness, and biomechanical stability as compared to nonlocking implants, resistance to cyclic fatigue, and the general versatility offered by plate design [1]. These principles have been discussed in previous chapters but some bear repeating, as they are particularly relevant to internal fixation in large animals.

6.1.1 Comfort

Immediate restoration of limb function and return to weight bearing is of critical importance in large-animal patients. Prolonged overbearing on the contralateral (support) limb leads to laminitis in the horse, laminitis or interdigital ligament breakdown in the cow, and angular limb deformity in the skeletally immature (developing) animal. The greater construct stiffness and stability achieved with the use of locking plates helps enable earlier return to function.

Excessive rigidity of fixation has been implicated in delayed or nonunion complications with fracture healing [2]. This is rarely a problem in large-animal patients because of the large cyclic loading imposed by their high body weights. It can be an issue in very young animals, but the superior healing characteristics of young bone usually overcome this disadvantage.

6.1.2 Implant Geometry

Very few implants are designed specifically for use in large animals. As such, large animal surgeons often operate at the limits of the tolerances of the plates and screws available. Locking implants offer increased strength through advances in construct strength but also, in some cases, simply by offering more metal. The 5.5 locking compression plate (LCP) is thicker (6.0 mm) than Dynamic Hip Screw and Dynamic Condular Screw system (DHS/DCS) by Synthes (5.8 mm), and the finer threads of the locking head screws (LHS) offer a

Locking Plates in Veterinary Orthopedics, First Edition.
Edited by Matthew D. Barnhart and Karl C. Maritato.

substantial increase in proportional core diameter as compared to cortex screws. More metal translates to an increase in area moment inertia and thus increases in implant rigidity and ultimate strength.

The head of a locking screw cannot rotate or toggle in the plate, virtually eliminating pullout failure [1]. With conventional plating, the nonthreaded head of the cortex screw can toggle in the smooth plate hole, allowing a *crowbar effect* under bending load (i.e. the plate acts like a crowbar and the screw is like a nail being pried straight out of the substrate). Application of force in this manner potentiates pullout failure. In this scenario, only the bone that is between the threads of the cortex screw needs to fail for the screw to pull out. In a fixed-angle construct, the threaded head cannot toggle in the threaded plate hole so there is no crowbar effect. An entire swath of bone would need to fail in compression, or the bone would have to fracture for failure of the plate/screw/bone construct to occur. This allows for use of much smaller threads on a locking screw. Smaller threads yield a bigger core shaft diameter and thus a stronger screw. For example: the core diameter of a 5.5 mm cortex screw is 4.0 mm, whereas the core diameter of a 5.0 mm locking screw is 4.4 mm (DePuy Synthes catalog 2017). The area moment inertia of the larger core diameter is 1.6 times greater, increasing substantially the bending and shear strength of the implant.

The LCP has "cut-outs" along its underside, which homogenizes its cross-sectional area, normalizing the area moment of inertia for the length of the plate. This eliminates internal stress risers and allows smooth bending when contouring the plate. One end is rounded, allowing for juxta-articular applications, while the other end is tapered, facilitating minimally invasive application.

Another significant improvement increasing LCP versatility is the combi-hole. The threaded potion of the hole is the root of its fixed-angle advantages, but without the dynamic compression unit (DCU) portion of the hole, the plate would function only as a pure internal fixator. The DCU portion of the combi-hole allows application in dynamic compression fashion, increasing exponentially the versatility and surgical value of the LCP. The DCU portion also allows angulation of cortex screws toward free fragments or away from neurovascular structures, joints, fracture gaps, and other implants. The combi-hole of the 4.5 and 5.5 LCP can accommodate 4.5 and 5.5 mm cortex screws and 6.5 mm cancellous screws. The DCU portion of the hole allows 40° of longitudinal angulation and 7° of transverse angulation of a 4.5 mm cortex screw. It allows 25° of longitudinal angulation with a 5.5 mm cortex screw. Another improvement is the coaxial, or "stacked," combi-hole. This perfectly round hole is smooth at the top and threaded at the bottom, allowing use of a cortex or locking head screw. This hole configuration takes up less space within the plate than a regular combi- or DCU hole, which allows it to be located closer to the end of the plate, thus permitting closer approximation of the end screw to a joint.

6.2 Clinical Applications

The increased rigidity and fixed-angle stability of locking plates and screws make them a clearly superior choice over nonlocking implants for arthrodesis and fracture repair in large animals.

6.2.1 Arthrodesis

Arthrodesis requires rigid fixation for bone fusion and for patient comfort. Construct rigidity results in less callus formation, decreasing the risk of impingement on the periarticular tissues and improving the cosmetic result.

6.2.1.1 *Proximal Interphalangeal Joint*

An LCP designed specifically for arthrodesis of the equine proximal interphalangeal joint is available (DePuy Synthes Vet, Paoli, PA). In this application, two abaxial (nonplate) transarticular screws engage the palmar/plantar processes of the middle phalanx and the plate is applied dorsally (Figure 6.1).

The specifics of plate application in this scenario warrant discussion because the technique differs from the original compression plating technique. The two transarticular screws are inserted and tightened compressing the palmar/plantar aspect of the joint. Countersinking

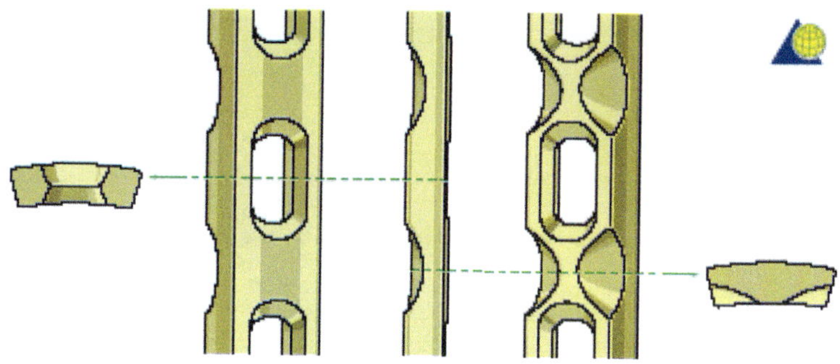

Figure 6.1 Locking compression plate (LCP) geometry. The underside of the LCP has undercuts that limit the surface area of bone contact. These cutouts occur at the points in between holes, helping to homogenize cross-sectional area for the length of the plate. (Source: Image credit: AO Foundation.)

is performed, taking care to remove bone proximally but not distally to prevent screw bending with asymmetrical contact between the screw head and bone when tightened. The plate is oriented with the stacked hole distally. The distal end is held firmly against the bone because the locking screw will not compress the plate to the bone surface in lag fashion. It can be held manually or with a push-pull device in the middle hole. A locking screw is inserted and tightened. A cortex bone screw is placed in the central hole in the load position and tightened, compressing the dorsal aspect of the joint. A locking screw is placed in the proximal hole.

The stacked hole and rounded end of the plate help prevent contact of the extensor process of the distal phalanx with the distal aspect of the plate at full extension of the distal interphalangeal joint. The LCP has been evaluated *in vitro* and demonstrated to be stiffer than an limited-contact dynamic compression plate (LC-DCP) construct [3]. The fact that less displacement was seen with the LCP construct during cyclic loading should translate to less callus formation *in vivo*. This is of particular importance in this location since horses are often expected to return to athletic performance after pastern arthrodesis. Excessive callus results in impingement on the soft tissues, most notably restriction of the long or common digital extensor tendon.

In the author's experience, a minimally invasive approach is preferable (when feasible) in cases of severe PIPJ arthritis. Preexisting cartilage destruction obviates arthrotomy and luxation. The PIP plate is introduced via subtendinous tunnel and all screws are inserted through stab incisions.

6.2.1.2 Metacarpo- / Metatarsophalangeal Joint

Fetlock arthrodesis in the horse is a challenging endeavor. The most common reasons for failure are not directly related to the implants or surgical procedure. They include subluxation of the proximal interphalangeal joint, vascular trauma at the time of injury, infection, and contralateral limb laminitis [4]. Locked plating increases construct rigidity and reduces surgical time [5]. The LCP is applied in the same general manner as nonlocking plates. Since the plate is applied dorsally, on the bending surface of the construct, a tension band must be placed at the palmar/plantar aspect of the joint (Figure 6.2). A cortex screw is used near the joint space and is angled proximally into the dense bone of the condyles.

6.2.1.3 Carpus

The specific advantage of the LCP in arthrodesis of the carpal joint(s) is engagement of the small carpal bones with a stronger screw at a fixed angle. It can be difficult or impossible to get more than one plate screw into the radial and ulnar carpal bones. The large core of the locking screw reduces the chances of implant failure. Additionally, the locking head eliminates the rotation and toggling that is possible with the smooth head of a cortex screws, reducing chances of implant loosening and increasing rigidity.

Locked plating for pancarpal arthrodesis is initiated with a standard technique. The fracture(s) are reduced and the articular cartilage is removed. The craniomedial plate is

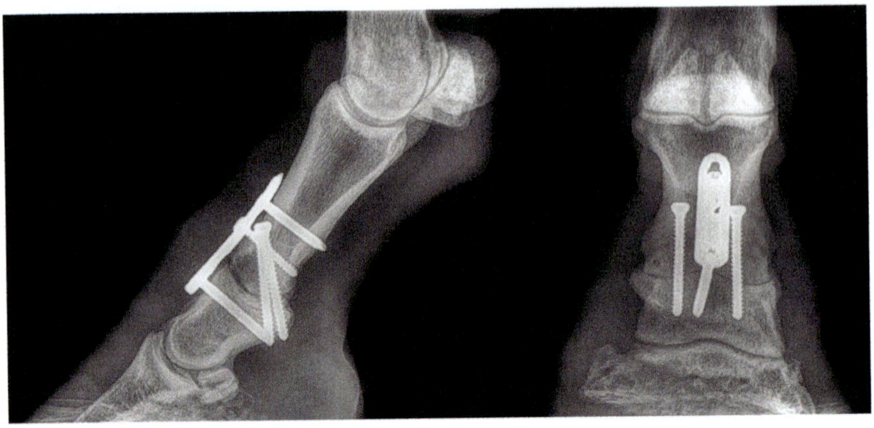

Figure 6.2 Plate/screw PIPJ arthrodesis. A three-hole 4.5 mm narrow (PIPJ-specific) LCP was applied dorsally for arthrodesis of the proximal interphalangeal joint. Abaxial transarticular screws were placed in lag fashion to compress the palmar aspect of the joint.

positioned with the locking units of the central two combi-holes directly over the radial and third carpal bones. A cortex screw is inserted through the plate in load position into the proximal aspect of the third metacarpal bone but not tightened. A second cortex screw is inserted in the load position into the distal aspect of the radius. These two screws are tightened to compress the carpal joints. The craniolateral plate is applied at this point with the same pattern of screw insertion. The craniolateral plate can be applied through the same incision. Some fracture configurations necessitate more lateral positioning of the craniolateral plate. Significant contouring is needed for adequate plate/bone contact in a nonlocking construct and a second incision is often required. Herein lies another advantage of the LCP, as perfect contouring is not required for stability and the second plate can be applied in a minimally invasive fashion. However, some contouring is still required – otherwise, skin closure will be very difficult. An additional cortex screw can be placed in load position on each side of the carpus in each plate. Locking screws are inserted into the remaining holes of both plates.

Partial carpal arthrodesis is performed most commonly for comminuted fracture of small carpal bone(s) or collapse secondary to advanced osteoarthritis. As such, plates are applied to buttress the joints(s), preventing collapse. Locking plates are applied to the dorsomedial and dorsolateral aspects of the carpus (Figure 6.3). The

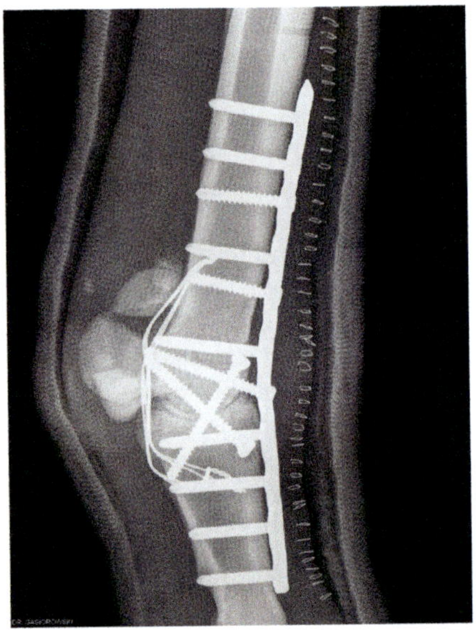

Figure 6.3 Tension band wire used in metacarpophalangeal arthrodesis. Due to anatomical constraints the LCP must be applied dorsally, on the bending surface of the joint. Here, a palmar tension band wire was used to mitigate cyclic bending forces on the plate.

dorsolateral plate is applied through the same incision or via minimally invasive approach. Locking screws are used when the small bones are intact or severely comminuted. If the small carpal bones have repairable damage (i.e. two-piece fracture), cortex screws placed (through the plate) in lag fashion are used to stabilize the fracture. The advantages gained from stabilization of the fracture outweigh the advantages of a locking screw in this position. If the small bone fracture can be compressed with a screw outside of the plate, then a locking screw is used in this plate hole.

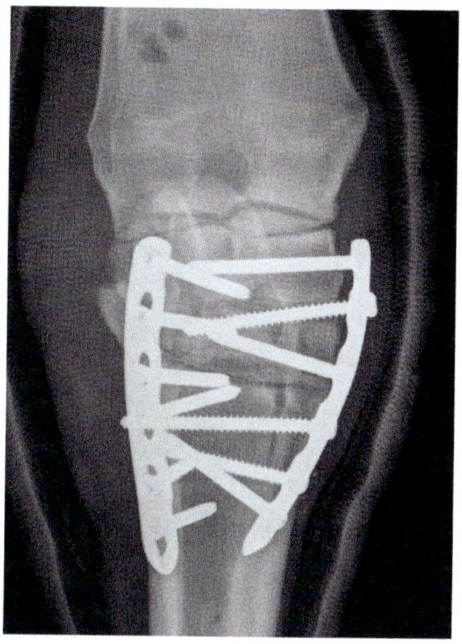

Figure 6.4 Partial carpal arthrodesis. 4.5 mm narrow locking compression plates (LCPs) were applied dorsomedially and dorsolaterally.

6.2.1.4 *Tarsus*

Arthrodesis of the tarsometatarsal and distal intertarsal joints is performed for treatment of fracture, luxation, or osteoarthritis. A T-plate (4.5 mm locking T-plate, DePuy Synthes Vet, Paoli, PA) is available and well-suited for this purpose [6]. The plate is applied dorsomedially (Figure 6.4) and three locking screws are inserted into the central tarsal bone through the "T" portion of the plate. These three screws tend to converge, so care must be taken when selecting screw length. A cortex screw is placed in the third tarsal bone in the load position and tightened. A cortex screw is placed into the proximal metatarsus in the load position and tightened. Locking screws are placed in the remaining plate holes. In the case of comminuted fracture of the small tarsal bones, the plate serves to buttress the joint and dynamic compression is not applied. In this case, cortex screws are used only to stabilize large fragments amenable to repair in lag fashion.

Axially unstable tarsal fracture and luxation of the proximal intertarsal joint are treated with a locking plate applied to the plantar lateral aspect of the tarsus. A 4.5 mm broad LCP is positioned to span the tarsus, extending from the calcaneus to the proximal third of the metatarsus, engaging the fourth metatarsal bone (Figure 6.5). Screw selection and placement

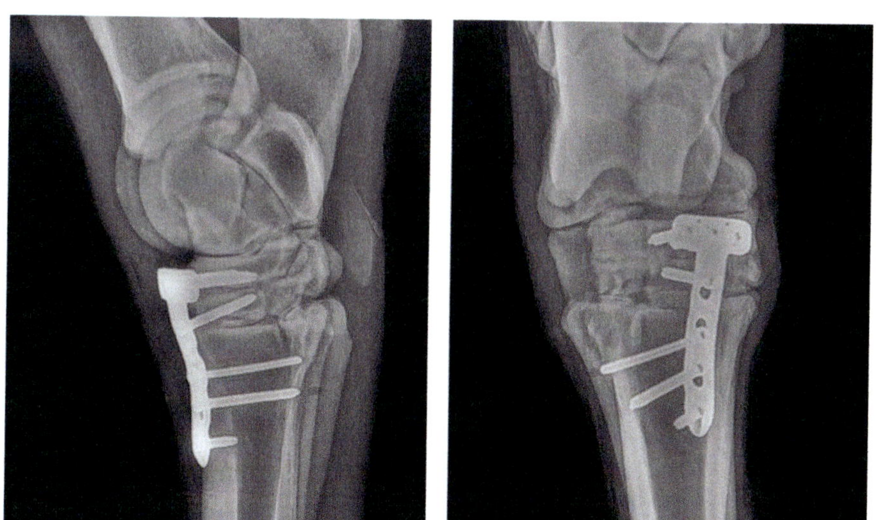

Figure 6.5 Distal tarsal arthrodesis. Locking head screws were placed through the horizontal portion of the locking T-plate into the central tarsal bone. A cortex screw was placed in the third hole in the load position to compress the DITJ and TMTJ before inserting another locking screw in the third tarsal bone.

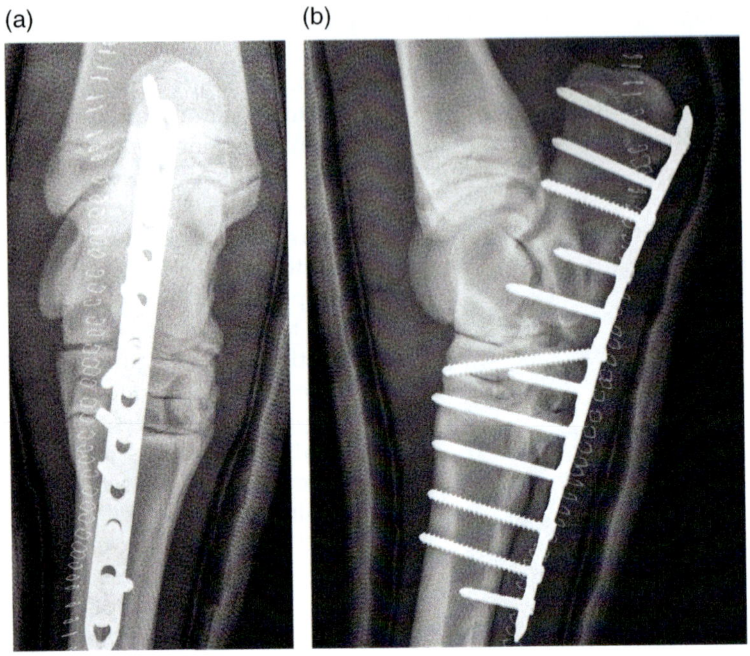

Figure 6.6 Luxation of the distal tarsal joints. (a, b) A 12-hole 4.5 mm narrow LCP was applied to the plantarolateral aspect of the tarsus to stabilize the distal tarsal joints after luxation. (Source: Image credit: McCormick [7].)

varies and is predicated on the injuries being addressed. Horses treated with this method of fixation have returned to athletic capacity [7].

6.2.1.5 *Cervical Vertebrae*

Fusion of cervical vertebrae for treatment of cervical spinal cord compression is performed most commonly with a kerf cut cylinder (KCC) [8] (Figure 6.6). Fusion has also been achieved with use of the LCP [9, 10] (Figure 6.7). *In vitro* comparison of KCC and LCP ventral fusion of the fourth and fifth cervical vertebrae demonstrated similar stiffness and moment to failure of the two constructs in four-point bending to failure. [8] The sixth and seventh cervical vertebrae were successfully fused with a broad seven-hole LCP in a three-month foal with cervical stenotic myelopathy [9]. The main advantage of the LCP construct is greater immediate stability, allowing definitive repair of cervical vertebral fractures and potentially decreasing the incidence of construct failure during recovery from general anesthesia. The disadvantages of locked plating in this application are the

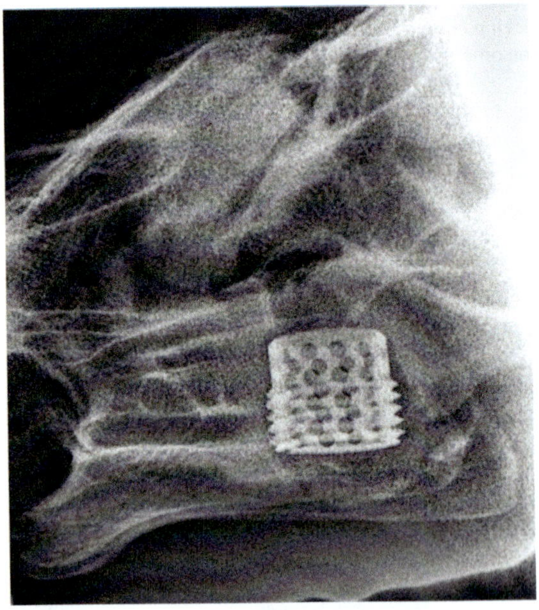

Figure 6.7 Cervical vertebral instability/malformation. The kerf cut cylinder (KCC), a partially threaded modification of the original Bagby Basket, was used for fusion of sixth and seventh cervical vertebrae.

need for greater exposure, the inability to expose adequately the caudal cervical vertebrae, and greatly increased need for intraoperative imaging. The KCC may be preferable in cases of spinal cord compression secondary to cervical vertebral compressive myelopathy or cervical facet arthritis. Locked plating may be preferable for treatment of instability secondary to cervical spinal fracture. As demonstrated by the model used by Reardon et al., locked plating does not increase significantly the stability of the construct when the vertebrae are intact. The cervical spinal column stabilizes itself. In the case of cervical vertebral fracture, it stands to reason that inherent stability of an internal fixator would be a specific advantage. This hypothesis has not yet been examined.

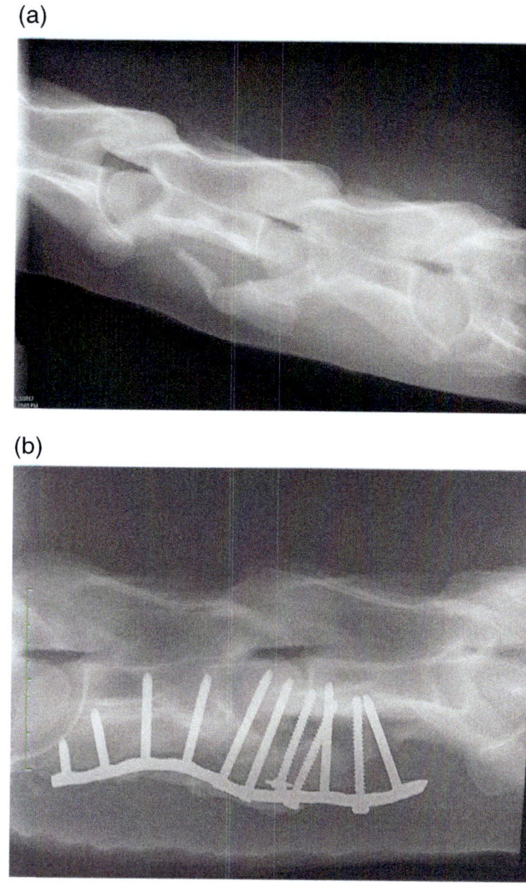

Figure 6.8 (a) Fourth cervical vertebra fracture and LCP fixation. Fracture of the caudal body of the fourth cervical vertebra. (b) A 10-hole 4.5 mm narrow LCP was applied ventrally for fusion of the fourth and fifth cervical vertebrae. (Source: Courtesy of Dr. Dean Richardson [4].)

6.2.2 Fracture Repair

6.2.2.1 Middle Phalanx

Repair of comminuted fracture of the middle phalanx often combines anatomic reconstruction with arthrodesis of the proximal interphalangeal joint (Figure 6.8). Implants are subject to immense static and cyclic loading in bending, shear, and torsion. The stability of a fixed-angle construct and the versatility of the combi-hole make the LCP an ideal implant for this type of repair. Repair is initiated with luxation of the joint and removal of the articular cartilage. After preliminary reconstruction of the fragments, two four- or five-hole 4.5 mm narrow locking plates are applied. The plates are positioned abaxially and oriented with the round end and stacked hole distally. The distal aspect of the plates is contoured to be slightly convex, so the screws will engage rigidly the medial and lateral palmar/plantar eminences of the middle phalanx. This is critical for the stability of the repair and for compression across the palmar/plantar aspect of the joint. It is important that the distal aspect of the plates not impinge on the extensor process of the distal phalanx during extension of the distal interphalangeal joint. The joint is compressed by insertion of cortex screws in the load position into proximal plate holes. The most proximal plate hole and the hole just proximal to the joint space should be reserved for locking screws. A cast is applied for recovery from general anesthesia and maintained at least until the incision(s) are healed. In highly comminuted fractures and all fractures with complete loss of axial integrity, an external skeletal fixator or transfixation pin cast should be applied to transfer the forces of weight bearing proximal to the site of injury.

6.2.2.2 Proximal Phalanx

Much like the middle phalanx, locked plating is ideal for repair of multifragment fractures of the proximal phalanx, for similar reasons. Anatomic reduction and accurate reconstruction of the joint surfaces (especially proximal) are critical. Incongruity in the articular surface

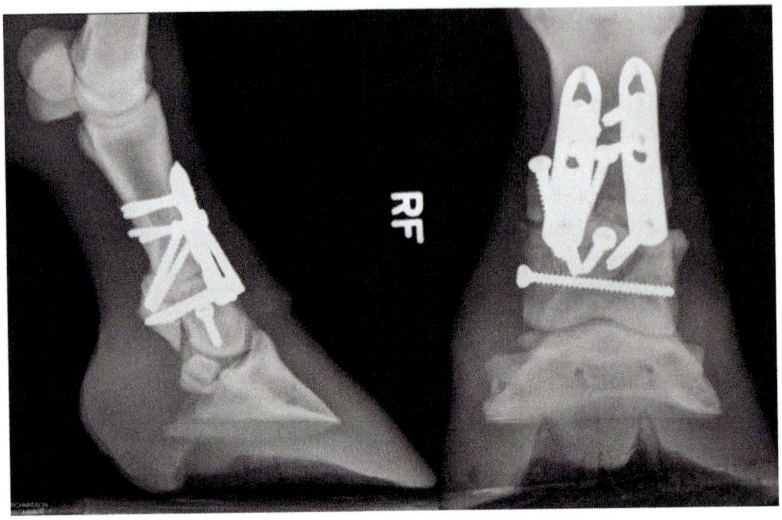

Figure 6.9 Comminuted fracture of the middle phalanx. The fractures were reduced and stabilized with cortex screws in lag fashion, then plated with two 4.5 mm narrow locking compression plates (LCPs) applied dorsally. Arthrodesis of the PIPJ was performed due to the high likelihood of development of arthritis but also to make use of the distal aspect of the proximal phalanx for plate application and construct stability. (Source: Courtesy of Dr. Dean Richardson [4].)

results in large bending moments applied to the screws and precipitates implant failure. Even if the construct holds, articular imperfections will lead to early onset of osteoarthritis.

The proximal joint surface is reconstructed with cortex screws placed in lag fashion. The surgeon must consider future plate application when selecting cortex screw position. Dorsomedial and dorsolateral plates are applied. Locked screws are used proximally across fractures that have already been compressed with independent cortex screws. Cortex screws are placed in distal plate holes in the load position to generate compression across the transverse fracture component. The rest of the holes are filled with locking screws. A cast is applied for recovery from general anesthesia and maintained at least until the incisions are healed.

Most multifragment transverse fractures without an intact vertical strut of bone are not amenable to plate fixation. These fractures are reconstructed as accurately as possible with cortex screws before external skeletal fixation is applied. A cast is insufficient coaptation, even with excellent anatomic reduction. A transfixation pin cast (Figure 6.9) or purpose-built external skeletal fixation device [11] (Figure 6.10) is

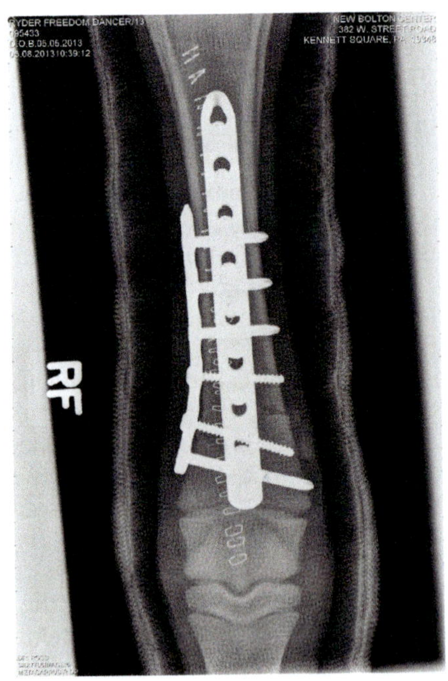

Figure 6.10 Distal diaphyseal MCIII fracture in a foal: 4.5 mm narrow LCPs were applied dorsally and laterally. The stacked combi-hole at the distal aspect of nine-hole plate allowed for close approximation of the plate to the distal physis.

required. In some cases with large proximal bone fragments, double-plate fixation (similar to that described for complex fractures of the middle phalanx) is possible. The proximal interphalangeal joint is fused and the middle phalanx is used for distal plate/screw purchase. With severe destruction of the distal aspect of the proximal phalanx, the plates buttress a large span and will fail under cyclic loading. Long-term protection of the construct with external skeletal fixation is required.

6.2.2.3 *Mc/MT3*

In vitro testing has shown the LCP to be superior to the LC-DCP in resisting overload in static bending and torsion and in resisting cyclic fatigue under four-point bending in osteotomized equine third metacarpal bones [12]. The lack of significant contour of the equine third metacarpal/metatarsal bone facilitates minimally invasive plating. An internal fixator (locking plate) is the most appropriate type of implant for this application: it does not rely on plate bone compression for stability and does not crush the periosteum beneath it.

Fractures of the medial condyle propagate proximally and are prone to catastrophic exacerbation in the absence of internal fixation. Repair with the LCP has been successful but has not been compared directly to repair with the LC-DCP or to internal fixation with screws alone. Repair with cortex screws applied in lag fashion alone is possible, but postoperative vertical propagation of the fracture beyond the level of internal fixation is a risk. It is hypothesized that plate augmentation of the repair may decrease the incidence of postoperative catastrophic exacerbation of the fracture.

Locked plating is the standard of care for diaphyseal fractures of the cannon bone. In small foals a single broad LCP may be sufficient (Figure 6.11). In most cases, double plating is required. The LCPs are applied using standard internal fixation technique. Cortex screws are placed across oblique fractures in lag fashion and are used for dynamic compression of transverse fractures. All cortex screws are placed and tightened fully before locking screws are inserted. Locking screws are also superior to cortex screws for stabilization of large, isolated cortical fragments in comminuted fractures.

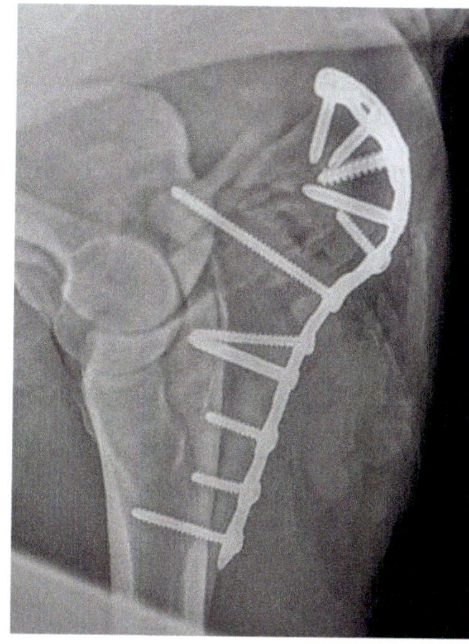

Figure 6.11 Comminuted fracture of the olecranon. An 11-hole 4.5 mm narrow locking compression plate (LCP) was applied caudally. The plate is loaded in almost pure tension.

Locked plates have distinct advantages for repairing Salter-Harris fractures. The epiphysis offers very little bone for screw/plate purchase. The superior stability and resistance to cyclic fatigue offered by the fixed-angle construct and larger core diameter of the locking screw is of tremendous value. Locked plating may also aid in the preservation of physeal viability.

6.2.2.4 *Ulna*

Ulna fracture repair in the horse is predicated on the tension band principle and has been described using tension band wiring, hook plating, and both DCP and LCP fixation techniques. A recent retrospective analysis of repairing 18 ulnar fractures with the LCP found 83% of horses sound for their intended purpose [13].

Several unique anatomic characteristics of the ulna warrant specific mention. The caudal spine of the ulna is straight, but profound medial concavity is present at the proximal aspect of the body. The caudal aspect of the medial humeral epicondyle enters this concavity during extension of the elbow. The LCP must be aligned so that fixed-angle screws avoid the medial concavity. This position centers the plate over the ulna but places it in a considerably lateral location relative to the proximal radius. The fixed angle of the distal plate holes aims the drill bit toward the lateral cortex of the radius. Catastrophic postoperative fracture of the radius has been reported in cases of penetration of the lateral radial cortex in this manner [14, 15]. This complication is avoided by correct positioning or the use of a cortex screw in this hole, angled medially. The surgeon should drill with keen awareness for the sudden advance of the drill bit that is associated with penetration of the near cortex and entry into the medullary cavity. If that sudden penetration does not happen, drilling should cease and the direction should be evaluated with craniocaudal fluoroscopic imaging.

Ulnar plates are loaded predominantly in tension, so a single narrow LCP is often adequate (Figure 6.12). Broad plates are recommended in horse over 500 kg. Augmentation of the construct with a lateral LCP is recommended for comminuted fractures. The caudal plate is applied first.

In foals less than seven months of age, transfixation of the ulna and radius with the distal plate screws must be avoided. Continued skeletal growth at the proximal radial physis will result in distal subluxation of the humeroulnar joint.

6.2.2.5 *Radius*

Repair of radius fractures is limited to those in which anatomical reconstruction is feasible. Inadequate reconstruction of the cortices guarantees failure; therefore, perfect reconstruction of the caudal cortex is imperative. Double-locked plate fixation is the treatment of choice and use of 5.5 mm LCPs, 5.0 mm locking screws, and 5.5 mm cortex screws is recommended (Figure 6.13).

Proximal physeal fractures happen concomitant with diaphyseal fracture of the ulna. This combination results in cranial or craniomedial displacement of the proximal metaphysis of the radius. Such displacement can cause irreversible damage to the radial nerve and paresis of the limb. Due to the typical "dropped elbow" presentation, radial nerve damage can be difficult to recognize preoperatively. This fracture is repaired with two LCPs, one positioned over the caudal aspect of the ulna and a second over

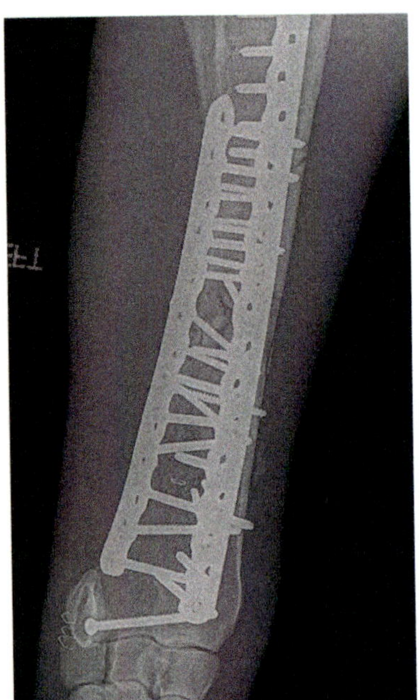

Figure 6.12 Comminuted mid-diaphyseal radial fracture: 5.5 mm broad LCPs were applied dorsally and laterally.

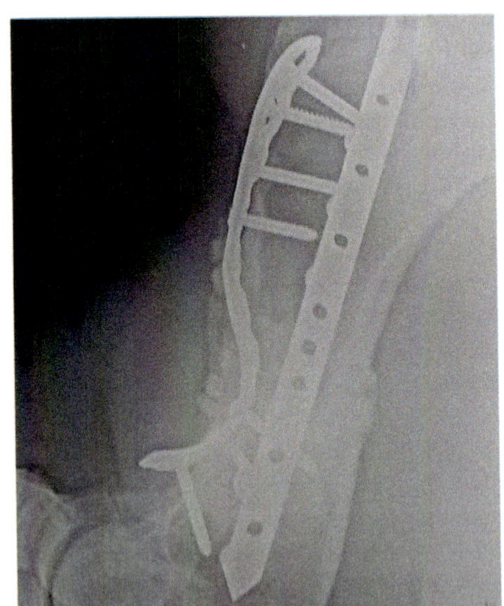

Figure 6.13 Mid-diaphyseal humeral fracture. An intramedullary interlocking nail was combined with cranial application of a 5.5 mm LCP. (Source: Image credit Dr. Jeffrey Watkins.)

the lateral aspect of the radius. Reduction is difficult and can be aided by the lag effect of a long cortex screw placed through the caudal plate at the level of the radial metaphysis. Maintenance of reduction can also be aided by lateral application of a transphyseal screw and tension band wire. The lateral plate is applied after initial stabilization of the fracture with four screws in the caudal plate, and the plate is oriented with the stacked hole proximal. Cortex screws are placed across the metaphyseal fracture component in lag fashion. Locking screws are inserted after the cortex screws are tightened fully. Screws are then inserted into the rest of the ulnar plate. The distal screws in the caudal plate engage the radius between the screws of the lateral plate as transfixation of ulna to the radius helps stabilize the construct. Unlike ulnar fracture repair, transfixation is not contraindicated in young foals since the proximal radial physis is damaged and bridged by the lateral plate.

Diaphyseal fractures of the radius are repaired with two broad LCPs. One plate is always applied cranially and the other is applied medially or laterally, depending on fracture configuration and status of the soft tissue envelope. The plates should span the entire length of the diaphysis. Screws can be inserted into the proximal and distal plate holes via stab incisions to minimize incision length. No coaptation should be applied for recovery from general anesthesia or in the postoperative period. With cast coaptation, the caudal cortex becomes the tension surface, precipitating construct failure. Repair in foals carries a good prognosis [16]. Adult horses should be supported in a sling in the postoperative period. The survival rate of adult horses after displaced fracture of the radius requiring open reduction and internal fixation is low [16, 17].

6.2.2.6 *Humerus*

Limited data exists on locking plate fixation of humeral fractures in the horse. Repair typically involves cranial and lateral dynamic compression plates. Locking implants are larger (5.5 broad plate and 5.0 mm LHS), and locked plating should increase construct stiffness and resistance to cyclic fatigue. A locking intramedullary nail combined with a cranial LCP has also been used successfully (Figure 6.14).

6.2.2.7 *Scapula*

Supraglenoid tubercle fractures have been repaired with bone screws placed in lag fashion in combination with tension band wires. Use of the LCP with successful outcome was recently described for repair of this fracture [18]. The fixed-angle construct allowed transverse positioning (Figure 6.15) of the implant(s) and engagement of the tubercle without biceps brachii tenotomy. The technique was simple, and three of the four horses returned to athletic function. The human distal femoral locking plate can also be used; the main advantage being the option to insert multiple screws into the distal fragment [19].

Scapular neck fractures have been repaired with two locking compression plates [20] and with the distal femoral locking plate (personal communication; J. Watkins and A. Watts) (Figure 6.16). The broad distal end of the femoral locking plate allows for robust engagement of the distal fragment with multiple screws. The plate is positioned craniolaterally in the groove between the spine and the flat portion of the bone. It is contoured by twisting it along its long axis to orient the locking screws caudomedially through the spine and into the caudal aspect of the flat portion of the scapula. This positioning affords maximum screw-bone purchase, and the narrower proximal aspect can be placed underneath the suprascapular nerve or contoured to pass over it. The prognosis for a return to athletic function is good [21].

6.2.2.8 *Tibia*

Salter Harris type-II fracture of the proximal tibia typically has a lateral metaphyseal spike. Reduction is critical for future limb function. Adequate engagement of the proximal epiphysis is the crux of the repair. Based on the direction of displacement, the medial aspect is the tension surface. The 4.5 mm locking T-plate (DePuy Synthes) was designed specifically for repair of this fracture in the horse. Reduction is maintained with bone forceps or an independent medial tension band. Three stacked holes in the horizontal portion of the plate allow solid engagement of the proximal epiphysis with 5.0 mm locking head screws. Compression is achieved with insertion of a 5.5 mm cortex screw in the load position of the second to last

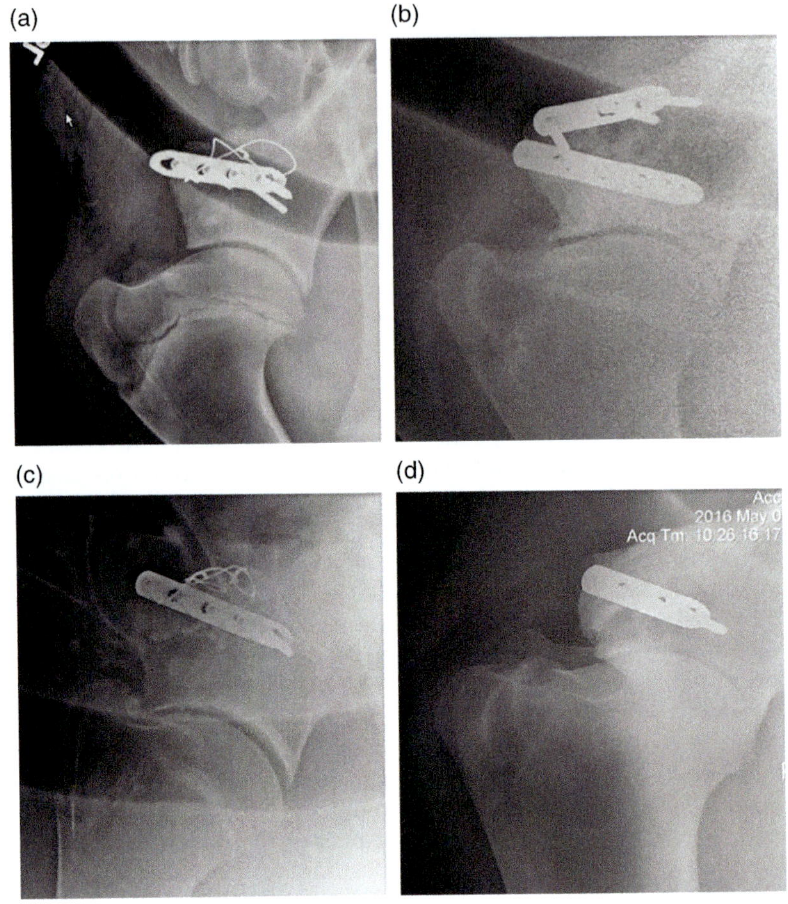

Figure 6.14 Supraglenoid tubercle fracture case series. One (a, c, and d) or two (b) 4.5 mm narrow LCPs were applied in transverse orientation with (a and c) or without (b and d) a tension band wire. (Source: Image credit Ahern et al. [18]).

combi-hole. One or two 5.5 mm cortex screws are inserted in the neutral position through the hole(s) just distal to the physis. These screws can be placed in lag fashion to secure the lateral metaphyseal spike. Locking head screws (5.0 mm) are then inserted into the remaining plate holes and tightened.

Diaphyseal fracture repair is difficult and usually successful only in foals weighing less than 200 kg. The tibia is subject to bending and torsional stress during normal loading and experiences enormous strain during recovery from anesthesia [22]. Double plating is required and currently the LCP is the best choice (Figure 6.17). One plate must be applied to the craniolateral tension surface of the bone. The position of the second plate is dictated by the fracture configuration or condition of the overlying soft tissues. In oblique fractures one plate should be applied over the distal aspect of the proximal fragment. In multifragment fractures at least one plate should buttress the isolated fragment or the region of comminution. Plates should span as much of the diaphysis as possible and are staggered to avoid stress concentration at the plate ends and to allow bicortical purchase of all locking head screws. All screws crossing the fracture should be placed in lag fashion.

6.2.2.9 *Femur*

Salter-Harris type-II fracture of the distal femur can occur in foals. The most challenging aspect of this repair is the relative paucity of bone in the distal fragment and the proximity of the

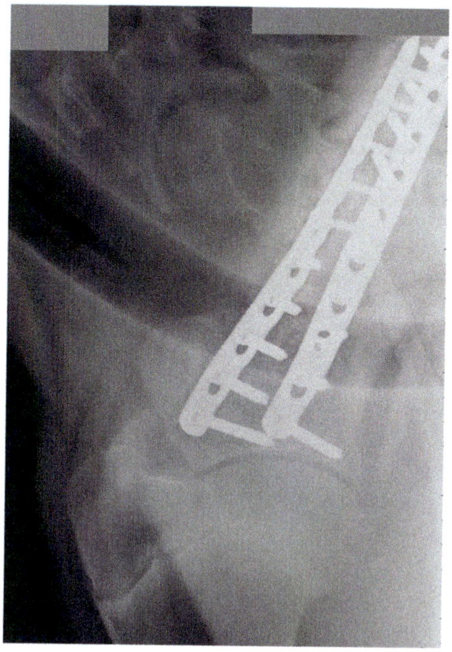

Figure 6.15 Distal femoral locking plate for scapular neck fracture repair. The broad head of the DFLP implant allows for engagement of the distal fragment with more screws. (Source: Image credit Drs. Jeffrey Watkins and Ashley Watts.)

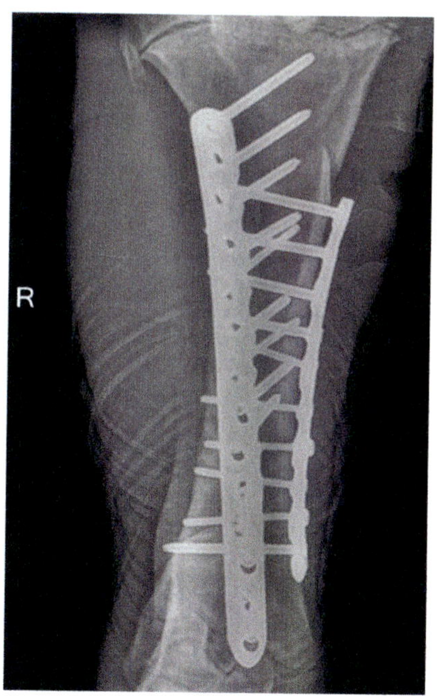

Figure 6.16 Comminuted mid-diaphyseal tibial fracture in a weanling. A 14-hole 5.5 mm broad LCP was contoured and applied from the dorsolateral cortex proximally to the dorsal cortex distally and a 10-hole 4.5 mm broad LCP was applied medially.

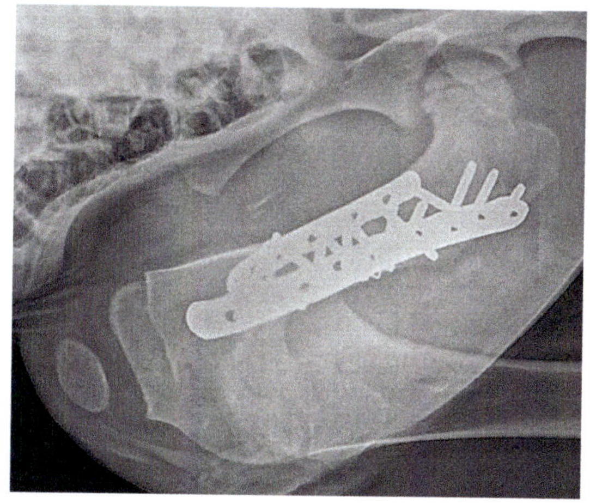

Figure 6.17 Mid-diaphyseal femoral fracture in a foal. This fracture was double plated with a 4.5 mm broad LCP laterally and a 4.5 mm narrow LCP cranially.

femoropatellar articulation. Double-plate fixation using the dynamic condylar screw plate (lateral) and the dynamic hip screw plate (cranial) has been the standard of care, however, standard locking compression plates can be used as well. More recently, successful repair of a distal femoral fracture in a donkey using a human distal femoral locking plate was described [23]. The advantages of the distal femoral locking plate include the option for insertion of up to seven locking screws into the distal fragment and ease of use as compared to DCS and DHS plates.

Mid-diaphyseal femoral fractures in foals have been successfully repaired with double plate fixation (lateral and cranial) (Figure 6.17). The increased stiffness of the LCP and locking screws, and the increased yield strength of the locking plate-screw-bone construct should increase the success rate of the procedure, especially in larger/older foals. That said, seroma formation and postoperative infection are the main reasons for failure [24] and are unlikely to be affected by the use of locking instrumentation.

6.3 Conclusion

Large animals, especially horses, must return immediately to weight bearing on all four limbs after fracture repair. Considering the inability to protect the biomechanical construct from cyclical loading, locked plating has arguably had a more significant influence on fracture repair in large animals than it has on the small animal field. The LCP offers increased construct rigidity, resistance to cyclical fatigue, and ultimate load to failure. Improvements in geometry make it the most versatile bone plate suitable for use in large animal orthopedics. Increased cost remains the only disadvantage.

References

1. Egol, K.A., Kubiak, E.N., Fulkerson, E. et al. (2004). Biomechanics of locked plates and screws. *Journal of Orthopaedic Trauma* 18 (8): 488–493.
2. Rahn, B.A., Gallinaro, P., Baltensperger, A. et al. (1971). Primary bone healing. An experimental study in the rabbit. *The Journal of Bone and Joint Surgery (American)* 53 (4): 783–786.
3. Ahern, B.J., Showalter, B.L., Elliott, D.M. et al. (2015). In vitro biomechanical comparison of a 4.5 mm narrow locking compression plate construct versus a 4.5 mm limited contact dynamic compression plate construct for arthrodesis of the equine proximal interphalangeal joint. *Veterinary Surgery* 42 (3): 335–339. doi: 10.1111/j.1532-950X.2013.01111.x.
4. Richardson, D.W. (2008). Complications of orthopaedic surgery in horses. *The Veterinary Clinics of North America Equine Practice* 24 (3): 591–610, viii. doi: 10.1016/j.cveq.2008.11.001.
5. Carpenter, R.S., Galuppo, L.D., Simpson, E.L. et al. (2008). Clinical evaluation of the locking compression plate for fetlock arthrodesis in six thoroughbred racehorses. *Veterinary Surgery* 37 (3): 263–268. doi: 10.1111/j.1532-950X.2008.00375.x.
6. Keller, S.A., Fürst, A.E., Kircher, P. et al. (2015). Locking compression plate fixation of equine tarsal subluxations. *Veterinary Surgery* 44 (8): 949–956. doi: 10.1111/vsu.12400.
7. McCormick, J.D. and Watkins, J. (2014). Plate fixation for management of plantar instability of the distal tarsus/proximal metatarsus in 5 horses. *Veterinary Surgery* 43 (4): 425–429. doi: 10.1111/j.1532-950X.2014.12149.x.
8. Reardon, R.J.M., Bailey, R., Walmsley, J.P. et al. (2010). An in vitro biomechanical comparison of a locking compression plate fixation and kerf cut cylinder fixation for ventral arthrodesis of the fourth and the fifth equine cervical vertebrae. *Veterinary Surgery* 39 (8): 980–990. doi: 10.1111/j.1532-950X.2010.00733.x.
9. Reardon, R., Kummer, M., and Lischer, C. (2009). Ventral locking compression plate for treatment of cervical stenotic myelopathy in a 3-month-old warmblood foal. *Veterinary Surgery* 38 (4): 537–542. doi: 10.1111/j.1532-950X.2009.00523.x.
10. Rossignol, F., Brandenberger, O., and Mespoulhes-Rivière, C. (2015). Internal fixation of cervical fractures in three horses. *Veterinary Surgery* 45 (1): 104–109. doi: 10.1111/vsu.12425.
11. Nunamaker, D.M. and Richardson, D.W. (1986). A new external skeletal fixation device that allows immediate full weight bearing application in the horse. *Veterinary Surgery* 15 (5): 345–355. doi: 10.1111/j.1532-950X.1986.tb00242.x.
12. SOD, G.A., Mitchell, C.F., Hubert, J.D. et al. (2008). In vitro biomechanical comparison of locking compression plate fixation and limited-contact dynamic compression plate fixation of osteotomized equine third metacarpal bones. *Veterinary Surgery* 37 (3): 283–288. doi: 10.1111/j.1532-950X.2008.00378.x.
13. Jacobs, C.C., Levine, D.G., and Richardson, D.W. (2017). Use of locking compression plates in ulnar fractures of 18 horses. *Veterinary Surgery* 46 (2): 242–248. doi: 10.1111/vsu.12607.
14. Jackson, M., Kummer, M., Auer, J. et al. (2011). Treatment of type 2 and 4 olecranon fractures with locking compression plate osteosynthesis in horses: a prospective study (2002–2008). *Veterinary and Comparative Orthopaedics and Traumatology* 24 (1): 57–61. doi: 10.3415/VCOT-10-02-0020.
15. Kuemmerle, J.M., Kühn, K., Bryner, M. et al. (2013). Equine ulnar fracture repair with locking compression plates can be associated with inadvertent penetration of the lateral cortex of the radius. *Veterinary Surgery* 42 (7): 790–794. doi: 10.1111/j.1532-950X.2013.12059.x.
16. Stewart, S., Richardson, D., Boston, R., and Schaer, T.P. (2015). Risk factors associated with survival to hospital discharge of 54 horses with fractures of the radius. *Veterinary Surgery* 44 (8): 1036–1041. doi: 10.1111/vsu.12412.
17. Auer, J.A. and Watkins, J.P. (1987). Treatment of radial fractures in adult horses: an analysis of 15 clinical cases. *Equine Veterinary Journal* 19 (2): 103–110.
18. Ahern, B.J., Bayliss, I.P.M., Zedler, S.T. et al. (2017). Supraglenoid tubercle fractures repair with transverse locking compression plates in 4 horses. *Veterinary Surgery* 46 (4): 507–514. doi: 10.1111/vsu.12600.
19. Frei, S., Fürst, A.E., Sacks, M. et al. (2016). Fixation of supraglenoid tubercle fractures using distal femoral locking plates in three warmblood horses. *Veterinary and Comparative Orthopaedics and Traumatology* 29 (3): 246–252. doi: 10.3415/VCOT-15-10-0164.
20. Kamm, J.L., Quinn, G., and van Zwanenberg, D. (2015). Fixation of a complete scapular neck fracture in a foal using two 3.5 mm locking compression plates. *Equine Veterinary Education* 29 (4): 180–183. doi: 10.1111/eve.12464.

21. Auer, J. (2017). Fractures of the scapula. *Equine Veterinary Education* 29 (4): 184–195. doi: 10.1111/eve.12496.
22. Rybicki, E.F. and Mills, E.J. (1977). In vivo and analytical studies of forces and moments in equine long bones. *Journal of Biomechanics* 10 (11/12): 701–705.
23. Bumbacher, S., Bryner, M.F., Fürst, A.E. et al. (2013). Treatment of a femoral fracture with a titanium locking compression plate distal femur (LCP-DF) in a young donkey. *Equine Veterinary Education* 26 (1): 27–31. doi: 10.1111/eve.12037.
24. Hance, S.R., Bramlage, L.R., Schneider, R.K. et al. (1992). Retrospective study of 38 cases of femur fractures in horses less than one year of age. *Equine Veterinary Journal* 24 (5): 357–363.

Section III

Current Veterinary Locking Plate Instrumentation and Implants

7 The Advanced Locking Plate System (ALPS)

Tomás Guerrero

The Advanced Locking Plate System (ALPS) (Kyon AG® Zurich, Switzerland) is a locking plate system developed for veterinary use [1–3]. ALPS was developed based on research performed on the point-contact fixator (PC-Fix) at the AO Research Institute, in Davos, Switzerland, aiming mainly to preserve blood supply [3–5]. This was accomplished by shaping the underside of the plate for minimal contact with the bone (Figures 7.1 and 7.2), and using only monocortical screws to protect the endosteal blood supply. Stoppers in the drill bits are used to reduce damage to endosteal vasculature.

The Sherman-shape of the plate is meant to provide uniform bending strength along the plate length and allows for contouring in all planes (Figure 7.3). The screw holes allow for insertion of locking and nonlocking screws. Locking screws must be inserted at a right angle to the plate while nonlocking screws can be angulated 30° in the longitudinal plane and 5° in the transverse plane. Additionally, nonlocking screws can be used to position the plate in compression or neutral functions. If needed, nonlocking screws can be replaced, once fixation is achieved, by the diameter larger locking screws using the same plate holes. The screwheads lock into the plate-holes by a combination of two mechanisms: (i) partial threads in the plate-hole that lock with the most proximal thread of the screw (Figure 7.1), and (ii) conical shape of both the screwhead and the plate hole.

The plates are made of grade 4 titanium and the screws are made of a titanium-aluminum-vanadium alloy (Ti-6A1–4V). Four size-systems, named based in the width of the plates, are available. Each system has two different sizes of plates fitting the same-size screws: mini (3.5/4 mm), small (5/6.5 mm), medium (8/9 mm), and large (10/11 mm). Details of plate size, locking and cortical screw sizes, and common applications of each system are provided in Table 7.1. A dedicated implant chart is used to evaluate proper implant size (Figure 7.4).

ALPS-specific instrumentation includes drilling guides for locking and nonlocking screws (Figure 7.5). Different from other locking systems, the guides for locking screws cannot be fixed to the plate and must be held in position by hand. Dedicated drill stoppers can be used to prevent damage to endosteal blood supply when using monocortical screws. Two different guides for nonlocking screws can be used: a compression sleeve used to apply eccentric screws for fracture compression and a guide

Locking Plates in Veterinary Orthopedics, First Edition.
Edited by Matthew D. Barnhart and Karl C. Maritato.

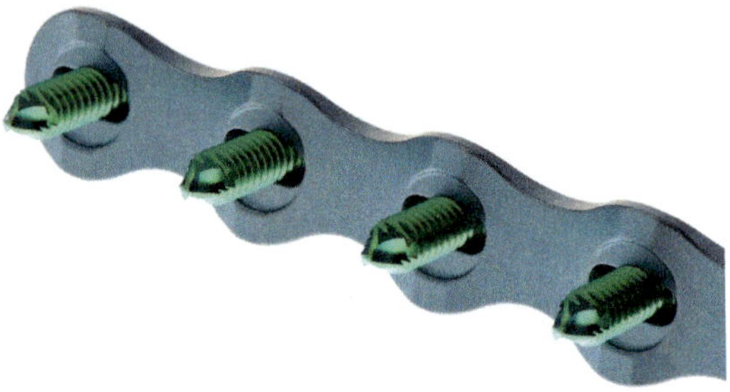

Figure 7.1 Detail of the back side of a plate showing its shape aimed to minimize plate to bone contact. The locking mechanism between the last screw-thread and the plate hole is also observed.

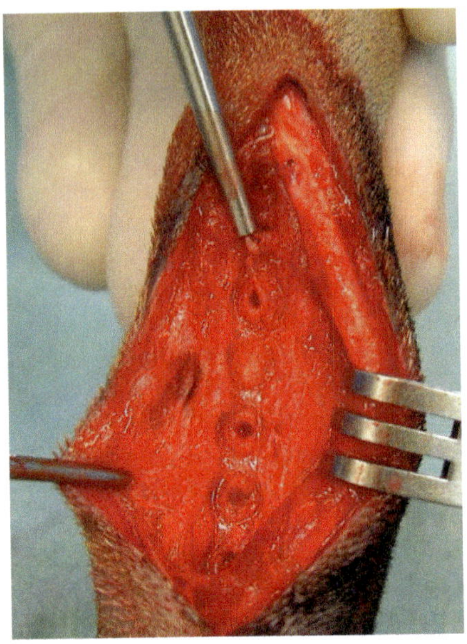

Figure 7.2 Good vascularized periosteum is observed after plate removal in a radius. (Source: Courtesy of Dr. Junga Ogawa)

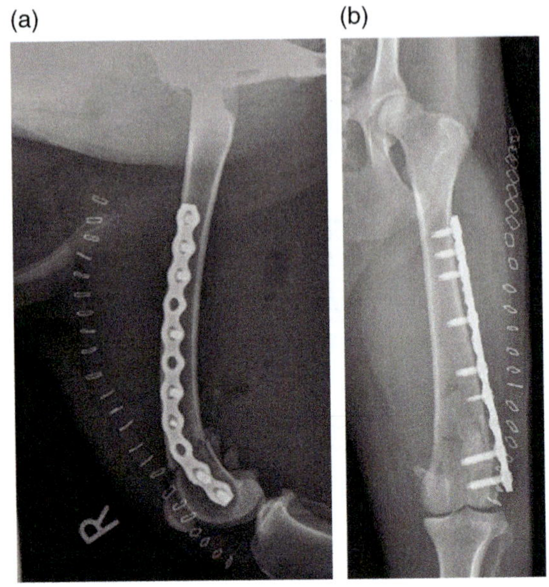

Figure 7.3 (a) and (b) Clinical application of an ALPS plate in a femur. The Sherman-shape of the plate allows for contouring it in all planes.

that centers the screw hole in the plate hole. This guide allows for the limited angulation described above.

Cutting irons for plates 3.5–9 mm and bending irons are also needed. Each size of plate has a proper size of cutting and bending iron. For in-plane bending, a special bending instrument is used. Plate holes are protected from deformation with plugs positioned before bending.

Clinical application of the system has been reported [1–3], showing an overall good outcome and good handling characteristics. There are no reports about the newest 3.5–4 mm plate system developed for miniature breeds. Dedicated ALPS plates are also used to perform tibial plateau leveling osteotomy (TPLO) and proximal abducting ulnar osteotomy (PAUL) to treat cranial cruciate disease and elbow medial compartment disease, respectively. Based on published reports [1, 6] showing that mono cortical screw fixation is in some cases insufficient, longer locking screws have been recently developed, increasing the longest length to 34 mm for the ALPS 10/11 system. There are no available reports on use of the new long bicortical locking screws.

Different from other plate–systems, plate-to-bone contact is needed when working with ALPS [1]. After contouring the plate to the bone, the proximal, and distal ends of the plate are fixed with nonlocking screws to the bone fragments. Further stabilization is provided using the locking screws. After the locking screws are placed, the initially placed nonlocking screws can be replaced by locking screws using the same screw holes (depending on bone quality redrilling to the proper drill bit size may be necessary). Locking screws can be positioned in mono or bicortical mode depending on bone quality and location in the bone. Bicortical

Table 7.1 Showing the available ALPS sizes and its common applications.

System		Plate sizes	Locking screws		Cortical screws		Common application
	(wide in mm)	Length: Plates 3.5–9 mm are cuttable in length	Diameter (mm)	Length (mm)	Diameter (mm)	Length (mm)	
Mini	3.5 4	20 holes / 79.5 mm 20 holes / 89–5 mm	1.6	5–10	1.0	5–12	Distal radius for small/toy breeds, maxillofacial, and exotics
Small	5 6.5	43 holes / 236.5 mm 34 holes / 238 mm	2.4	5–16	1.5	6–30	Feline and small-breed canine tibia fractures, distal radius fractures in medium breeds
Medium	8 9	26 holes / 234 mm 22 holes / 234 mm	3.2	6–30	2.4	10–32	Femur fractures in cats and as a complementary plate in larger patients
Large	10 11	2 holes / 23 mm–12 holes / 143 mm 4 holes / 51.5 mm–18 holes / 233.5 mm	4.0	10–34	2.7	10–34	Long bone fractures in medium to large and even giant (ALPS 11) breed dogs

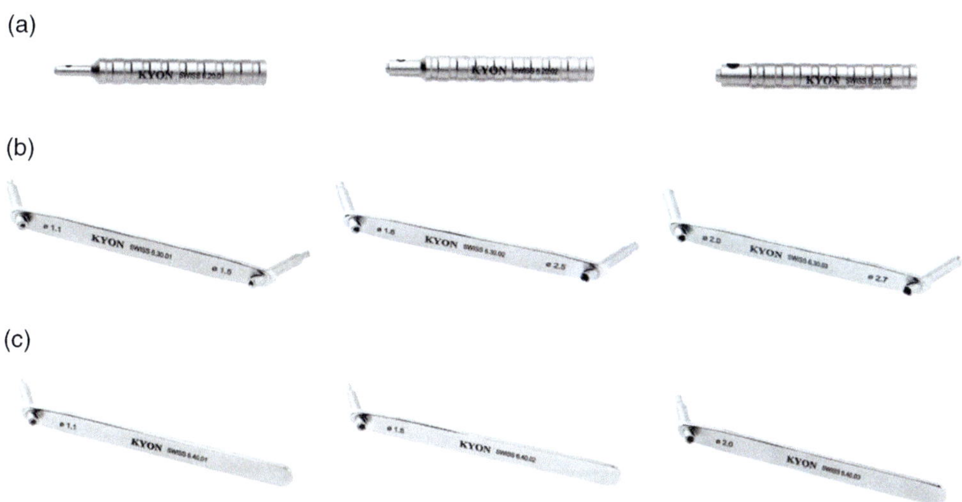

Figure 7.4 The different drill guides are shown. The guides for locking screws (a) must be held by hand in position during the drilling. (b)The guides for cortical screws allow for angulation in both planes, centering the screws in the plate hole. These guides are also used to position lag screws. The guides in the lower row (c) are used to drill the bone holes eccentrically in the plate hole and in this manner to create interfragmentary compression.

screws should be used in very young patients, metaphyseal areas of the bone, and in dogs with poor bone quality. ALPS screws are larger in diameter in comparison with other plate systems (e.g. ALPS 10, the equivalent to the dynamic compression plate [DCP] 3.5 system, takes 4.0 mm locking screws). Care must be taken to avoid creating a fracture using this large-diameter screw size. In dogs with adequate bone quality and in the diaphyseal section of the bone, short screws positioned in monocortical fashion are preferentially used. In these cases, drilling is performed using a drill stopper attempting to protect the endosteal blood supply. To prevent screw pullout, the cutting flutes must penetrate the cortex completely. In miniature dogs with small endosteal cavities and insufficient intramedullary space for the cutting flutes, bicortical screws should be used to prevent risk of transcortical fracture. Close to

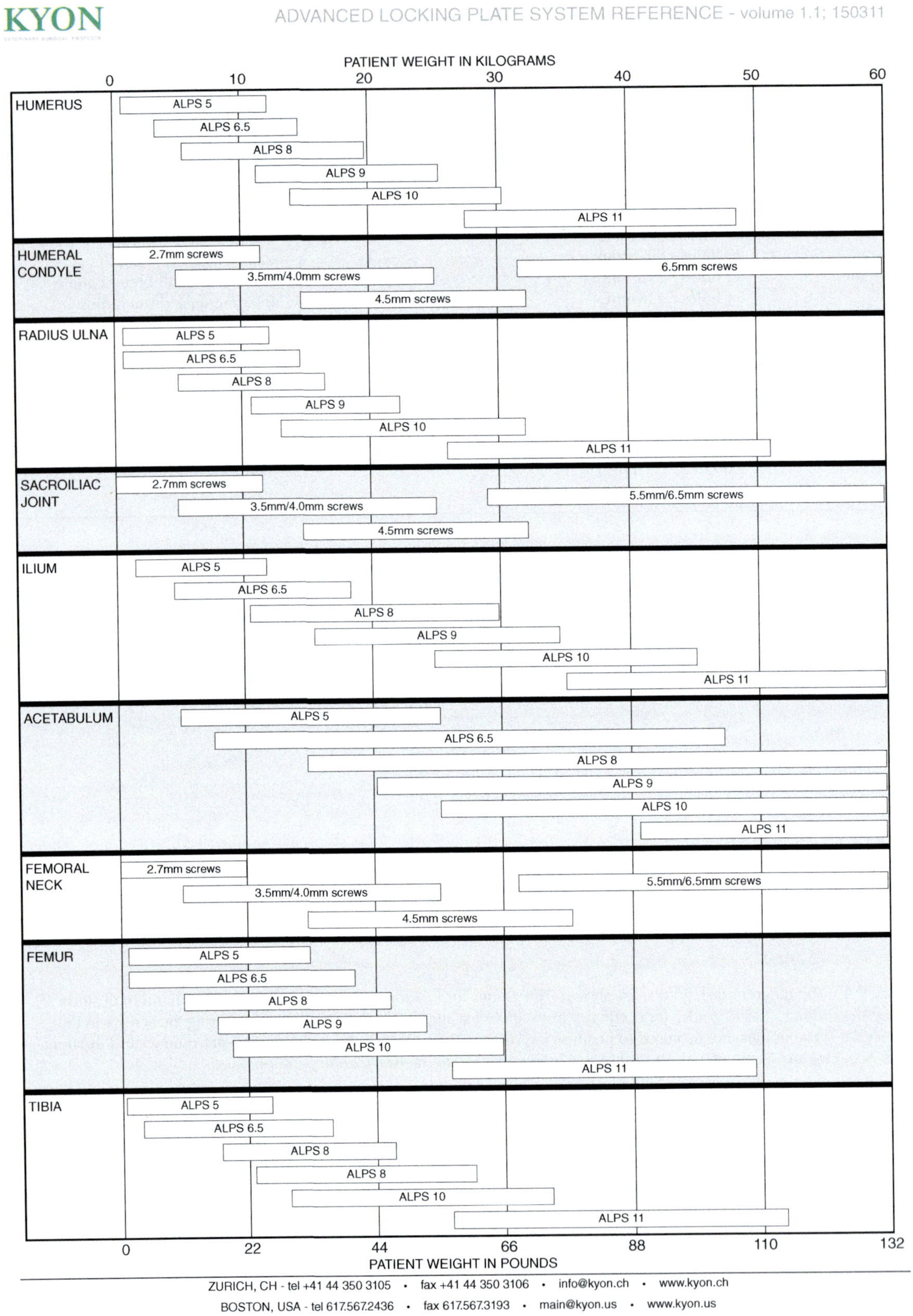

Figure 7.5 Reference chart for clinical application of ALPS.

joints, when angulation is needed, nonlocking screws can be used. Nonlocking screws may also be used in cases where larger locking screws may risk a fracture. Distal fixation of carpal and tarsal arthrodesis are examples of this type of fixation [1].

References

1. Guerrero, T.G., Kalchofner, K., Scherrer, N. et al. (2014). The advanced locking plate system (ALPS): a retrospective evaluation in 71 small animal patients. *Vet. Surg.* 43 (2): 127–135.
2. Inauen, R., Koch, D., and Bass, M. (2009). Arthrodesis of the tarsometatarsal joints in a cat with a two hole advanced locking plate system. *Vet. Comp. Orthop. Traumatol.* 22 (2): 166–169.
3. Nojiri, A., Nishido, T., Horinaka, O. et al. (2015). Initial clinical application and results of the advanced locking plate system (ALPS) in small animal orthopedics: two hundred eighty two procedures. *Int. J. Appl. Res. Vet. M* 13 (1): 64–79.
4. Perren, S.M. (2002). Evolution of the internal fixation of long bone fractures. The scientific basis of biological internal fixation: choosing a new balance between stability and biology. *J. Bone Joint Surg. Br.* 84 (8): 1093–1110.
5. Tepic, S., Remiger, A.R., Morikawa, K. et al. (1997). Strength recovery in fractured sheep tibia treated with a plate or an internal fixator: an experimental study with a two-year follow-up. *J. Orthop. Trauma* 11 (1): 14–23.
6. Boudrieau, R.J. (2016). Complications specific to locking plates. In: *Complications in Small Animal Surgery* (ed. D. Griffon and A. Hamaide), 714–726. Wiley Blackwell.

8 The Fixin Implant System

Kevin P. Benjamino and Massimo Petazzoni

The Fixin system differs from other locking systems because it is a locking screw-insert (bushing)-plate construct [1–4]. Locking is achieved between the screwhead and the bushing by a conical coupling locking mechanism. The bushing is an intermediary insert that screws into the plate and couples with the screwhead (Figure 8.1). Fixin screws have a 1.0° and 1.5° (large and mini system, respectively) conical head that will lock into a corresponding tapered cone within the bushing [2–4]. The screw-bushing coupling is achieved by friction, micro-welding, and elastic deformation between the screwhead and the bushing insert [1, 2] (Figure 8.2). An advantage of the screw-bushing-plate construct is that it allows for an easier option if the implant needs to be removed, as opposed to both nonlocking and locking screw to plate interfaces. In other systems, if the screw has deformed (cold welding) to the screw hole or the screwhead does not engage the screwdriver, many times the screw cannot be removed without cumbersome methods such as burring the screwhead. If the screwhead is no longer able to engage the screwdriver the bushing-screw complex can be removed with the bushing extractor. The bushing construct also allows for even force distribution over the screwhead. If the screw hole is not filled with a screw, the bushing still maintains even force distribution, decreasing the risk of plate failure over this site, in comparison to previous plate designs (dynamic compression plates, combination locking compression plates, etc.). The addition of the bushing increases the screws resistance to shear forces and also allows for a thinner plate design overall. With the bushing–plate construct, the bushings allow for the plate design to be decreased in thickness and of comparable strength to other, thicker locking plate systems. Due to the decreased thickness, the plate allows for more elasticity (elastic deformation), which promotes earlier callous formation around the fracture or osteotomy and earlier clinical and radiographic union. Also, a thinner plate design allows for less irritation and impingement on surrounding soft tissue structures (proximal tibia, distal tibia, carpus, tarsus, and other distal extremities) [2–4].

8.1 Fixin Implants and Instrumentation

8.1.1 Standard and Mini Fixin Systems

The plates are constructed of AISI 316LVM stainless steel, the bushing inserts and screws are composed of titanium alloy Ti-6Al-4 V, and

Locking Plates in Veterinary Orthopedics, First Edition.
Edited by Matthew D. Barnhart and Karl C. Maritato.

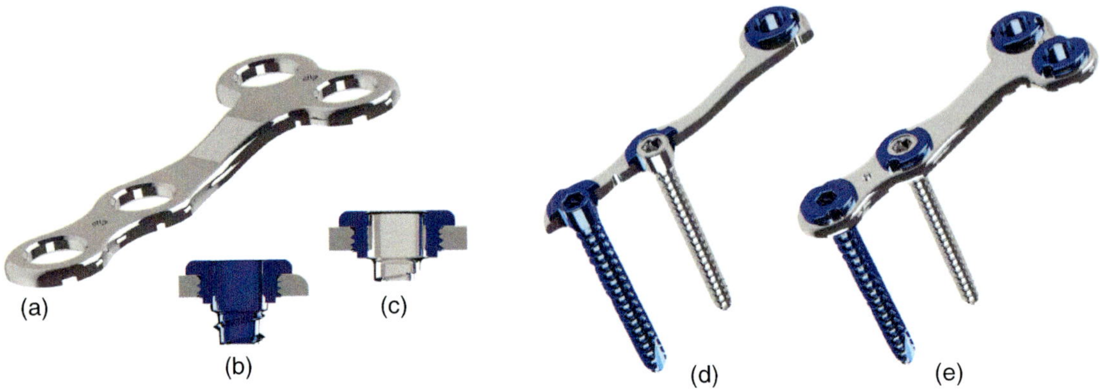

Figure 8.1 Note the conical-shaped head within the bushing that is threaded into the plate. The coupling/locking mechanism is engaged via divergent angles. (Source: Courtesy of Massimo Petazzoni.)

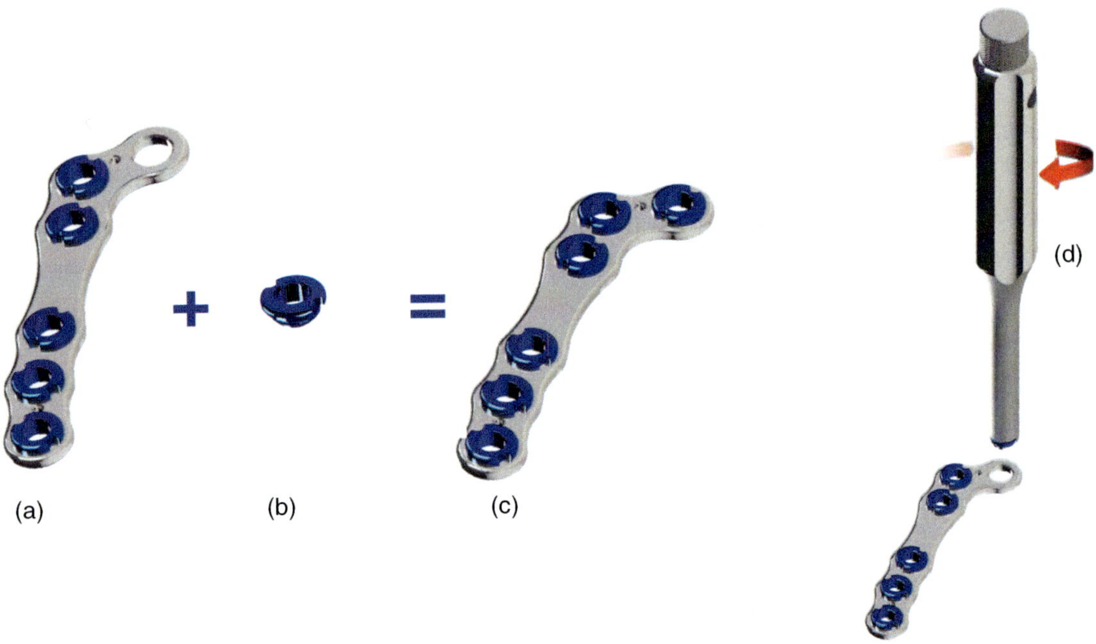

Figure 8.2 This demonstrates the plate and bushing combination. D refers to the designated bushing extractor for ease of replacing or removing the bushings. (Source: Courtesy of Massimo Petazzoni.)

the screws are self-tapping. As noted, the Fixin system combines two different metals, providing a titanium-to-stainless-steel interface. While historically there has been concern for the occurrence of galvanic corrosion when two different types of metal are combined, recent studies have demonstrated that this does not occur between titanium and stainless steel. In one study, which evaluated galvanic corrosion in different interfaces (stainless steel to stainless steel, stainless steel to titanium, and titanium to titanium) during cyclic loading in saline, it was shown that the stainless-steel-to-titanium interface had less evidence of corrosion than the other interfaces [5]. In another study evaluating cyclic loading in serum, the mixture of metal implants did not cause metal release or loss when compared to a single metal construct, further demonstrating the safety of titanium-to-stainless-steel interface [6].

The plates are made with variable thickness, from 1.2 mm to 3 mm. The number of holes in each plate varies from four to eight holes, and the plate length varies as well, with the exception of cuttable mini and micro plates [2–4]. Specialty plates (precontoured) are available for specific procedures – such as tibial plateau leveling osteotomy (TPLO), distal femoral osteotomy (DFO), center of rotation and angulation (CORA)-based leveling osteotomy (CBLO), double pelvic osteotomy (DPO), pancarpal and pantarsal arthrodeses, and acetabular fractures [7] (Figures 8.3 and 8.4).

The screw sizes allow for flexibility in application. The standard Fixin system accepts 3.0 mm (2.5 mm drill bit) and 3.5 mm (2.8 mm drill bit) screws that are interchangeable within the bushing. The mini Fixin system accepts 1.9 mm (1.5 mm drill bit) and 2.5 mm (2.0 mm drill bit) screws that are also interchangeable within the bushing. All Fixin screws are self-tapping and have smaller threads and an increased core diameter compared to nonlocking cortical screws, which is similar to other

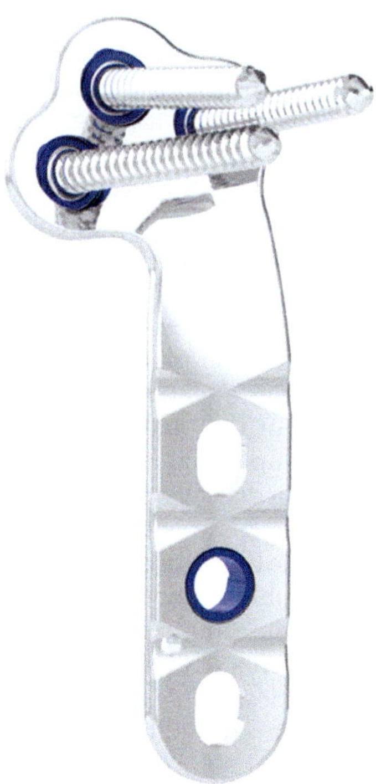

Figure 8.3 Combination compression and locking tibial plateau leveling osteotomy (TPLO) plate. (Source: Courtesy of Intrauma.)

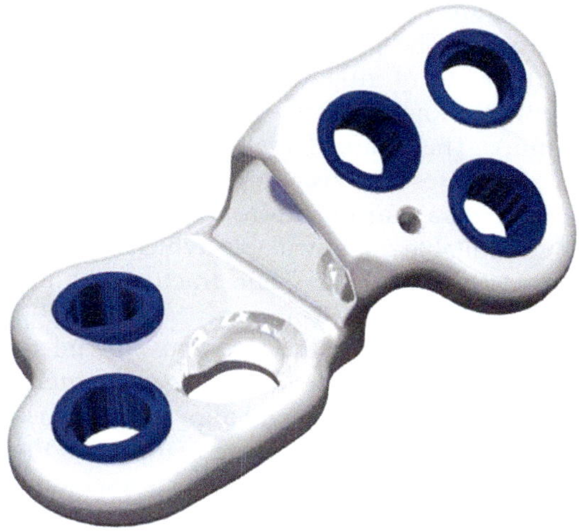

Figure 8.4 Double pelvic osteotomy (DPO) plate. Note the compression screw hole. (Source: Courtesy of Intrauma.)

locking screw designs. These features allow for increased resistance to screw bending and increased resistance to shear forces due to an increased cantilever effect [2–4].

Fixin-specific instrumentation includes the bushing extractor, temporary stabilizing screws, and pin stoppers [2]. There is a specific plate bender manufactured for the standard and mini Fixin systems exclusively. The dedicated recesses in the plate bender provide bushing protection against deformation during contouring of the plate.

8.1.2 Micro Fixin System

The micro Fixin system is conceptually the same as the standard and mini systems; however, some of the materials are different. The micro system was designed to decrease the incidence of stress protection of the bone that was observed when using the mini Fixin system in toy-breed dogs and cats (<4 kg) [8]. The advantages (as is evident in the design and experienced by the authors) of the micro system in smaller patients are the decreased thickness of the implant (more "elasticity" of the implant) and the decreased diameter of the screws (decreasing the stiffness of the construct). Additionally, like other locking systems, minimal screw numbers (two to three) per bone fracture segment are necessary to maintain adequate stability [8]. The plates, bushings, and screws are all made of titanium alloy (Ti-6Al-4 V), and the thicknesses of the plates are uniform (1.2 mm). There are T-plates, L-plates, and straight plates for osteotomy correction or fracture repair application. There is also a 26-hole cuttable plate available, which has been particularly useful for feline fractures or toy breed dog osteotomy fixation.

Similar to the other Fixin systems, the micro system has a drill guide that engages the bushings in the same fashion and allows for the use of a 1.3 mm drill bit. The depth gauge is on the surface of the drill guide, and there is a window in the drill guide that allows for visualization of the drill bit, as well as a laser line on the drill bit that corresponds to measurements on the drill guide to give an accurate measurement (Figure 8.5). A star screwdriver is used that corresponds to the star recess within the screwhead. A conventional mini depth gauge (1.5/2.0 DCP standard set) is also compatible.

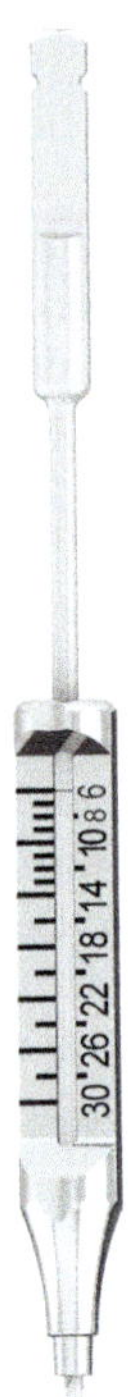

Figure 8.5 Note the micro system drill guide and the corresponding laser line on the 1.3 mm drill bit. (Source: Courtesy of Intrauma.)

8.2 Surgical Technique

There are several methods in which the plate can temporarily be stabilized against the bone to ensure proper position prior to screw placement. There are small holes within the plates (trauma and specialty plates) that allow for small Kirschner-wire (K-wire) placement (0.045 in., or 1.2 and 1.0 mm for the micro system). The wire should be placed in bicortical fashion and then bent over the plate to provide plate stability during drilling for screws. Another method is using the pin stopper method; this utilizes a K-wire placed within a screw hole. A drill guide is placed in the desired screw hole and a smooth or threaded K-wire is placed through the drill guide in the *cis* cortex (or bicortically). Next, a pin stopper is placed over the wire and flush with the drill guide and subsequently tightened. This method can be employed and placed at both ends of the plate [1–4]. A third technique would be to use a temporary fixation screw, which is a monocortical or bicortical screw that does not engage the locking mechanism. The temporary fixation screw is placed in the screw hole and engages the bone; however, the head is larger than the bushing and it sits on top of the bushing. The locking screwheads should be either flush with the bushing or slightly protruding. If the head is not appropriately seated within the bushing, the locking mechanism is not properly engaged [2].

It is advisable when either stabilizing or inserting the first screws to utilize the holes at the periphery of the plate. This will ensure that the other holes are appropriately lined up over the length of the bone. If the peripheral screws do wind up lying off the major portion of bone and bicortical screw placement is impossible and plate position cannot be changed, then the bushing can be removed and the largest possible cortical screw should be placed in the hole (not exceeding 25% of the bone diameter). This screw should be angled to engage both cortices.

The precontoured Fixin TPLO and DPO plates do allow for compression of the osteotomy site. This is achieved by placing standard cortical screws before placing the locking screws, in the dedicated compression holes present in these plates (Figure 8.3).

The Fixin system affords the veterinary surgeon the ability to handle most of the different types of fracture repairs and osteotomy procedures. There are key advantages to this system. The system has a strikingly easy application to bone and fracture segments with simple placement of the drill guide into the bushings (conical coupling versus threaded placement). Screw/implant removal, when needed, has been simplified as well. The implants accommodate minimally invasive applications very well with their solid plate design, decreasing or eliminating the risk of implant breakage at screw hole left unfilled. One advantage noted by the authors is the ease of plate contouring and how this applies to dogs that have both a cranial cruciate ligament rupture and medial patella luxation. The five- to six-hole TPLO plates allow for easy contouring and accommodate medialization of the proximal segment of a TPLO, thus lateralizing the tibial tuberosity and patellar tendon. Other advantages include the ability to use different-diameter screws with the same plate when needed and the low-profile nature (decreased thickness) of the plates, which facilitates positioning in distal, limb fractures where muscle and skin coverage is limited.

References

1. Petazzoni, M. and Nicetto, T. (2015). Stifle arthrodesis using a locking plate system in six dogs. *Vet. Comp. Orthop. Traumatol.* 28: 288–293.
2. Petazzoni, M., Urizzi, A., Verdonck, B. et al. (2010). Fixin internal fixator: concept and technique. *Vet. Comp. Orthop. Traumatol.* 23: 250–253.
3. Valentini, R., Martinelli, B., Cosmi, F. et al. (2007). Mechanical behavior of one internal fixator (O'Nil plate and screws system): a finite element study and clinical experiences. *Tech. Orthop.* 22: 173–180.
4. Nicetto, T., Petazzoni, M., Urizzi, A. et al. (2013). Experiences using the Fixin locking plate system for the stabilization of appendicular fractures in dogs. *Vet. Comp. Orthop. Traumatol.* 26: 61–68.
5. Serhan, H., Slivka, M., Albert, T. et al. (2004). Is galvanic corrosion between titanium alloy and stainless steel spinal implants a clinical concern? *Spine J.* 4 (4): 379087.
6. Hol, P.J., Moister, A., and Gjerdet, N.R. (2008). Should the galvanic combination of titanium and stainless steel surgical implants be avoided? *Injury* 39 (2): 161–169.
7. Petazzoni, M. and Nicetto, T. (2014). Rapid prototyping to design a customized locking plate for pancarpal arthrodesis in a giant breed dog. *Vet. Comp. Orthop. Traumatol.* 27: 85–89.
8. Petazzoni, M., Nicetto, T., and Urizzi, A. (2012). Riassorbimento osseo da sospetta protezione da stimolo meccanico dopo applicazione di un impianto a stabilita angolare. *Veterinaria* 26 (2): 31–36.

9 The Liberty Lock System

Karl C. Maritato

In 2012, a new form of polyaxial screw placement in locking plates was introduced with liberty lock plates. The benefit of polyaxial plate design is the ability to angle the screws in the screw hole of the plate, where traditional locking plates require 0° of angulation (true perpendicularity to the plate). Without polyaxial design, angulation of the screws in the screw holes results in inadequate screw locking and difficult insertion and removal. In addition, being confined to 0° of angulation in the plate limits use in certain clinical situations, such as near fracture sites, joints, and growth plates. Lastly, because locking plates are frequently used with an IM pin, it can be easier to avoid the pin if one is able to angulate the screw.

The liberty lock polyaxial mode of action is different than other reported poly-axial systems [1, 2], as the screws do not cut the threads into the screw holes. The locking holes and screws are manufactured to work together to provide for a polyaxial locking mechanism. The screw holes are manufactured with "interrupts" in the thread, allowing the bone screw four entry points into the threaded hole of the plate. The bone screw has two entry points in the locking thread on the screwhead. By combining these two features, the screw can be angled up to 15° in any direction, while virtually eliminating any potential cross threading of the locking screws.

The plates and screws are made of 316LVM stainless steel, which is austenitic. Austenitic stainless steel is more resistant to corrosion and is very formable, making it a good choice for locking plates. The screwheads utilize the hexalobe (aka *stardrive*) drive mechanism. This drive allows for increased torque, which has been shown to allow for a stronger locking mechanism in locking plates [1].

The pushout strength of the 3.5 mm screws has been investigated in the laboratory at various angles up to 15° within the 3.5 mm plate. With 2.5 Nm of insertion torque, the push-out force (N) was noted to be as follows: 0°, 3320 N; 5°, 3087 N; 10°, 2778 N; 15°, 2500 N.

Currently, liberty lock plates designed for fracture repair are available in three sizes: 3.5, 2.7, and 2.4 mm, with corresponding screw sizes, as well as a variety of specialty plates (hybrid T-plates, arthrodesis plates, double pelvic osteotomy [DPO] plates, distal femur plates, and acetabular plates). The 2.4 plates can be used with either 2.7 or 2.4 mm screws. They are

Locking Plates in Veterinary Orthopedics, First Edition.
Edited by Matthew D. Barnhart and Karl C. Maritato.

also available are 3.5 mm mini, 3.5 mm regular, and 3.5 mm broad tibial plateau leveling osteotomy (TPLO) plates.

It is important to differentiate these locking screws from traditional compression screws, as the drill bits used are different and correlate with the inner core screw diameter. For 3.5 mm screws, a 2.8 mm drill bit is used; with 2.7 mm screws, a 2.1 mm drill bit is used; and with 2.4 mm screws, a 1.8 mm drill bit is used. In order to ensure proper alignment of the screw-head threads and the plate hole threads, there are threaded drill guides that fit into the threaded plate holes, defining the angle at which the screw can be inserted and allowing for the screws to be inserted properly. It is very important to not make drill holes for locking plates without using the proper drill bit guide, as it can result in an improper locking mechanism and weakness in the screw-plate construct.

The author has successfully used liberty lock plates in both open and minimally invasive fashions. They are particularly well suited to combination plate-rod constructs, because of the angulation degrees allowable, making it easier to avoid the IM pin (see Figure 9.1a and b). The 3.5 and 2.7 mm plates are relatively low profile and have a node-internode design fashion. This allows the surgeon to place plate benders along the internode, avoiding damage to the node that can result in deformation of the screw hole and poor locking mechanism. This also allows for rotational bending of the plates as well. The 2.4 plates are not node-internode in shape, but rather, cuttable and similar to the shape of nonlocking cuttable plates, making them very useful in smaller-animal long bones (Figure 9.2a and b), as well as in the mandible (Figure 9.3a and b).

The author has also successfully used the TPLO plates available (See Figure 9.4a and b). The TPLO plates have a cloverleaf design proximally, allowing for solid plate coverage in the proximal segment, while allowing maneuverability for those wishing to use a jig to complete the procedure. The screws in the proximal plate are also angled at 6° distally, assisting the surgeon to avoid the joint. The plate is low profile compared to other locking

(a) (b)

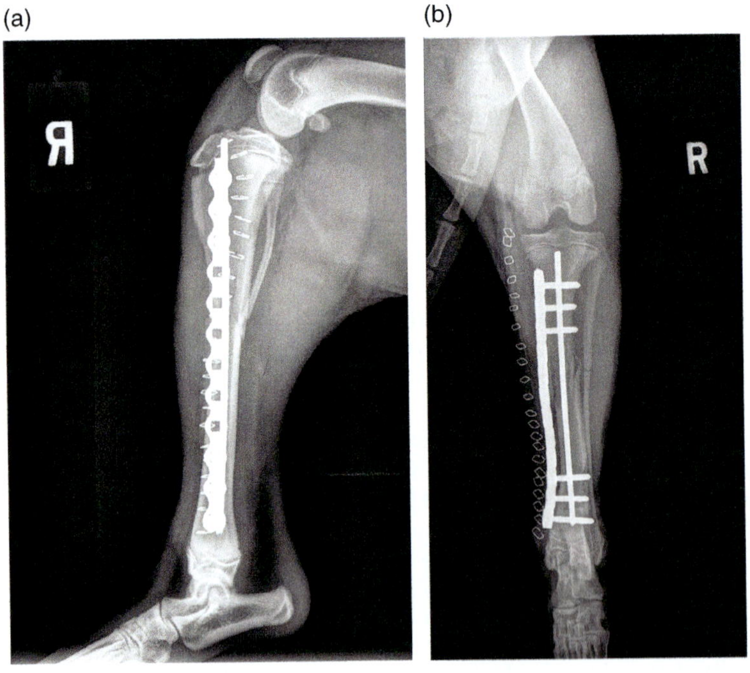

Figures 9.1 (a) and (b) Postoperative lateral and craniocaudal radiographic projection of a repaired tibia fracture.

TPLO plates, yet maintains over 400 N of stiffness. The plates are precontoured based on contouring performed during surgery during the design phase of the implant, with the average contoured shape used. They can be further contoured as needed.

In conclusion, the strength and flexibility afforded to the surgeon by liberty lock plates has proven to be very useful for the treatment of many different fracture types and anatomic locations in both dogs and cats, as well as for the correction of joint abnormalities.

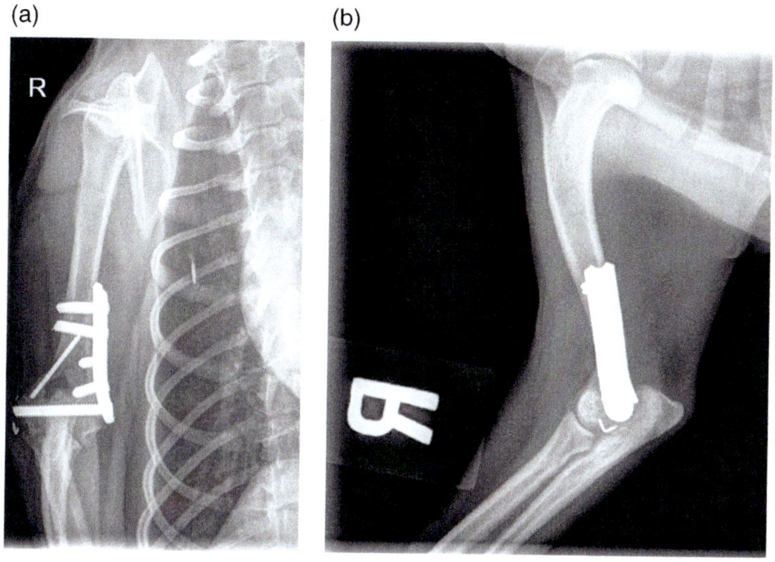

Figures 9.2 (a) and (b) Postoperative lateral and craniocaudal radiographic projection of a repaired humeral condylar fracture. (Source: Courtesy of Dr. Casey Havemann.)

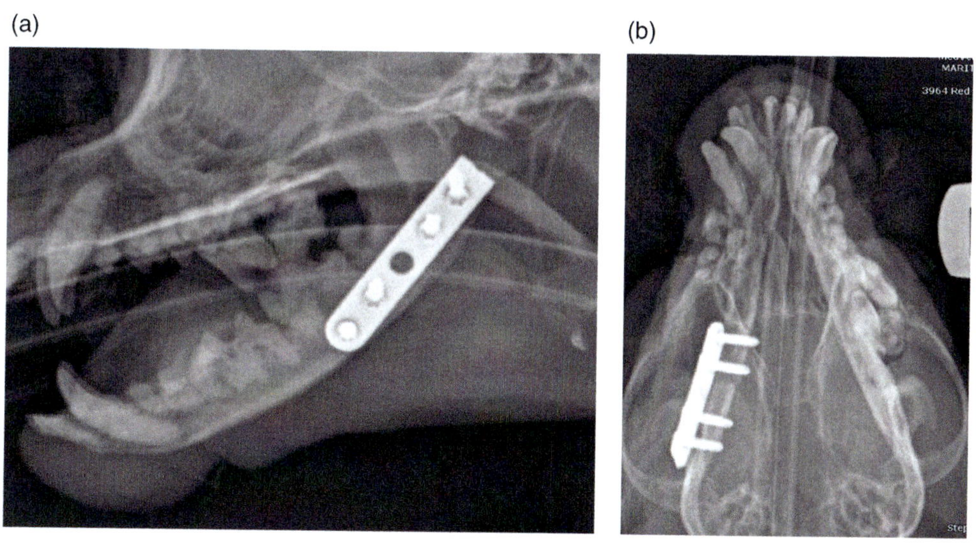

Figures 9.3 (a) and (b) Postoperative lateral and ventrodorsal radiographic projection of a repaired mandibular fracture.

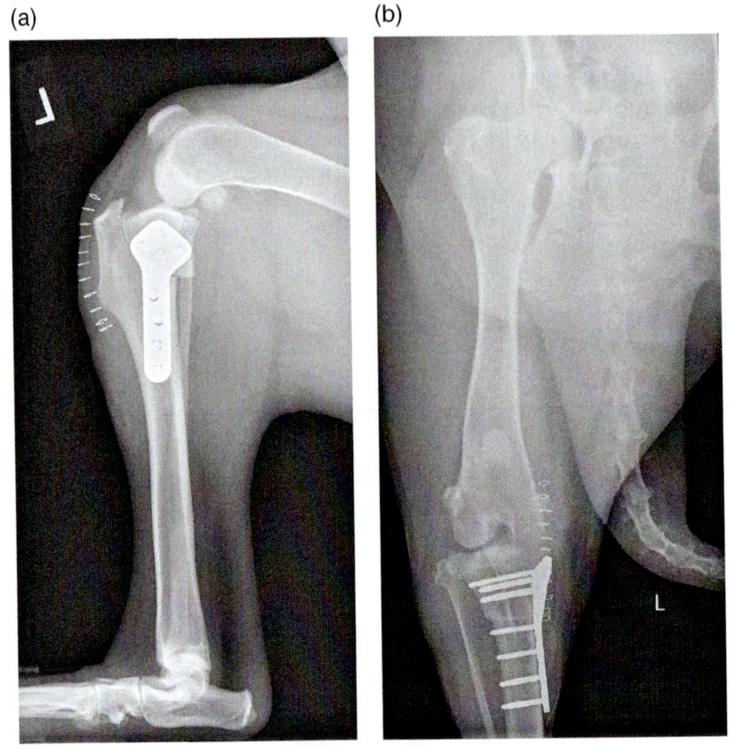

Figures 9.4 (a) and (b) Postoperative lateral and craniocaudal radiographic projection of a tibial plateau leveling osteotomy (TPLO). (Source: Courtesy of Dr. Casey Havemann.)

References

1. Bufkin, B.W., Barnhart, M.D., Kazanovicz, A.J. et al. (2013). The effect of screw angulation and insertion torque on the push-out strength of polyaxial locking screws and the single cycle to failure in bending of polyaxial locking plates. *Vet. Comp. Orthop. Traumatol.* 26 (3): 186–191.
2. Tomlinson, A.W., Comerford, E.J., Birch, R.S. et al. (2015). Mechanical performance in axial compression of a titanium polyaxial locking plate system in a fracture gap model. *Vet. Comp. Orthop. Traumatol.* 28 (2): 88–94. doi: 10.3415/VCOT-14-03-0046 Epub 2015 Feb 23.

10 The Polyaxial (PAX) Advanced Locking System

Matthew D. Barnhart

There are now many different locking plate systems available to veterinarians. While they differ from each other in a variety of ways, the majority have in common the fact that they are fixed-angle locking systems. Screwhead and plate threads are machined precisely such that the screws must be inserted into the plate at a predetermined angle in order to achieve a locked coupling. Failure of precise placement can result in compromised screw locking and/or cross threading between the plate hole and screwhead threads, causing incomplete insertion and challenging screw removal. The fixed angle also limits flexibility for screw placement when there is a need to avoid joints, fracture lines, and other implants. Additionally, some fracture locations (e.g. acetabulum) can be difficult to insert drill guides at 90° to the bone because of regional anatomic constraints. By contrast, only two multidirectional locking systems, which offer freedom from fixed-angle insertion requirements, have been reported in the veterinary literature [1, 2].

In 2009, the Polyaxial (PAX) Advanced Locking System was introduced into the veterinary market in order to provide the benefits of locking plate technology with a unique multidirectional angle stable (i.e. polyaxial) screw insertion option. The PAX screws are made of a titanium alloy that is approximately twice the hardness of the titanium PAX plate. Locking coupling is achieved by structural deformation of the vertical plate hole ridges by the sharp, cutting threads of the harder screwhead that occurs during tightening. PAX screws can be inserted multidirectionally up to 5° within the plate without a significant loss of push-out strength. At an insertion angle of 10° the push-out strength does decrease significantly; however, it is still higher than the pull-out strength of 3.5 mm cortical screws in bone [3] (Figure 10.1). While successful screw-plate coupling can still occur at insertion angles in excess of 10°, push-out strength progressively decreases. Using the PAX drill guide helps to prevent drilling at an excessive angle as it will fulcrum out of the plate hole if placed at an angle of greater than 15°.

Generating adequate torque is particularly important when inserting PAX screws in order to achieve complete coupling. The greater the depth of screwhead engagement, the more resistance to screw push-out is generated. A minimum insertion torque of 2.5 Nm has been recommended, with 3.5 Nm being ideal [3–5]. The author recommends using a large-handled

Locking Plates in Veterinary Orthopedics, First Edition.
Edited by Matthew D. Barnhart and Karl C. Maritato.

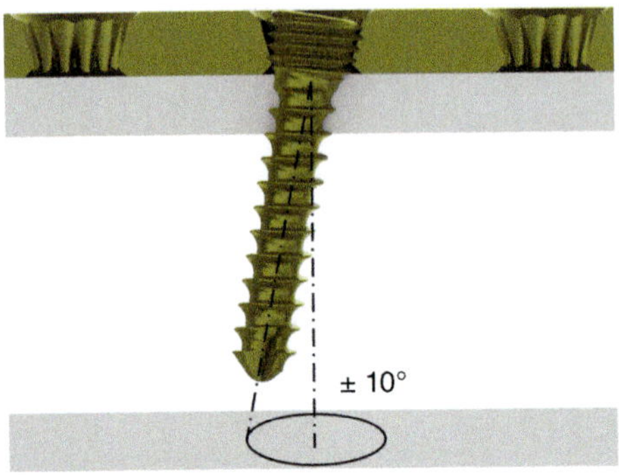

Figure 10.1 Illustration of multidirectional stability of polyaxial (PAX) screw within plate.

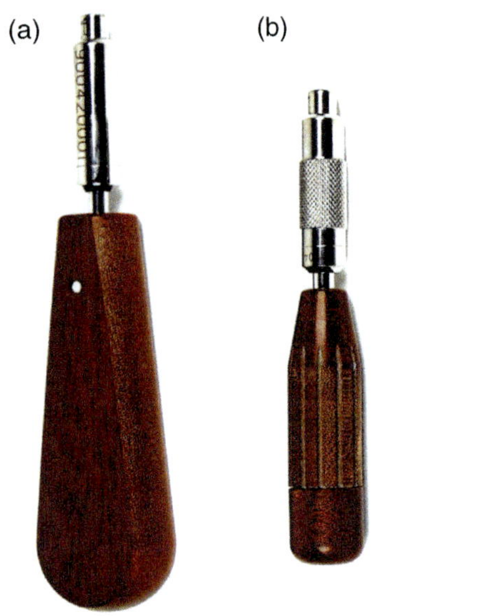

Figure 10.2 Example of a large-handled driver (a) compared to a palm-sized (b). The former should be used with the PAX system to help ensure adequate insertion torque is generated by hand.

driver for the 2.7 and 3.5 mm screws in order to maximize hand-generated torque and ensure adequate depth of insertion (Figure 10.2). Screwheads should appear flush to slightly countersunk within the plate when properly inserted. Fortunately, there's little danger of applying too much torque since the screwheads have the same ability to "cut" their way out as they do in (i.e. no cold welding).

The PAX trauma plates come in three types: reconstruction (RP), extension (EP), and limited-contact straight plates (SP) (Figure 10.3a and b).

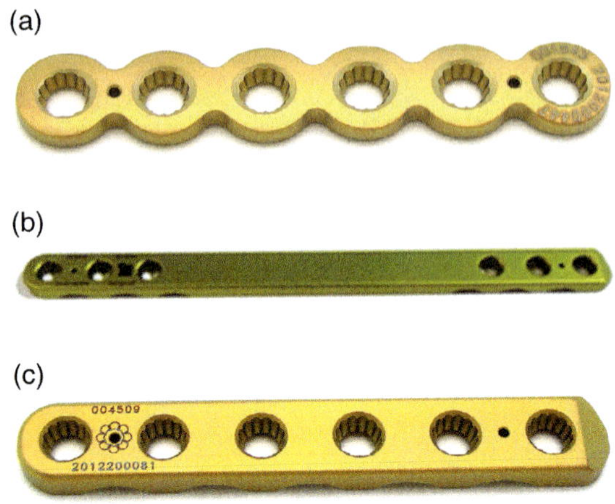

Figure 10.3 PAX trauma 3.5 mm reconstruction (a), extension (b), and limited contact straight (c) plates.

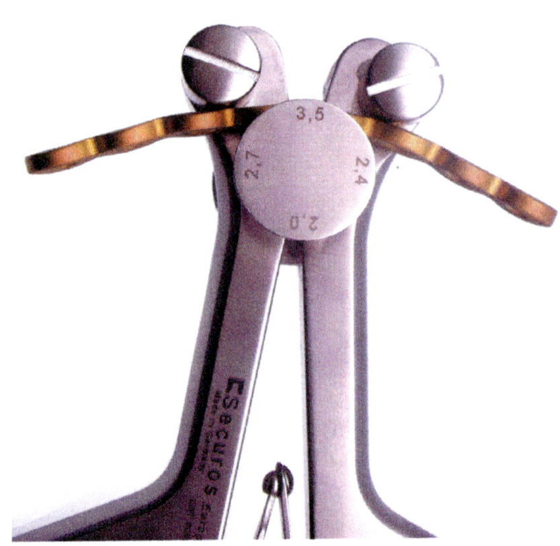

Figure 10.4 PAX plate benders are adjustable to all sizes of PAX plates and reconstruction-style plates can be contoured in all planes.

The RPs can be easily contoured in all planes with the use of specialized plate benders (Figure 10.4). All the plates have holes at both ends to accommodate a Kirschner wire (K-wire) if the surgeon desires to affix the plate to help maintain plate position and to prevent the *helicopter effect*, which can occur in locking plates when the first screw is tightened (0.035″ K-wire for 2.0/2.4 mm plates and 0.045″ K-wire for 2.7/3.5 mm plates). The author recommends against using RPs in a buttress fashion

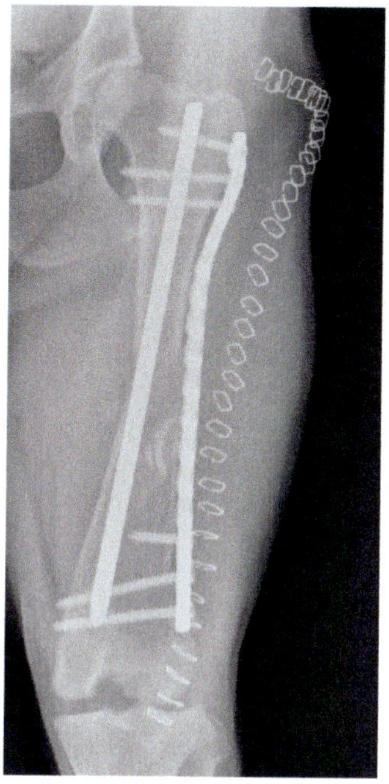

Figure 10.5 A highly comminuted fracture stabilized with a 3.5 mm polyaxial straight plate (PAX SP) and intramedullary pin. Note the multiple bicortical screw placement despite the relatively large IM pin size. This was possible because of the ability to angle the screws in multiple directions as need to avoid the pin.

in appendicular fractures unless combined with a stiff intramedullary implant. The SP and EPs are a stiffer design and can be used to bridge fracture gaps. The mechanical characteristics of the SP compare favorably with similarly sized dynamic compression plates (DCPs), locking compression plates and limited contact-DCPs [3, 6]. Additionally, the PAX screws are interchangeable between 2.0/2.4 and 2.7/3.5 mm systems (e.g. 2.7 mm screws can be used in 3.5 mm plates and vice versa, etc.), which could be advantageous when a stiffer plate is desired for a smaller diameter bone. Noteworthy is that the core diameters of the 2.0 and 2.4 mm PAX screws are slightly smaller than the cortical screw counterparts. The drill bits for the 2.0 and 2.4 mm PAX screws are 1.3 and 1.7 mm, respectively.

The utility of PAX system for the successful management of numerous fracture types and for the treatment of atlantoaxial luxations, using a specially designed butterfly plate, has been reported [1, 7] (Chapter 24). Additionally, the PAX locking design is offered in double pelvic osteotomy and tibial plateau leveling osteotomy plates.

Like other locking plate systems, PAX is highly amenable to plate/ rod constructs. However, the ability to angle locking screws away from intramedullary implants allows for more flexibility with bicortical screw placement and the use of large intramedullary implants if desired (Figure 10.5). A shared potential disadvantage with other the locking plate systems is the inability to achieve interfragmentary compression of simple transverse fractures with the PAX implants. PAX plates do accommodate cortical screws of similar size. Anecdotally, when such a screw is eccentrically placed within the plate hole, up to 0.5 mm of axial compression can occur during tightening by following the AO principles recommended for DCP placement. Additionally, the use of cortical screws will compress the plate to the bone in order to facilitate fracture reduction before locking screws are applied, if desired.

In conclusion, the PAX system has been found to be suitable for the treatment of a wide variety of veterinary orthopedic applications. The ability to angle screws provides additional options for screw placement adjacent to articular surfaces, fracture lines, or other implants. The author and numerous colleagues have taken advantage of the PAX multidirectional insertion capability and thoroughly appreciate the intraoperative flexibility it offers.

References

1. Barnhart, M.D., Rides, C.F., Kennedy, S.C. et al. (2013). Fracture repair using a polyaxial locking plate system (PAX). *Vet. Surg.* 42: 60–66.
2. Tomlinson, A.W., Comerford, E.J., Birch, R.S. et al. (2015). Mechanical performance in axial compression of a titanium polyaxial locking plate system in a fracture gap model. *Vet. Comp. Orthop. Traumatol.* 28: 88–94.
3. Bufkin, B.W., Barnhart, M.D., Kazanovicz, A.J. et al. (2013). The effect of screw angulation and insertion torque on the push-out strength of polyaxial locking screws and the single cycle to failure in bending of polyaxial locking plates. *Vet. Comp. Orthop. Traumatol.* 26: 186–191.
4. Boudreau, B., Benamou, J., von Pfeil, D. et al. (2013). Effect of screw insertion torque on mechanical properties of four locking systems. *Vet. Surg.* 42: 535–543.

5. Baroncelli, A.B., Reif, U., Bignardi, C. et al. (2013). Effect of screw insertion torque on push-out and cantilever bending properties of five different angle-stable systems. *Vet. Surg.* 42: 308–315.
6. Blake, C., Boudrieau, R., Torrance, B.S. et al. (2011). Single cycle to failure in bending of three standard and five locking plates and plate constructs. *Vet. Comp. Orthop. Traumatol.* 24: 408–417.
7. Dickomeit, M., Alves, L., Pekarkova, M. et al. (2011). Use of a 1.5 mm butterfly locking plate for stabilization of atlantoaxial pathology in three toy breed dogs. *Vet. Comp. Orthop. Traumatol.* 24 (3): 246–251.

11 The String of Pearls (SOP) System

Malcolm G. Ness

11.1 Introduction

The *string of pearls* (SOP) is a veterinary locking plate system developed specifically for veterinary use [1, 2]. Since its inception in 2006, SOP has been used in well over 100,000 clinical cases, thoroughly evaluated, and reported in many clinical research presentations and papers published internationally in the peer-reviewed veterinary literature. The system was designed by a small group of veterinary surgeons and engineers to address the problems and limitations they had encountered using first-generation locking systems.

11.2 Description of the System

The SOP system is manufactured in three sizes, 2.0, 2.7, and 3.5 mm (corresponding to the cortical bone screw size) and available in surgical stainless steel (316 LVM) or titanium alloy (Ti-6Al-4 V) [4].

The "plates" have a circular cross-section with a repeating pattern of cylindrical "internodes" and spheroid "pearls." Each pearl is threaded in the base to accept a standard cortical bone screw, with a proximal aperture just wide enough to accept the screw's head. The screw-head impinges within the pearl, producing an interference fit – a secondary lock between the plate and screw (Figure 11.1).

Size-specific bending irons are used. The "bending end" imparts four-point bending and a "twisting end" twists the plate evenly along the length of the internode [2–4].

Specific drill guides position the drilled hole central and perpendicular to the pearl. Finally, small, reusable screw-like "bending tees" placed into each pearl preserve the locking function despite contouring.

11.3 Design Features of the SOP Locking Plate System

Specific design features of the SOP system include the following:

1. The SOP is slightly stiffer and stronger than the corresponding standard 2.0, 2.7, and 3.5 self-compressing plates [1].
2. The design of the four-point bending irons minimizes the inevitable weakening that

Locking Plates in Veterinary Orthopedics, First Edition.
Edited by Matthew D. Barnhart and Karl C. Maritato.

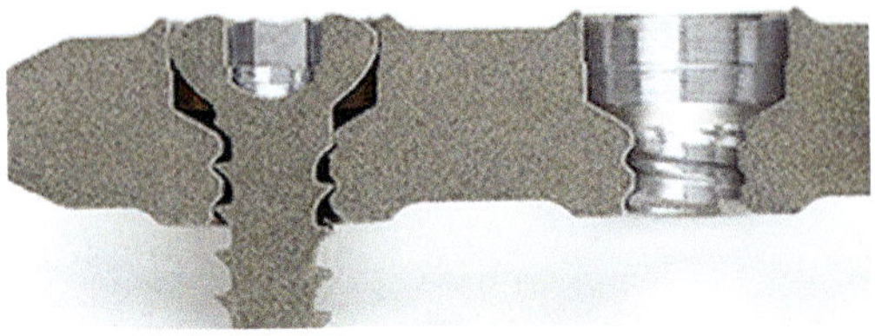

Figure 11.1 Cut-away section of a 3.5 string of pearls (SOP) plate, with screw in situ. The base is threaded to accept a standard cortical bone screw and the inner surface of the pearl features a small ridge – the aperture reduces from 6.00 to 5.85 mm diameter – against which the 6.00 mm screwhead will impinge and lock.

follows the bending or twisting of any metallic implant [2, 4].

3. The SOP plate's circular cross-section facilitates complex contouring of the implant [5, 6].
4. The locking function is preserved without compromise following bending and/or twisting of the plate.
5. There is a secure double-locking mechanism – a conventional "thread-in-thread" feature and a second interference fit between screwhead and pearl.
6. Screw holes are not weak points – empty screw holes can be left over a fracture or elsewhere, according exclusively to clinical need [7].
7. SOP has a relatively consistent stiffness profile, which mitigates damaging stress concentration under bending loads and optimizes the biomechanical environment at the fracture site [8].
8. The plates can be cut to any length and without compromising locking function using only the bending irons.
9. The SOP system utilizes standard cortical bone screws.

11.4 Perceived Limitations/Controversies

11.4.1 Screws Cannot Be Angled through the SOP Plate

While the design of the SOP precludes the use of angled screws, the SOP plate is easily and precisely contoured, allowing screws to be effectively directed into underlying bone without compromise (Figures 11.2 and 11.3).

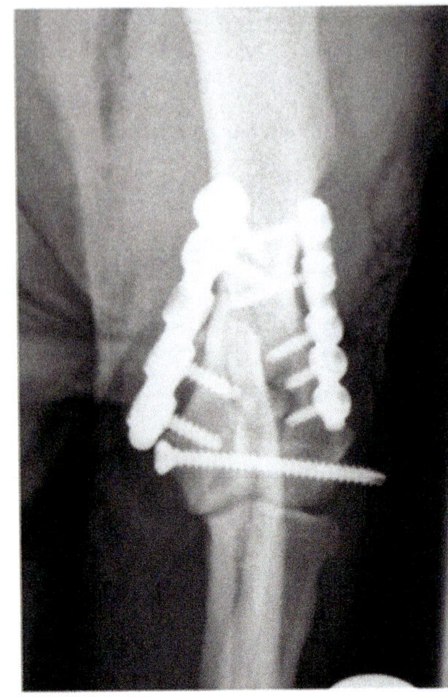

Figure 11.2 Cranio-caudal radiographs of a Y-T fracture of the distal humerus of a 36 kg Labrador retriever fixed with two string of pearls (SOP) plates (one 3.5 and one 2.7) and 11 screws.

11.4.2 Conventional Bone Screws Have Inadequately Thin Cores

Inevitably, locked screws will be exposed to cyclic loading and may fail by metal fatigue. Increasing the core diameter of a screw will increase its fatigue life, but this observation applies only to a single isolated locked screw – a situation that should not be encountered in clinical applications. SOP guidelines require three screws in each major fragment such that they *load-share,* and cumulatively protect one another from damaging bending loads.

11.4.3 You Can't Compress the Fracture with SOP

This is a deliberate design feature. Locked plate systems act as "buttress" fixation – angle-stable implants that transmit load <u>*past*</u> the fracture – and in that scenario, load sharing through

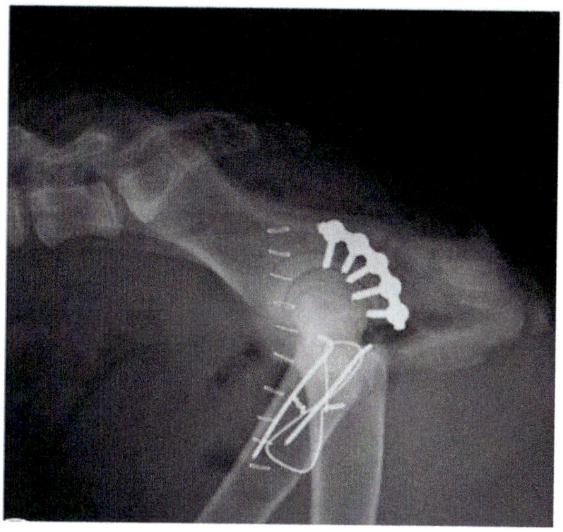

Figure 11.3 Lateral radiograph of an acetabular fracture in a 48 kg cross breed fixed with a single 2.7 string of pearls (SOP) and five screws. (Source: Courtesy of Prof. Karl Kraus.)

interfragmentary compression is irrelevant. Furthermore, the inevitable viscoelastic relaxation, dieback, and then remodeling of living bone after surgery impair the functionality of nonlocked screws, leaving any locked screws mechanically exposed.

11.4.4 The SOP Has a High Profile

The 3.5 SOP plate with screws is "taller," but narrower, than a comparable standard self-compressing plate and screws. However, even in locations with minimal soft tissue coverage, this is rarely more than a minor cosmetic issue.

11.5 Range of Clinical Application

The SOP system has been used on more than 100,000 patients treating a wide variety of orthopedic conditions, including diaphyseal fractures of the femur, humerus, antebrachium, and tibia/fibula [9, 10, 11] (Figures 11.2 and 11.4); metaphyseal fractures, notably the Y-T fracture of the distal humerus [6] (Figure 11.2); and fractures of the maxilla or mandible and pelvic fractures – both iliac and acetabular injuries (Figure 11.3). SOP has proved effective in arthrodesis, notably of the shoulder [5] but also the stifle, elbow, and hock, and it is frequently used in revision fracture surgery or to resolve complications following joint replacement [10]. Spinal applications include fracture repairs, distraction-fusion, and stabilizations [7, 12] (Figure 11.5). Finally, specially developed SOP implants have been widely used in triple pelvic osteotomy (TPO) and tibial plateau leveling osteotomy (TPLO) surgery.

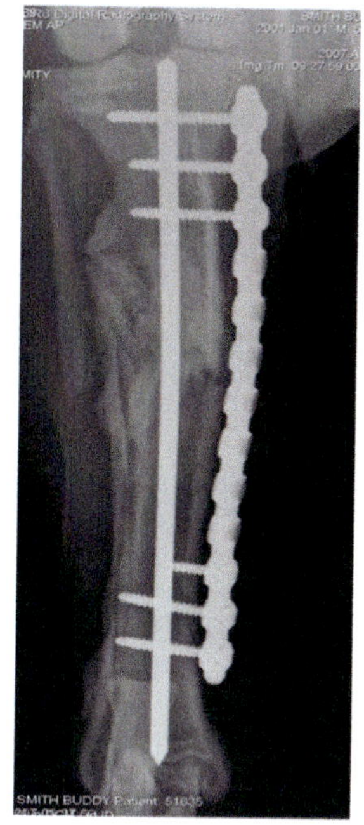

Figure 11.4 Seven weeks follow-up cranio-caudal radiographs of a comminuted fracture of the tibia and fibula fixed using the string of pearls (SOP)-rod technique. (Source: Courtesy of Dr. Brian Beale.)

11.6 Clinical Guidelines

While participation in a dedicated SOP course and workshop is considered an essential prerequisite, the clinical guidelines for SOP application are summarized below:

1. **Diaphyseal fractures of the major long bones, femur, humerus, tibia/fibula**. SOP-rod technique: select and insert an intramedullary pin with a diameter similar to the internode of the chosen SOP. Fix the SOP using three adjacent screws in the proximal major fragment and three screws in the

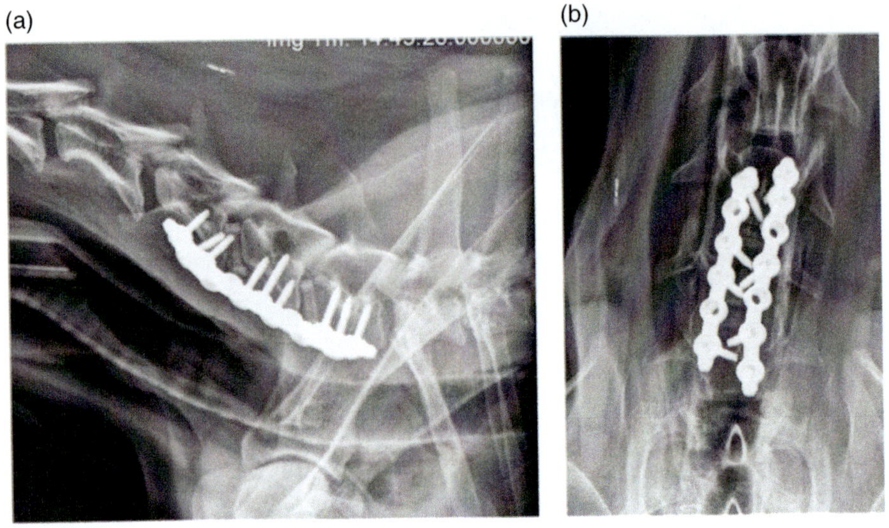

Figures 11.5 (a) and (b) Lateral and ventro-dorsal radiographs of a two-space (C5–6 and C 6–7) distraction-fusion surgery fixed with two, 2.7 string of pearls (SOP) plates and nine screws. (Source: Courtesy of Dr. Peter Earley.)

distal major fragment, leaving at least three empty screw holes centrally. Make no attempt to reconstruct or fix any comminutions. Mono-cortical screws are acceptable, though at least one bi-cortical screw in each of the proximal and distal fragments is preferred [13–15] (Figure 11.4). For antebrachial fractures, the rod is placed in ulna and the SOP on the radius.

2. **Metaphyseal fractures.** Use two SOP plates with a total of four screws proximal to the fracture and four screws distal to the fracture. Mono-cortical screws are acceptable. The plates may both be the same size or of different sizes, as clinical needs dictate (Figure 11.2).
3. **Spinal fracture or distraction-fusion**. Use SOP in pairs to ensure a stiff, robust repair. Use the longest screws that the clinical/anatomical situation will permit and aim to have a total of three screws in each vertebral body. The SOP can be "stood-off" the bone to avoid and preserve essential neurovascular anatomy (Figure 11.5).

11.7 Conclusions

SOP is a novel locking plate system designed specifically for veterinary use. Locking plate mechanics and biomechanics in general, and those of SOP in particular, are not obvious, and extrapolation of knowledge relevant to standard self-compressing plates is inappropriate and potentially problematic. Blake et al. [16], writing about locking plate systems in veterinary orthopedics, referred to "these diverse implant systems" and noted "identical approaches to fracture management cannot be applied."

In relation to SOP, the necessary system-specific techniques are easily assimilated, allowing surgeons to use the system effectively on a remarkably wide and disparate range of orthopedic and spinal cases.

References

1. DeTora, M. and Kraus, K. (2008). Mechanical testing of 3.5 mm locking and non-locking bone plates. *Vet. Comp. Orthop. Traumatol.* 21 (4): 318–322.
2. Ness, M.G. (2009). The effect of bending and twisting on the stiffness and strength of the 3.5 SOP implant. *Vet. Comp. Orthop. Traumatol.* 22 (2): 132–136.
3. MacLeod, A.R., Simpson, A.H., and Pankaj, P. (2016 Nov). Age-related optimization of screw placement for reduced loosening risk in locked plating. *J. Orthop. Res.* 34 (11): 1856–1864. doi: 10.1002/jor.23193 Epub 2016 Oct 14.
4. Rutherford, S. and Ness, M.G. (2012). Effect of contouring on bending structural stiffness and

bending strength of the 3.5 titanium SOP implant. *Vet. Surg.* 41 (8): 983–987.
5. Fitzpatrick, N., Yeadon, R., Smith, T.J. et al. (2012). Shoulder arthrodesis in 14 dogs. *Vet. Surg.* 41 (6): 745–754.
6. Ness, M.G. (2009). Repair of Y-T humeral fractures in the dog using paired "String of Pearls" locking plates. *Vet. Comp. Orthop. Traumatol.* 22 (6): 492–497.
7. McKee, W.M. and Downes, C.J. (2008). Vertebral stabilisation and selective decompression for the management of triple thoracolumbar disc protrusions. *J. Small Anim. Pract.* 49 (10): 536–539.
8. Goodship, A.E., Cunningham, J.L., and Kenwright, J. (1998). Strain rate and timing of stimulation in mechanical modulation of fracture healing. *Clin. Orthop. Relat. Res.* 355 (Suppl): S105–S115.
9. Hespel, A.M., Bernard, F., Davies, N.J. et al. (2013). Surgical repair of a tibial fracture in a two-week-old grey seal (Halichoerus grypus). *Vet. Comp. Orthop. Traumatol.* 26 (1): 82–87.
10. Fitzpatrick, N., Nikolaou, C., Yeadon, R. et al. (2012). String-of-pearls locking plate and cerclage wire stabilization of periprosthetic femoral fractures after total hip replacement in six dogs. *Vet. Surg.* 41 (1): 180–188.
11. Kim, S.E. and Lewis, D.D. (2014). Corrective osteotomy for procurvatum deformity caused by distal femoral physeal fracture malunion stabilised with string-of-pearls locking plates: results in two dogs and a review of the literature. *Aust. Vet. J.* 92 (3): 75–80.
12. Early, P., Mente, P., Dillard, S. et al. (2015). In vitro biomechanical evaluation of internal fixation techniques on the canine lumbosacral junction. *PeerJ* 3: e1094.
13. Rutherford, S., Demianiuk, R.M., Benamou, J. et al. (2015). Effect of intramedullary rod diameter on a string of pearls plate-rod construct in mediolateral bending: an in vitro mechanical study. *Vet. Surg.* 44 (6): 737–743.
14. Benamou, J., Demianiuk, R.M., Rutherford, S. et al. (2015). Effect of bending direction on the mechanical behaviour of 3.5 mm string-of-pearls and limited contact dynamic compression plate constructs. *Vet. Comp. Orthop. Traumatol.* 28 (6): 433–440.
15. Demianiuk, R.M., Benamou, J., Rutherford, S. et al. (2015). Effect of screw type and distribution on the torsional stability of 3.5 mm string of pearls locking plate constructs. *Vet. Surg.* 44 (1): 119–125.
16. Blake, C.A., Boudrieau, R.J., Torrance, B.S. et al. (2011). Single cycle to failure in bending of three standard and five locking plates and plate constructs. *Vet. Comp. Orthop. Traumatol.* 24 (6): 408–417. doi: 10.3415/VCOT-11-04-0061 Epub 2011 Sep 21.

12 The Synthes Locking Compression Plate (LCP) System

Jessica A. Dahlberg and Kenneth A. Bruecker

The Synthes Locking Compression Plate (LCP) with its patented combination plate holes (*combi-holes*) that accommodate conventional or locking screws was released in 2001 [1, Chapter 2]. Cortical or cancellous screws can be inserted in the dynamic compression unit (DCU) of the combi-hole to provide axial compression. The other half of the combi-hole is threaded and conical to accept a locking screw, allowing for fixed-angle stability. As such, an LCP can be applied in two manners: as a compression plate or as a bridging "internal fixator" plate.

The strength of the locking fixation depends less on the integrity of the bone than on fixations using conventional compression plates. Locking plates allow rigid fixation of comminuted fractures using biological fixation and are ideal for fractures in weak bone. Furthermore, locking plates are the ultimate implant for minimally invasive plate osteosynthesis (MIPO).

The locking drill guide threads into the threaded portion of the combi-hole in the plate in a fixed direction (uniaxial) for an angle-stable construct (Figure 12.1). The threads of the locking screw are smaller than cortical screws, as they do not have to create compression between the bone and the plate. Locking screws also have a larger core diameter than conventional screws, allowing them to be stronger in bending and shear forces. The thread leads on the shaft and the head of the locking screw are 1 mm. The pitch on the threads in the head is 0.5 mm, or two threads per 1 mm of space, also known as a *2-start thread*. In a 2-start thread, there are two sets of threads 180° apart. During screw insertion, the shaft and head spin at the same rate but the threads in the head travel twice the distance. If the screwhead threads come in contact with the plate threads and become 90° out of phase, a height/distance of 0.25 mm is created. The plate/screw/bone will adjust to allow the screwhead to properly thread into the plate without stripping the threads into the bone. The leading screwhead thread will tend to compress the plate against the bone until the threads come into phase. When the threads mate together, the plate will release some of the built-up compression. Per the manufacturer, the Synthes stardrive screwhead design is 65% stronger in insertional torque than conventional hexagonal screwhead design (Synthes publication #036.001.395). Locking screws offer less risk of screw loosening than do conventional screws.

Locking Plates in Veterinary Orthopedics, First Edition.
Edited by Matthew D. Barnhart and Karl C. Maritato.

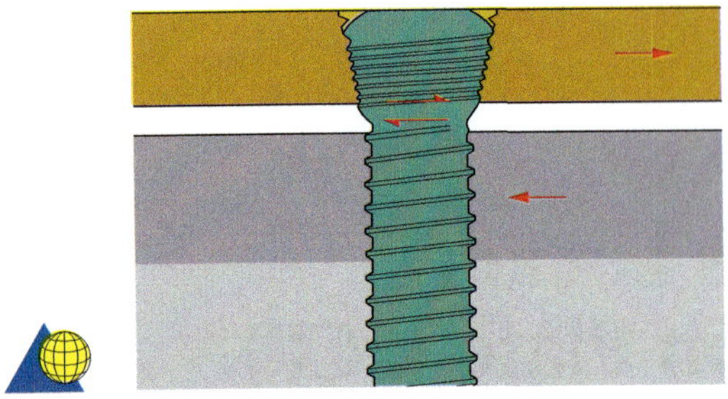

Figure 12.1 Synthes locking compression plate. (Source: Courtesy of AO foundation.)

12.1 Other Locking Compression Plate Manufacturers

Since its debut several years ago, many manufacturers have utilized the Synthes plate and screw design. However, most did not duplicate the 2-start thread design. In 2004, New Generation Devices introduced a similar locking plate design with combination holes with 2-start thread screwheads (Figure 12.2). The screw holes and heads are not conical, but the screwhead has a collar that prevents overinsertion (Figure 12.2).

12.2 Applications of Implants

If using both locking and nonlocking screws in a plate, the surgeon has options depending on need.

Locking exclusive application (Figure 12.3a):
Using only locking screws provides a buttress effect and produces no additional compression across a fracture or osteotomy. Reduction of fragments using lag screws may be performed before application of the plate, if so desired for the intended repair. Monocortical locking screws may be used in the plate because of the angle-stable construct, without danger of toggling occurrence as with nonlocking screws.

If using the plate as an internal fixator, precise contouring of the Synthes LCP is not required. However, contouring may be performed using bending instruments placed between holes to avoid large gaps beneath the plate. In a study of 4.5 mm LCP constructs, no loss of stability was noted with a 2 mm gap below the plate [2]. However, a 5.0 mm gap between the plate and bone did result in some compromise to stability. The plate holes allow a small degree of deformation. However, as the locking holes accept locking screws perpendicular to the plate, it is important not to

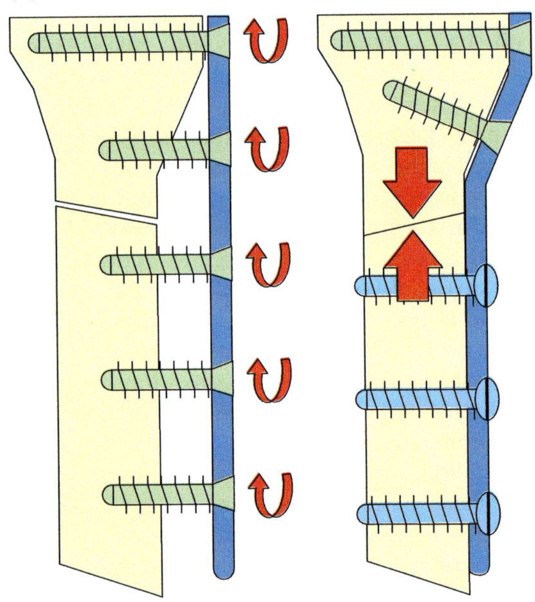

Figure 12.3 AO plate applications. Locking only (3a). Combination locking and compression (3b). (Source: Courtesy of AO foundation.)

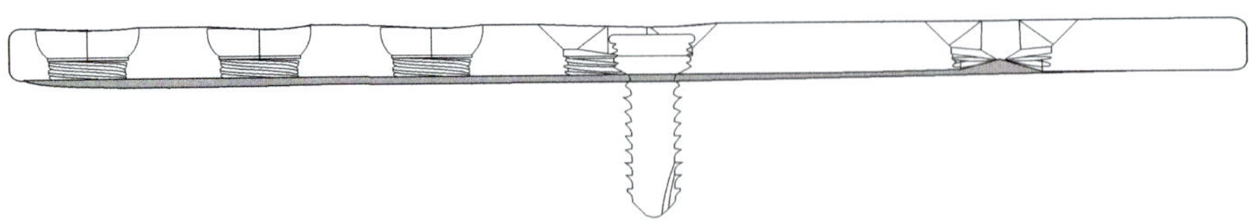

Figure 12.2 New Generation Devices locking plate. (Source: Courtesy of New Generation Devices.)

deform this portion of the combi-hole, as distortion will lessen locking effectiveness.

Plates may be secured to the bone using several techniques. The plate can be lightly secured with bone-holding forceps or temporary cortical bone screw. Additionally, a Synthes push-pull reduction sleeve or threaded plate holder may also be implemented. These instruments temporarily hold the plate to the bone through the plate hole. The push-pull device has a Synthes quick connection for power insertion within the cis-cortex only.

Locking screws (self-tapping) require utilization of a Synthes drill bit and threaded drill guides. The drill guides must be removed before using the depth gauge. Drill bit sizes for specific locking head screws are shown in Table 12.1.

Screws are tightened with the Synthes stardrive screwdriver. A Synthes torque-limiting attachment (1.5 Nm) should be used when using power. Screwheads should be checked to ensure that they are flush with the LCP. Cross-threaded locking heads will not fully seat into the plate, resulting in compromised stability.

Hybrid application (Figure 12.3b): Internal fixation with Synthes LCP can be achieved using a combination of locking and standard screws (us.synthesvet.com). If using an LCP to compress across a fracture or osteotomy, one option is to apply all locking screws to one segment first to secure that segment, then place a nonlocking (cortical or cancellous) screw in the other segment in DCU fashion. The remaining locking or nonlocking screws can then be placed. When using locking and nonlocking screws in the same segment, the nonlocking screws must be placed first, which will secure the plate to the bone. If the locking screw is placed first, it would fix the plate away from the bone and not allow the cortical screw to compress the plate down to the bone, resulting in a loss of stability. Improper screw placement order may result in rotational malalignment.

Table 12.1 Synthes drill bit and screw sizes.

Drill bit(mm)	Screw (mm)
1.5	2
1.8	2.4
2	2.7
2.8	3.5

12.3 Tips for Implant Removal

Unlock all screws in the plate by hand before removing any one screw. This prevents screw-head stripping and rotation of the plate on the bone while removing the last screws.

12.4 Locking Compression Plate Indications

FEMUR (Figure 12.4): This illustrates a three-year-old spayed female Rhodesian Ridgeback with a highly comminuted midshaft femoral fracture.

Procedure: Lateral Approach to Femur with minimal handling of comminuted fragments. A 1/8″ IM pin (approximately 40% of the medullary cavity diameter) was inserted in a normograde fashion). An eight-hole 3.5 mm LCP (Synthes) was placed on the lateral cortex with monocortical and bicortical locking screws.

RADIUS (Figure 12.5): Two-year-old, 4.8 kg intact male Terrier with short oblique distal diaphyseal radius and ulna fractures.

Procedure: Dorsomedial approach to radial diaphysis. Extensor mm retracted to expose diaphysis. Fracture reduced and seven-hole LCP with nonlocking and locking screws in a compression fashion.

HUMERUS (Figure 12.6): Three-year-old, 25.1 kg intact female Labrador with a reducible mid-diaphyseal humeral fracture with fissure fracture in distal segment.

Procedure: Medial approach to humerus. Three cerclage wires were placed around distal fissured segment. The fracture was reduced and stabilized with a plate-rod construct using an IM pin and an eight-hole 3.5 mm Synthes LCP in neutralization fashion on the medial aspect of the bone.

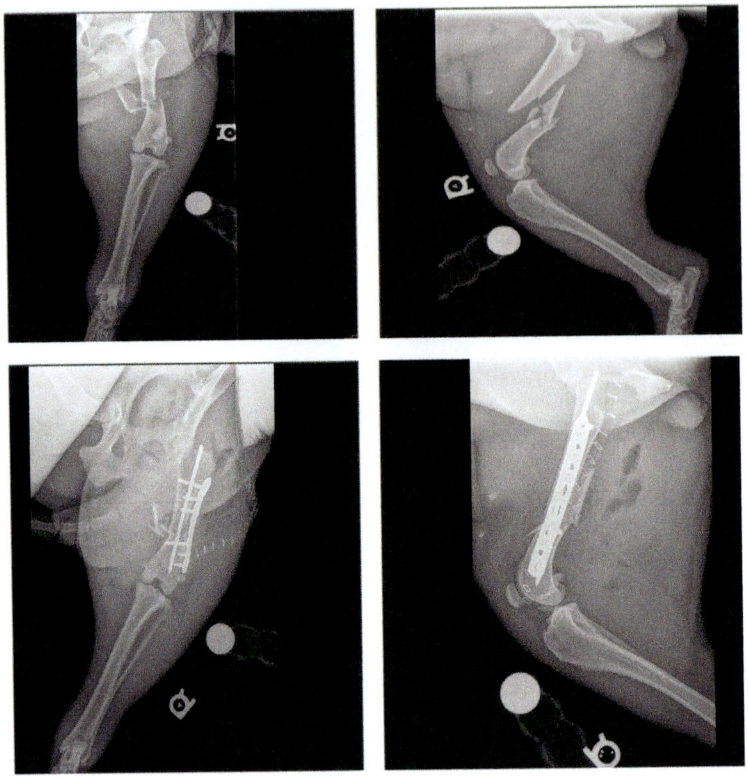

Figure 12.4 A three-year-old SF Rhodesian Ridgeback. Pre- and postoperative radiographs of a highly comminuted midshaft femoral fracture.

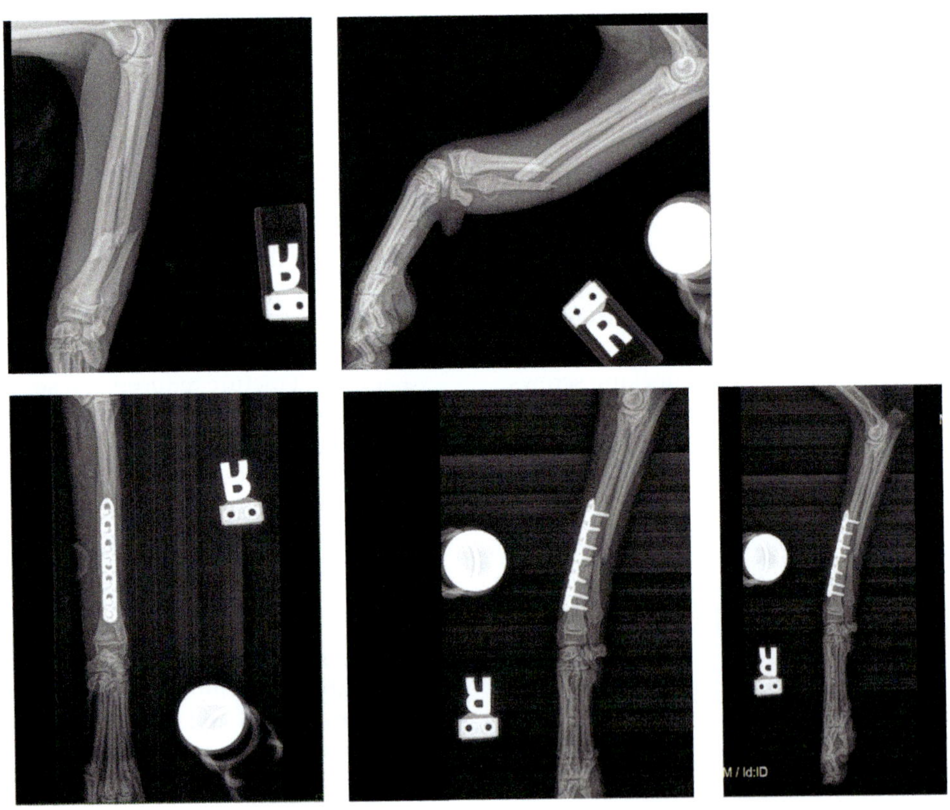

Figure 12.5 Two-year-old M Terrier 4.8 kg. Pre-, immediate post-, and three-week postoperative radiographs of a short oblique distal diaphyseal radius and ulna fractures.

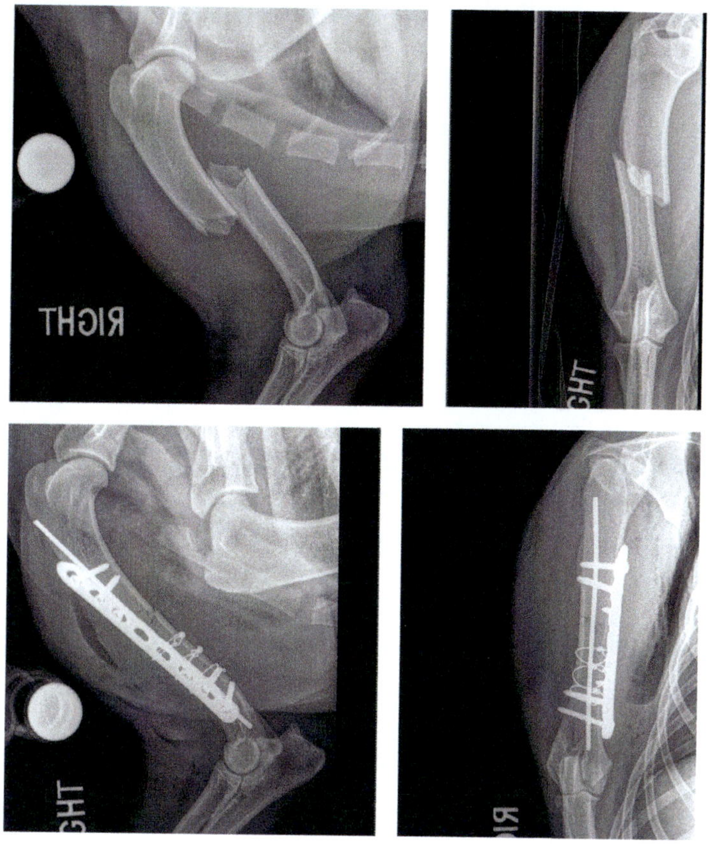

Figure 12.6 Three-year-old female Labrador 25.1 kg. Pre- and postoperative radiographs of a reducible mid-diaphyseal humeral fracture with fissure fracture in distal segment.

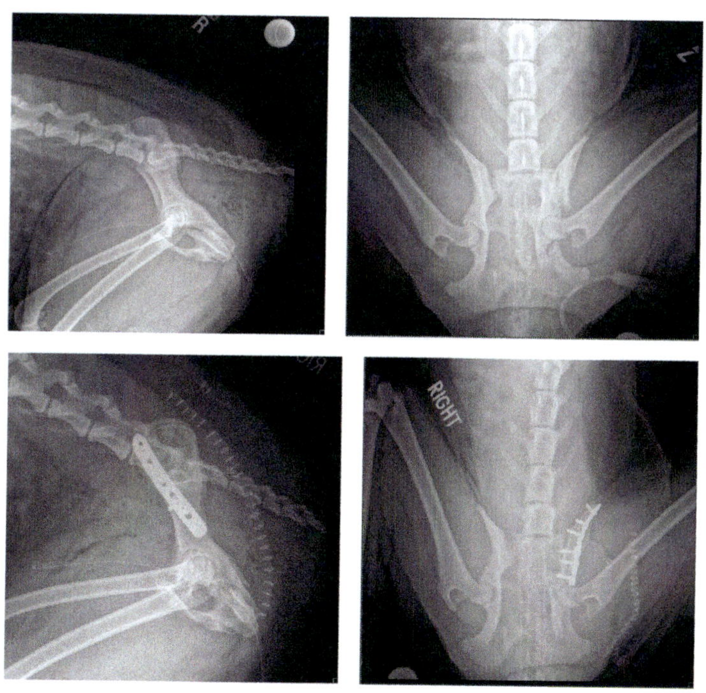

Figure 12.7 3 yo SF Rhodesian Ridgeback cross 26.7 kg. Pre- and postoperative radiographs of a midbody - oblique fracture of left ilium.

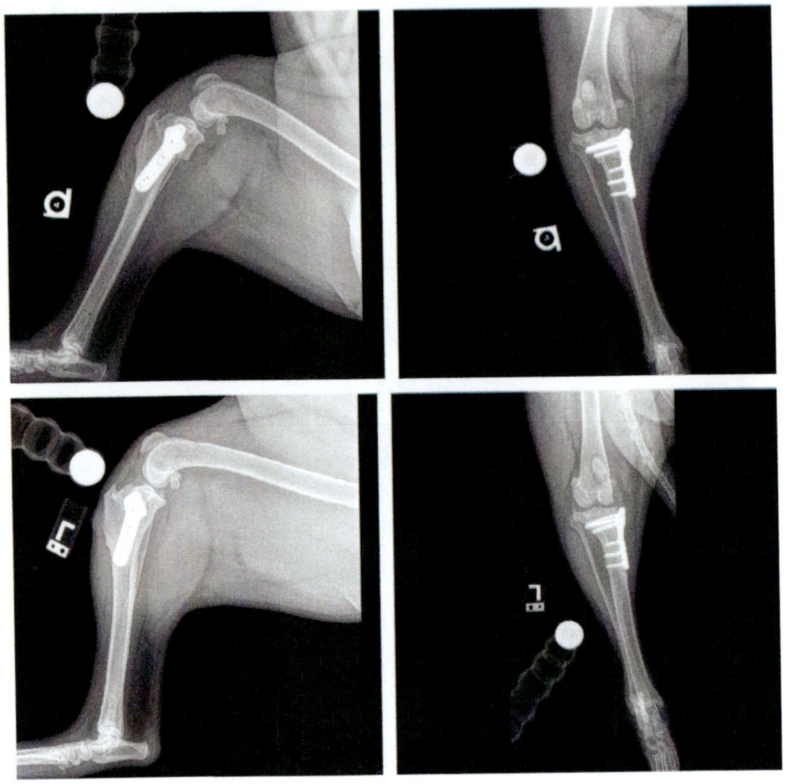

Figure 12.8 Two-year-old CM GSD 43.1 kg. One-month and 11-month postoperative radiographs.

ILIUM (Figure 12.7): Three-year-old, 26.7 kg spayed female Rhodesian Ridgeback cross with a midbody oblique fracture of left ilium.

Procedure: Dorsolateral approach. Six-hole 3.5 mm LCP applied across fracture and stabilized with two cortical and four 3.5 mm locking screws.

TPLO (Figure 12.8): Two-year-old, 43.1 kg castrated male German Shepherd Dog with a left rupture of the cranial cruciate ligament.

Procedure: Synthes LCP tibial plateau leveling osteotomy (TPLO) plates are placed in a Hybrid fashion to compress across the osteotomy. Screw sites four and six hold cortical screws. The other four holes are combi-holes and can accommodate either cortical or locking screws.

References

1. Johnson, A.L., Houlton, J.E.F., and Vannini, R. (2005). *AO Principles of Fracture Management in the Dog and Cat*. AO Publishing.
2. Ahmad, M., Nanda, R., Bajwa, A.S. et al. (2007). Biomechanical testing of the locking compression plate: when does the difference between bone and implant significantly reduce construct stability? *Injury, Int. J. Care Injured* 38: 358–364.

Section IV

Trauma Applications: Clinical Case Examples

IV-A Appendicular Skeletal Fractures

13 Humerus Fractures

David R. Mason

13.1 Introduction

Humerus fractures account for approximately 10% of all long bone fractures in dogs and cats [1–3], most of which occur secondary to trauma. Some fracture configurations are predictable based on the age of the patient, such as condylar fractures in young animals with open physes. The majority of fractures tend to involve the middle and distal thirds of the humerus [1].

13.2 Anatomy

The humerus has unique features that make it a challenging bone to approach and repair, in part due to its proximal location with a large surrounding muscle mass. Accurate knowledge of the relevant anatomy is essential for successful reduction of fracture fragments and application of a fixation apparatus (Figure 13.1). Differences in anatomy between dogs and cats can dictate the choice of fracture repair technique, along with the actual position of the chosen implants. Specific factors that are relatively unique to the humerus are the S-shaped nature with a twist moving distally. There are ridges proximally and distally, which make accurate plate contouring especially challenging. The radial nerve is located on the distolateral aspect, with the canine median and ulnar nerves being located on the medial aspect. The feline humerus differs in three ways. First, there is a supracondylar foramen; second, the median nerve and a branch of the brachial artery pass through the supracondylar foramen; and third, the communication between the olecranon fossa caudally and the radial fossa cranially is interrupted by bone across the supratrochlear foramen.

Supracondylar humeral fractures can be especially challenging due to the complex anatomy of the distal humerus. There are several important factors, the most notable being the presence of the supratrochlear foramen in the dog; a thin lateral epicondylar ridge; irregular surfaces of the metaphysis; and finally, the proximity to the elbow joint [4]. These factors in combination lead to challenging surgical repairs and a very small area for safe and effective implant placement.

13.3 Surgical Approach

It is possible to approach the humerus from lateral, cranial, and medial surfaces. The approaches are challenging because of the

Locking Plates in Veterinary Orthopedics, First Edition.
Edited by Matthew D. Barnhart and Karl C. Maritato.

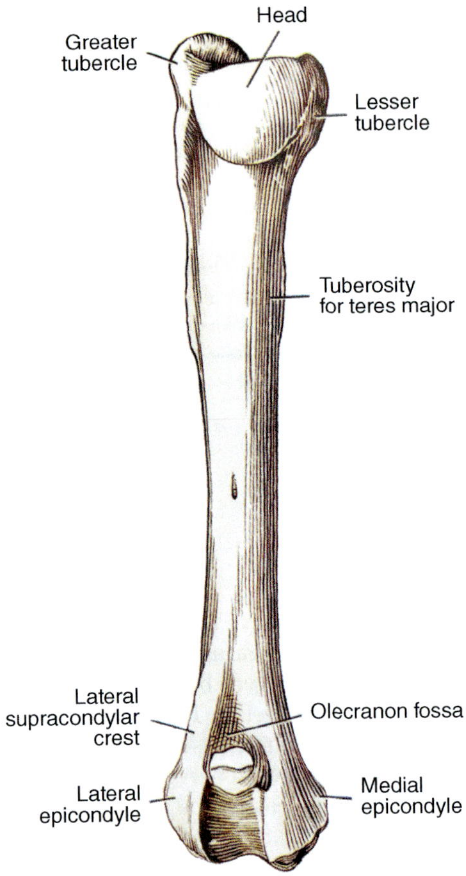

Figure 13.1 Normal anatomy of the humerus. (Source: *The Guide to the Dissection of the Dog,* 5th edition. Evans and deLahunta W·B Saunders Company. Page 11.)

plethora of neurovascular structures that can be encountered during dissection, along with the significant muscle bellies [5].

It is the opinion of the author that diaphyseal fractures are generally best approached from the medial aspect, with the exception of proximal fractures, which may be more accessible through a lateral approach. Medially, the humeral diaphysis is relatively straight and flat and the medial epicondylar crest is less pronounced than that of the lateral epicondyle. These features permit less plate contouring and thus a simpler application of a plate on the medial surface; particularly given that locking plates need not fit perfectly to the shape of the bone [1].

Medial approaches to the feline humerus are advantageous for visualization and protection of the median nerve and the brachial artery within the supracondylar foramen [1, 6]. (See Figure 13.2). This medial approach in itself is relatively straightforward. Depending on the patient and injury factors, it might require cutting of the pectoral muscle origins proximally, reflecting the biceps brachii muscle caudally and the brachiocephalicus muscle cranially. It is the author's experience that the overall soft tissue trauma and subsequent morbidity is significantly less when utilizing this particular approach. It is imperative to identify and protect the median and ulnar nerves along with the brachial vessels when performing a surgical approach to the medial aspect of the humerus in both species.

13.4 Biomechanics

There are limited clinical studies describing the biomechanics of the humerus; however, there are a few recent studies regarding locking plate (LP) technology used in this location. Short monocortical screws, 50% transcortical screws, and bicortical screws were compared in different regions of the humerus. The use of short monocortical screws was shown to contribute to failure of LP fixation of humeral fractures, especially when placed in the condyle. In fact, a linear relationship was noted between screw length and axial pullout strength. Thus the authors suggested that when bicortical screw placement is not possible, maximizing monocortical screw length might optimize fixation stability for distal humeral fractures [7]. A canine cadaveric humeral supracondylar fracture model was used to compare unilateral string of pearls (SOP) plating with bicortical screws versus bilateral plating with monocortical screws. The unilateral constructs had significantly lower stiffness in torsion and axial compression, and a significantly higher ultimate strength than bilateral constructs. All of the unilateral constructs failed by bending of the transcondylar screw and SOP plate. All bilateral constructs failed by axial pullout of the distal most screws. The incorporation of a transcondylar screw through the medial plate was found to be beneficial to construct strength [8].

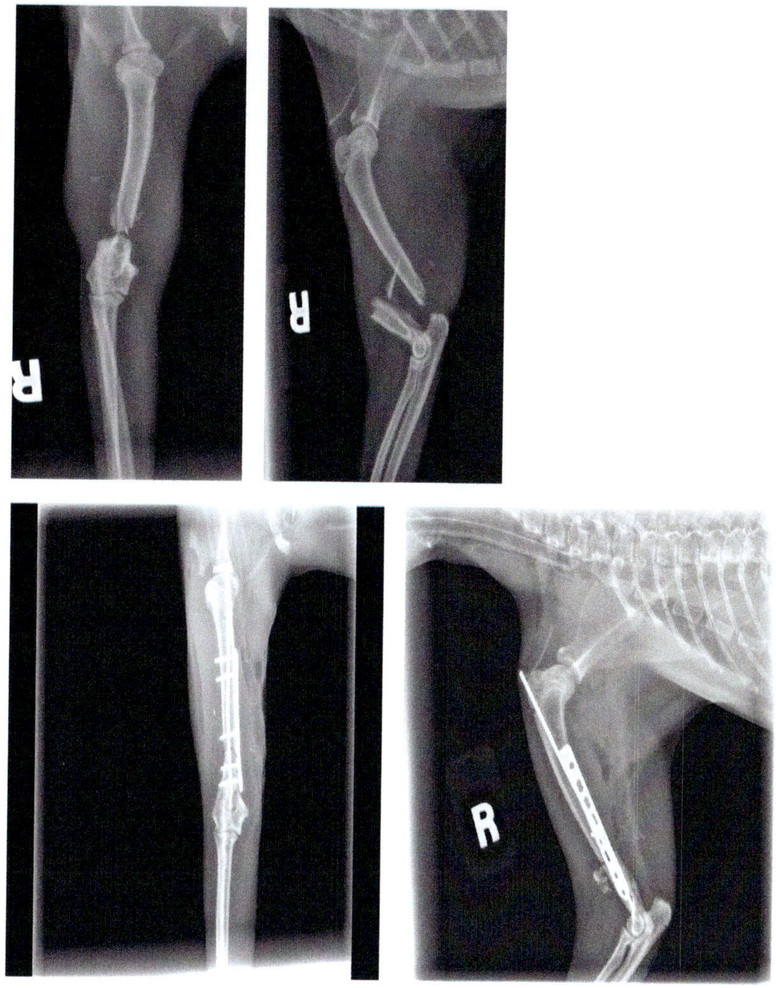

Figure 13.2 Pre- and postoperative radiographs of a feline humeral fracture. Postoperative radiographs show a combination repair with a 2.0 mm Synthes locking compression plates (LCP).

13.4.1 Material Considerations

Bone plating has been described, including medial or combined medial and lateral plating. Locking plates offer several advantages to conventional plate fixation when applied to the humerus. Due to the angle stable construct with traditional locking devices created by the screw interlocking with the plate, neither bicortical screw placement nor precise plate contouring is necessary. These attributes are useful, especially in application distally due to the need to avoid the supratrochlear foramen and articular surface, and because of the irregular surfaces of the distal humerus. The author uses a variety of LP systems for repair of humeral fractures. These include the PAX locking plate (Securos, Fiskdale, MA, USA), string of pearls (SOP Orthomed LTD, Huddersfield, UK), and Synthes (DePuy Synthes Vet, West Chester, PA). The choice of which implant to use is based on specific patient size and fracture configuration at the time of the procedure.

Additionally, the author commonly utilizes the combination plate and rod approach depicted in Figure 13.2. In general, the pin should fit to approximately 30% of the diameter of the medullary canal; however, since monocortical screw placement is a viable option with locking plates, larger-diameter pins can also be used [9].

A specific factor that relates to choice of the polyaxial stable (e.g. PAX) system is the ability to angle screws during screw insertion up to 10° while maintaining pullout strength [10, 11]. This gives additional flexibility to the construct when inserting screws close to the olecranon fossa or the distal humeral articular surface. The S-shaped diaphysis of the humerus, which is even more pronounced in brachycephalic breeds, makes the SOP plate particularly useful in many cases. This is due to the ability to contour the plate in three planes, where a straight plate might not align with the bone either proximally or distally.

In the case of diaphyseal fractures, the author attempts to use the longest bone plate possible and most commonly places two screws at the most proximal and distal ends and a third screw as close to the fracture site as is possible without violation of the fracture line itself. This is based on our own unpublished findings in combination with those of authors that

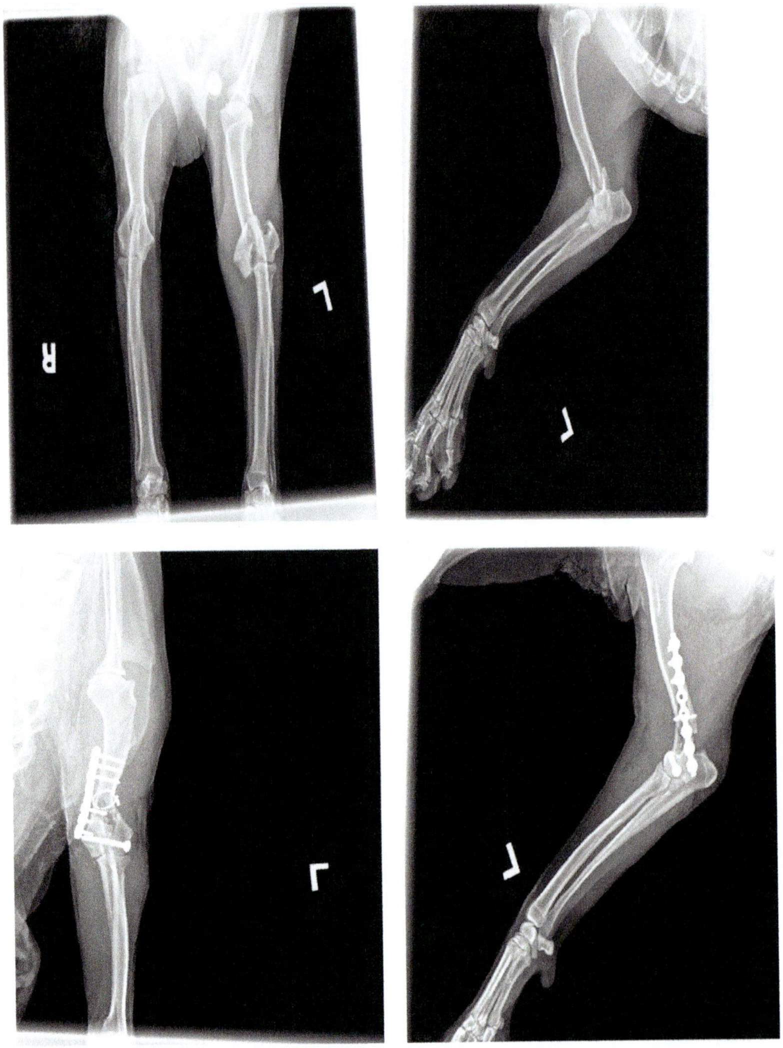

Figure 13.3 Pre- and postoperative radiographs of a distal condylar Y fracture in a dog. The condylar portion was repaired with a compression screw, and then a 2.0 mm string of pearls (SOP) plate was added with a combination of unilateral and bilateral cortical screws.

described this configuration in a Synthes eight-hole locking compression plate. A locking screw inserted adjacent to the fracture gap was similar under biomechanical testing to a plate where all eight holes had been filled with a locking screw [12].

13.5 Distal Humeral Fractures

The intent of this chapter is to highlight those fractures particularly amenable to repair with locking plates. The fracture region most benefited by the positive attributes of locking plates is the humeral epicondyle and condyle.

Fractures of the condyle that communicate with the articular surface through the medial and lateral epicondylar crests are commonly referred to as T or Y fractures and present a significant challenge to the surgeon. Intra-articular fractures require anatomic reduction and rigid fixation if joint function is to be restored [13]. Perfect reduction of the articular fracture, coupled with the need to reduce and repair the metaphyseal or diaphyseal component, is both mechanically and anatomically challenging (see Figures 13.3 and 13.4).

There are several well-described approaches to this region [14–17]. The author tends to perform a lateral approach with the addition of a tenotomy of the tendon of the triceps brachii muscle. This approach provides excellent ability to judge the reduction of the articular surface while providing access to the medial and lateral portions of the supracondylar region to secure a bone plate. The sequencing of the actual repair might vary, depending on the surgeon and the specific type of fracture configuration. The author will generally repair the condylar segment with a lag screw initially and then reduce this segment to the distal diaphysis. The surgeon will determine whether to place the medial or lateral plate first. The tendon can then be repaired using a three-loop pulley or similar tendon-specific suture pattern [18].

The author has not noted this tenotomy to cause any long-term issues and encourages early passive range of motion on the part of the owners to reduce the potential complication of fibrosis / contracture leading to loss of functional range of motion. In addition, the author typically prefers this technique because it negates the requirement of further implants and complications with physeal damage or bony union, as can be seen in the case of an olecranon osteotomy being performed. Bilateral approaches can also be used, which does not require surgery on the triceps tendon.

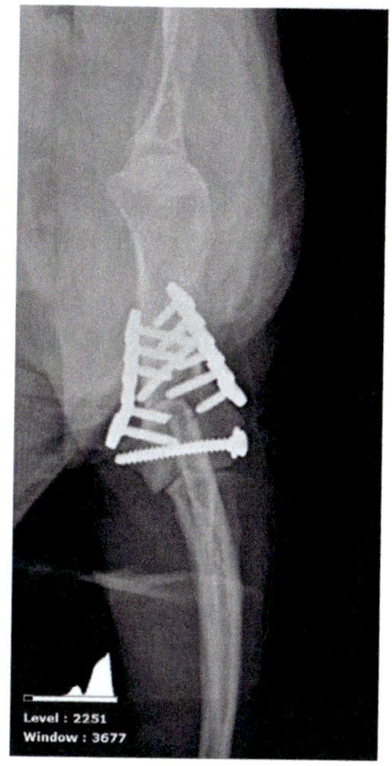

Figure 13.4 A postoperative radiograph demonstrating an alternative method of repairing a distal condylar Y fracture in a dog with a compression screw in the condylar fracture combined with the addition of a 2.7 mm Polyaxial Advanced Locking System (PAX) plate.

13.6 Conclusion

There are multiple options when it comes to implant choices for repair of humeral fractures, regardless of the configuration and causative factors. When used appropriately, locking plate constructs provide a more simple and effective means of rapid healing with successful return to function for both dogs and cats. These constructs are likely more expensive in the short term but provide improved construct strength, maintain fracture reduction, and likely lower the possibility of failure and the potential requirement for further costly and debilitating surgeries.

References

1. Harari, J., Roe, S.C., Johnson, A. et al. (1986). Medial plating for repair of middle and distal diaphyseal fractures of the humerus in dogs. *Vet. Surg.* 15: 45.
2. Hill, F.W. (1977). A survey of bone fractures in the cat. *J. Small Anim. Pract.* 18: 457.
3. Phillips, I.R. (1979). A survey of bone fractures in the dog and cat. *J. Small Anim. Pract.* 20: 661.
4. Macias, C., Gibbons, S.E., and McKee, W.M. (2006). Y-T humeral fractures with supracondylar comminution in five cats. *J. Small Anim. Pract.* 47: 89.
5. Wallace, M.K. and Berg, J. (1991). Craniolateral approach to the humerus with transection of the brachialis muscle. *Vet. Surg.* 20: 97.
6. Voss, K., Langley-Hobbs, S.J., and Montavon, P. (2009). *Humerus. Feline Orthopedic Surgery and Musculoskeletal Disease*, 343. Edinburgh: Saunders.
7. Vaughan, D.P., Syrcle, J.A., Ball, J.E. et al. (2016). Pullout strength of monocortical and bicortical screws in metaphyseal and diaphyseal regions of the canine humerus. *Vet. Comp. Orthop. Traumatol.* 29 (6): 466–474.
8. Hurt, R.J., Syrcle, J.A., Elder, S. et al. (2014). A biomechanical comparison of unilateral and bilateral string of pearl locking plates in a canine distal humeral metaphyseal gap model. *Vet. Comp. Orthop. Traumatol.* 27: 186–191.
9. Hulse, D., Hyman, W., Nori, M. et al. (1997). Reduction in plate strain by addition of an intramedullary pin. *Vet. Surg.* 26 (6): 451–459.
10. Bufkin, B.W., Barnhart, M.D., Kazanovicz, A.J. et al. (2013). The effect of screw angulation and insertion torque on the push out strength of polyaxial locking screws and the single cycle to failure in bending of polyaxial locking plates. *Vet. Comp. Orthop. Traumatol.* 26 (3): 186–191. doi: 10.3415/VCOT-12-03-0043.
11. Barnhart, M.D., Rides, C.F., Kennedy, S.C. et al. (2013). Fracture repair using a polyaxial locking plate system (PAX). *Vet. Surg.* 42 (1): 60–66.
12. Rowe-Guthrie, K.M., Markel, M.D., and Bleedhorn, J.A. (2015). Mechanical evaluation of locking, nonlocking, and hybrid plating constructs using a locking compression plate in a canine synthetic bone model. *Vet. Surg.* 44 (7): 838–842.
13. Ness, M.G. (2009). Repai of Y-T humeral fractures in the dog using paired "string of pearls" locking plates. *Vet. Comp. Orthop. Traumatol.* 22 (6): 492–497.
14. Bardet, J., Hohn, R., Rudy, R. et al. (1983). Fracture of the humerus in the dog and cat: a retrospective study of 130 cases. *Vet. Surg.* 12: 73.
15. Denny, H. (1983). Condylar fracture of the humerus in the dog: a review of 133 cases. *J. Small Anim. Pract.* 24: 185.
16. McKee, W.M., Macias, C., and Innes, J.F. (2005). Bilateral fixation of Y-T humeral condyle fractures via medial and lateral approaches in 29 dogs. *J. Small Anim. Pract.* 46: 217.
17. Mostosky, U., Cholvin, N., and Brinker, W. (1959). Transolecranon approach to the elbow joint. *Vet. Med.* 54: 560.
18. Moores, A.P., Owen, M.R., and Tarlton, J.F. (2004). The three-loop pulley suture versus two locking-loop sutures for the repair of canine Achilles tendons. *Vet. Surg.* 33: 131–137.

14 Radius/Ulna Fractures

Laurent P. Guiot and Reunan P. Guillou

14.1 Introduction

Traumatic radius and ulna (antebrachial) fractures are common in dogs and cats and often require surgical treatment for optimal outcome (Figure 14.1). The current standard-of-care techniques involve open reduction of the fracture and placement of either a bone plate (applied on the cranial or medial radial surfaces) or closed reduction with an external skeletal fixator (ESF) [1–3]. The choice of implants is dictated by patient size, fracture configuration, and surgeon preference. In particular, locking plates have recently become an attractive alternative to conventional plating for the treatment of radius and ulna fractures. In this chapter, we will review specificities of locking plate application for traumatic antebrachial fractures, including the types of approaches and fracture reduction techniques that can be used with this type of implant.

Conventional osteosynthesis (CO) of radius fractures has been associated with fair to good clinical outcomes with reported healing times of 54–90 days. Unfortunately, complication rates of up to 48%, including delayed healing, infection, pin track drainage (when using ESF) and implant failure, have been reported (Figure 14.2) [4–9]. Furthermore, 25% of these complications are severe and include catastrophic failure of the repair and nonunions. These shortcomings likely result from a combination of factors, including poor fracture biology and inappropriate mechanical environment. As a result, longer healing times may be expected, and, accordingly, relatively strong bone plates are often used in an attempt to prevent implant fatigue failure before bone union occurs [8, 10, 11]. This strategy, however, may result in significant osteopenia of the bone underneath the plate and increases the risk of secondary fracture. This risk is further potentiated with the use of open approaches that disrupt fracture biology, and during which relatively short plates are typically used, creating stress concentration at the proximal aspect of the plate.

Direct surgical approach of the fracture during CO has a negative impact on periosteal vascularization, and the use of conventional bone plates may further deplete the viability of the periosteum [12, 13]. The importance of periosteal vascularization during bone healing is critical in all breeds, but may be more so in small and toy breeds due to the paucity of

Locking Plates in Veterinary Orthopedics, First Edition.
Edited by Matthew D. Barnhart and Karl C. Maritato.

(a) (b)

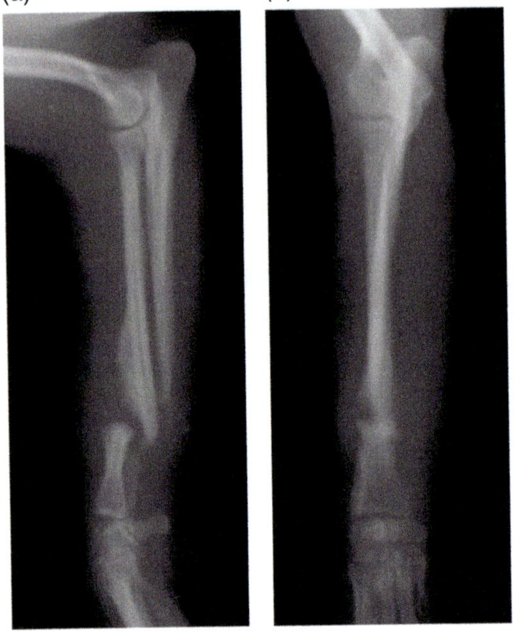

Figure 14.1 Medio-lateral (a) and cranio-caudal (b) radiographic images of a radius-ulna fracture treated with a splint for 16 weeks. There is a hypertrophic nonunion with moderate periosteal proliferation on the cranial aspect of the proximal radial fragment and obliteration of the medullary cavity at the fracture ends.

endosteal and medullary supply [14]. It has been reported that in dogs less than 6 kg, internal fixation or external coaptation are associated with complication rates ranging from 54% to 83% [15, 16]. In these cases, the use of locking implants could prove advantageous, as they significantly reduce damage to the periosteum, while providing mechanical advantages compared to standard plates. The preservation of periosteal blood supply should favor early formation of a callus and expedite healing of the fracture while limiting osteonecrosis under the bone plate. Faster bone healing may, in turn, allow for the safe use of relatively smaller implants, as the required implant fatigue life is decreased. While studies are lacking to support these hypotheses, it is our belief that locking implants have the potential to mitigate complications associated with internal fixation of radius fractures in all patients, and particularly in toy-breed dogs. The use of these implants in combination with adherence to biological osteosynthesis principles will likely offset some of the complications seen in CO of antebrachial fractures.

14.2 Biological Osteosynthesis in R-U Fracture Repair

Biological osteosynthesis principles emphasize preservation of the soft tissue envelope surrounding a fracture site to optimize bone healing capability [17]. When these principles are used to apply a bone plate, it is often referred to as minimally invasive plate osteosynthesis (MIPO) (Figure 14.3). While MIPO can be performed using conventional implants, locking plates are specifically designed for biological applications, and their full benefit is attained when used in combination with these techniques.

Available literature on biological osteosynthesis for the treatment of antebrachial fractures in dogs is very limited and includes one cadaveric anatomical study, a short comparative study using bone plates, and retrospective case series using ESF [18–22]. Our clinical experience suggests that MIPO of radius and ulna fractures is possible in a variety of patient sizes and represent an effective fixation method that could replace traditional techniques in the future. It is generally agreed by clinicians that the advent of locking implants facilitates MIPO in various fracture patterns but that the lack of direct observation of the fracture site during surgery makes restoration of alignment more challenging.

14.3 Reduction Techniques for Radius Fractures Stabilized with a Locking Plate

While it is possible to achieve and maintain the anatomical alignment with two bone forceps applied to the radial metaphyses through the small incisions used in MIPO, the forceps often impede the application of a bone plate, and they require constant manual control by a scrubbed assistant [23, 24]. In addition, locking implants require specific drilling guides that must adequately engage the locking mechanism of the plate in order to allow proper screw insertion. If the reduction instrumentation interferes with the drill-guides, there is a risk of

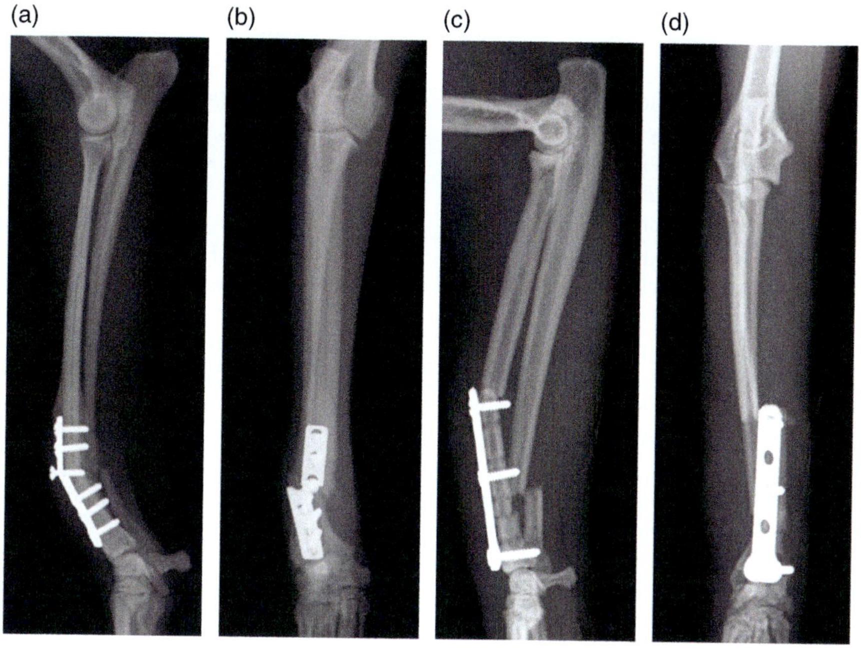

Figure 14.2 Construct failures in a dog (a, b) and a cat (c, d) with distal radius and ulna fractures. The short bone plate used in the dog failed through a screw hole adjacent to the fracture site, despite its adequate thickness. Fatigue failure can be explained by the high stress concentration at the level of the fracture site due to the short working length of the plate that functioned as a bridging implant in this case where a small defect was present on the caudal radial cortex postoperatively. In the cat (c, d), the bone fractured just proximal to the bone plate. This failure is partly explained by an abrupt change in construct strength and stiffness at the level of the plate extremity. This phenomenon is commonly observed in small-breed animals with distal radius-ulna fractures, where a short bone plate is selected. Note the presence of four holes beneath the plate on the lateral projection (c) corresponding to drill holes and subsequent repositioning of the bone plate due to suboptimal initial fracture reduction.

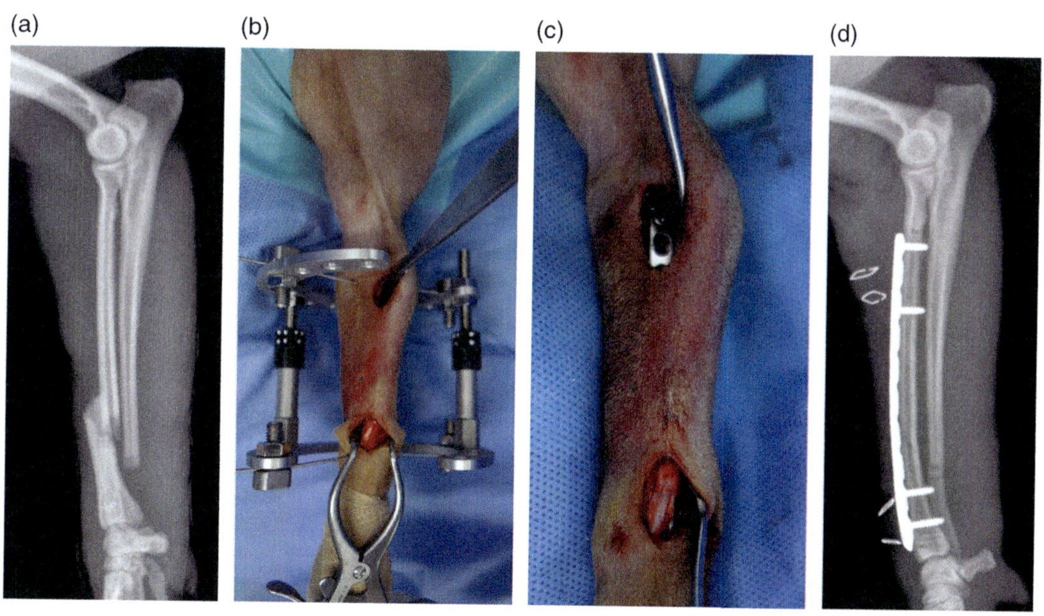

Figure 14.3 Preoperative radiograph (a), intraoperative images (b, c) and postoperative radiographs (d) of a radius and ulna fracture treated using minimally invasive plate osteosynthesis (MIPO) in a dog. A distraction frame using partial rings and two motors was secured to the radius with one transverse K-wire per fragment (b). Two small approaches to the proximal and distal radial metaphyseal regions were made on the cranial radial surface. A 2.0 locking compression plate was inserted into an epiperiosteal tunnel over the cranial radial surface (c). The extensor tendons were preserved during the procedure. Immediate postoperative radiographs (d) show adequate restoration of alignment and apposition. The plate bone ratio (PBR) is high (82%), and the plate screw density is low (0.4).

malpositioning the screw, which would negatively affect construct properties.

Alternatives to direct fragment manipulation with bone-holding forceps include the placement of a temporary distraction frame/device, the application of toothed reduction handles, and the use of a hanging leg technique or a traction table. The first two techniques provide direct control over the bone, as they anchor into the radius at locations remote from final fixation. Their downside is that they do result in minor trauma to the bone when compared to the latter two options. Nevertheless, we prefer the use of a distraction frame as our standard reduction technique for radius/ulna fractures for several reasons. First and foremost, the damage created to the bone and surrounding tissues is minimal, as the frame uses small-sized, percutaneously inserted Kirschner wires (K-wires) applied to metaphyseal regions. Next, it allows for progressive, controlled distraction of the fracture site and permits adjustments in varus/valgus, rotation and pro-recurvatum as necessary. Finally, it does not interfere with the placement of a locking plate if applied properly (Figure 14.4).

Key elements to proper application include the placement of K-wires within the metaphyseal regions of the radius. The wires should be applied in the frontal plane proximally and distally, parallel to each articular surface. The wires are then secured to partial, three-quarter circular-external-fixator rings, allowing unrestricted access proximally to the cranio-lateral and distally to the cranio-medial radial surfaces. Proper rotational alignment is restored; the rings are then connected with distraction motors. Distraction is applied to regain length, and any translation is adjusted by sliding the bone fragments along either wire. Once radial alignment is restored, fixation using a bone plate can take place, typically on the cranial radial surface. Plate insertion with MIPO requires the creation of an epiperiosteal tunnel.

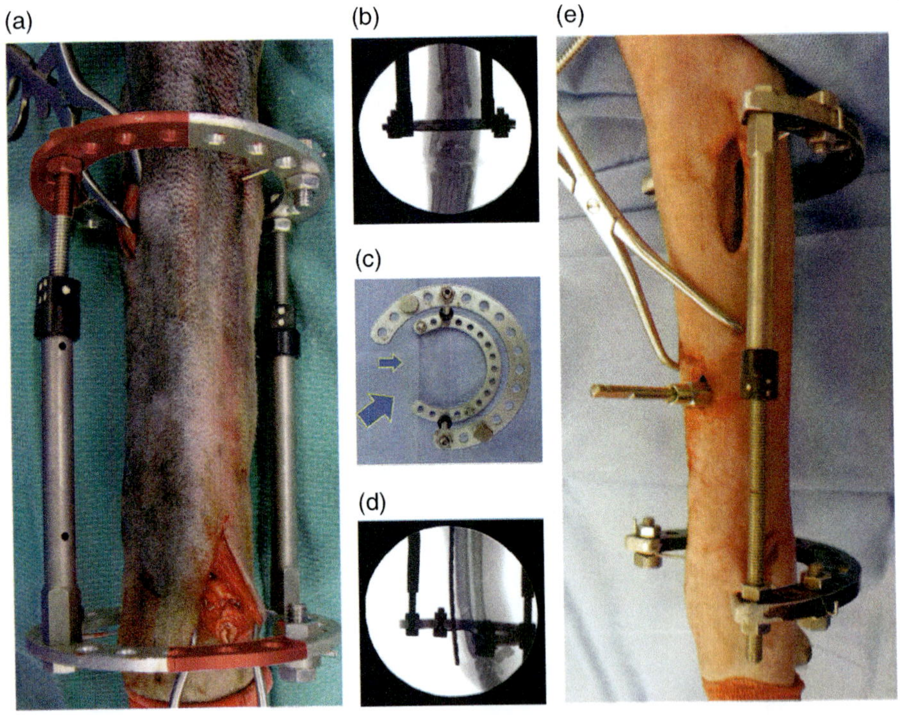

Figure 14.4 Distraction frame using full (a, b) or partial (c–e) rings can be used to restore radial alignment during minimally invasive fracture repair. Full rings, however, compromise access to the metaphyseal regions (a), making implant insertion and fixation difficult. Using partial rings can offset this issue, providing unrestricted access to the surgery sites if placed adequately (e). It is advisable to select the orientation of each ring based on the planned surgical approach (c). The proximal ring opening is better located cranio-laterally, while the distal ring opening should be placed cranio-medially.

The tunnel can be created with a blunt dedicated instrument or directly with the bone plate when the plate design allows it (e.g. locking compression plate [SynthesVet, Paoli, PA, USA] featuring a beveled tip). The plate is contoured based on preoperative radiographs of the contralateral side, and is then secured to the bone using two or three screws per fragment. Even when using locking plates, it is important to contour the plate appropriately in order to prevent interference with musculo-tendinous structures, particularly distally (Figure 14.5), as well as reducing the working length of the screws. A traction screw or a push-pull device can be used to approximate the bone to the plate (reduction onto the plate) in cases where alignment is not completely restored in the sagittal plane, prior to inserting the final locking screws. Using this technique, we found that anatomical alignment was consistently attained in an unpublished series of 10 cases [25]. In some cases, we elect to augment construct stiffness by using intermediate screws closer to the fracture site, which can be placed through stab incisions facing the plate hole of intended use (Figure 14.5). Defining the right amount of fixation is not an easy task and the guidelines we propose in the next section are somewhat empirical and based on our experience with this method of fixation.

(a)

(b)

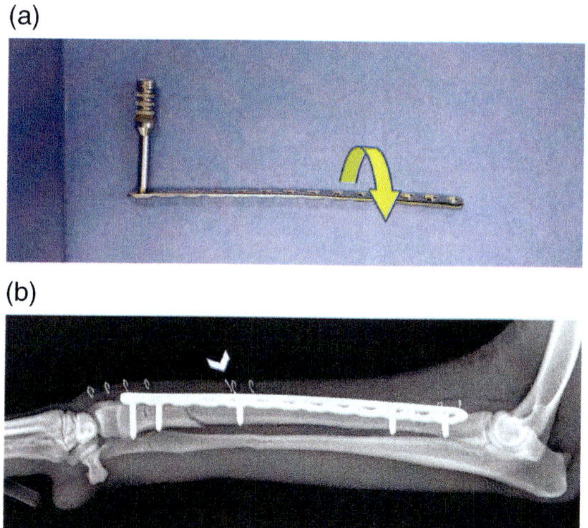

Figure 14.5 The radius features a slight cranial curvature with a mild rotation. When using long, it is advisable to contour the plate with a twist (a) to accommodate for the radial anatomy. The postoperative radiographs (b) show proper restoration of alignment and adequate apposition of the short oblique radial fracture. The locking plate was twisted and bent to follow the radial anatomy proximally. Note the presence of an intermediate screw (arrowhead) used to increase construct.

14.4 Mechanical Construct Consideration When Using Locking Plates for the Treatment of Radius-Ulna Fractures

While proximally, transarticular forces are evenly transmitted to both radius and ulna, the radius is the main load-bearing bone distally. This particularity is accounted for during construct design, and ulnar stabilization is given more and more consideration as the fracture location shifts proximally.

Radial fixation with bone plates is typically performed on the cranial or medial surfaces. Medial plating offers a theoretical greater resistance to bending moments in the sagittal plane, as the plate is bent "on edge." However, this configuration diminishes the error margin for screw placement as holes are being drilled in the smallest radial dimension and is limited to distal fractures because of the interference of the ulna proximally. When using a locking plate medially, these limitations can lead to improper screw anchorage due to the inability to choose screw orientation with fixed-angle locking plates. In addition, medial plating reduces plate span ratio (PSR or ratio between plate length and fracture length) and plate bone ratio (PBR or ratio between plate length and bone length) by confining the plate to the distal half of the radius. This limits the usefulness of medial plating for MIPO and makes the cranial location more desirable.

The benefits of locking technology on a biological perspective were discussed in Chapter 3. It is worth noticing that these benefits are potentiated in areas of lower healing capability such as the distal radius of small or toy breeds of dogs or in cases that have sustained severe comminution. In those patients, the limited bone stock for fixation is often the primary determinant of implant choice, and special locking plates, such as the notched or T-plate, can be advantageous. Regardless of fracture configuration and location, we advocate the use of plates with high PBR [26]. This translates into a need to contour the plate in torsion to follow the radius curvature, particularly in dogs (Figure 14.5). Imprinting torsion to the plate may deform screw holes, which can negatively affect the locking mechanism. Therefore, whenever possible, twisting of the plate should be applied in areas where screws are not intended to be used.

Screw type and distribution influence construct strength and stiffness. A minimum of three cortices is required per fragment. The use of at least one bicortical screw per fragment is recommended in order to increase the resistance to torsional forces, while the other screw(s) may be monocortical. The safe use of monocortical locking screws may be advantageous in the proximal radius because of the possible interference of bicortical screws with the ulna. This is particularly true when using monoaxial locking implants, as the drilling path is dictated by the bone plate.

The distance between the screws adjacent to the fracture site greatly influences the stiffness of the construct. When using bridging plates during MIPO, these screws are typically placed away from the fractures site, within one or two holes from the plate extremity through the same keyhole incisions as the ones used for the outermost screws [20, 27]. However, if a stiffer construct is deemed necessary, secondary stab-incisions can be made to insert screws closer to the fracture site. Ensuring proper drill-guide insertion through these small approaches is critical to prevent inadequate drilling orientation and suboptimal screw fixation. For comminuted fractures, bridging plates with screws at the plate extremities are recommended. For transverse fractures, we will tend to bring intermediate screws closer to the fracture site in order to decrease interfragmentary strain (Figure 14.6), particularly in mature patients. Care is taken to avoid the cephalic vein during intermediate screw insertion, as this vessel runs directly over the implant in the diaphyseal radial region.

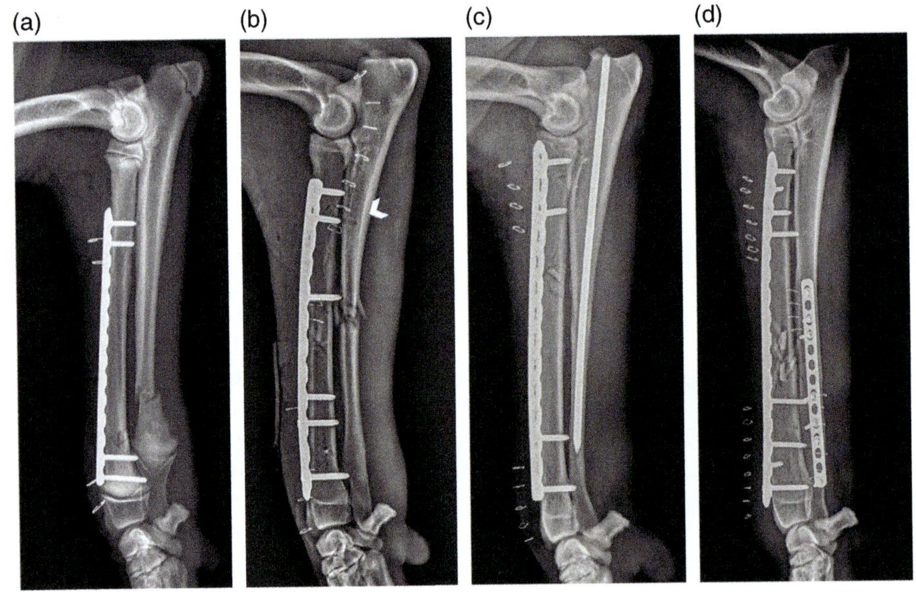

Figure 14.6 Postoperative radiographs of four different constructs using locking plates for the treatment of radius and ulna fractures. The construct stiffness is incremental from left to right. In the first case (a), a small (2.0 mm) plate was chosen with a long working distance between the innermost screws. A high compliance was selected in this young dog to foster rapid secondary bone healing and protect the bone–screw interfaces. A stiffer construct was created with the second case (b) by using intermediate screws, closer to the fracture site. Note the presence of a drill path (arrowhead) extending into the ulna at the level of the second screw. This technical mistake should be avoided, as it could result in postoperative complications. The addition of an ulnar intramedullary rod (c) further increases construct stiffness. The rod diameter should be chosen to maximize canal fill at the level of the fracture site. In larger patients like the Great Dane (d), we will often resort to bone plate fixation of the ulnar fracture to further increase construct stability.

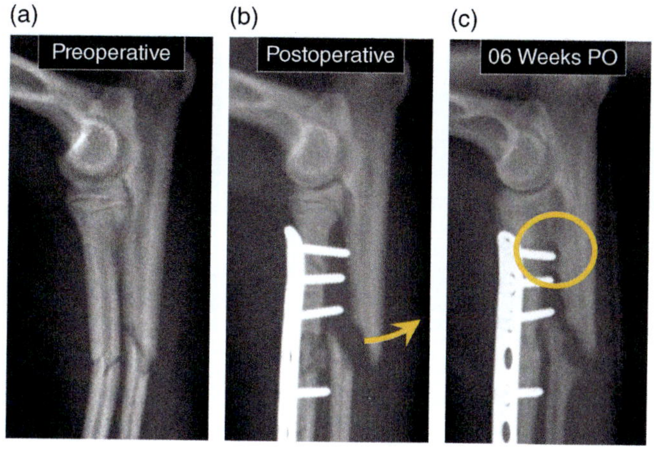

Figure 14.7 Preoperative (a), postoperative (b), and follow-up radiographs (c) of a proximal radius and ulna fracture treated with a bone plate and screw. The proximal screws were too long and created a displacement of the ulna during surgery (arrow). While the radius fracture healed adequately, the ulnar fracture presents with a delayed union sixweeks postoperatively, and there is a severe reaction of the cranial ulnar surface at the level of the proximal screw (circle), secondary to chronic mechanical interference. This phenomenon is responsible for residual lameness, and implant removal is necessary to allow full recovery.

One of the limitations of placing the plate on the cranial radial surface is the possible interference between the screws and the ulna, which may result in discomfort and could lead to premature loosening of the screw or focal osteolysis of the ulna at the site of interference (Figure 14.7). Using locking screws with monoaxial systems potentiates this risk, as the bone plate predetermines screw orientation; and as most screws used in locking configuration are self-tapping, the minimum protruding distance on the transcortical side is increased. Strategies to mitigate this shortcoming include (i) use of monocortical screws, (ii) placement of the plate along the lateral margin of the proximal radius, and (iii) use of a nonlocking, cortical screw aiming caudo-laterally.

14.5 Ulnar Fracture Fixation

Fixation of ulnar fractures may be recommended, depending on the location, degree of comminution, concurrent radial fracture, patient body weight, and other patient-related considerations such as the presence of additional lesions to the musculoskeletal system affecting other limbs (Figure 14.6). In our experience, proximal ulnar fractures tend to be painful, with significant lameness persisting during the healing process until clinical union is achieved, and for this reason, fracture fixation is often elected. Locking plates offer potential advantages over conventional plates for proximal ulnar fractures: when applied caudally, monocortical screws can be used to minimize risk of joint violation, and when applied on the lateral ulnar surface, the use of locking screws in a relatively thin bone could limit the risk of screw pullout.

14.6 Conclusion

Locking plates offer mechanical and biological advantages over traditional plates that are highly valuable in the treatment of antebrachial fractures. Since bone plates are the only realistic internal fixation method available for radial fractures involving the diaphyseal and metaphyseal regions, it is expected that surgeons will often resort to this implant. While there is a cost associated with the use of locking implants, there is enough evidence to support their use over nonlocking options [27]. This should prompt surgeons to consider locking plates as the gold standard for internal fixation of radial fractures. In doing so, surgeons must be aware

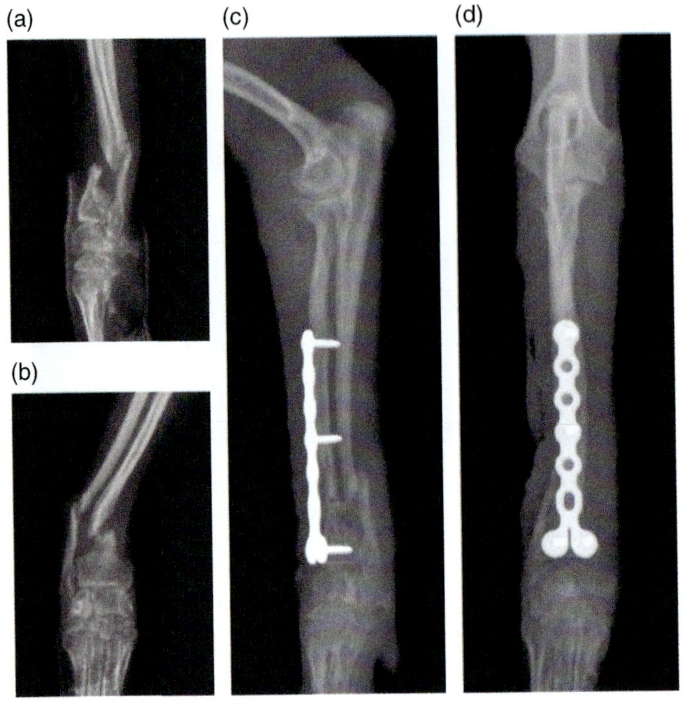

Figure 14.8 Preoperative radiographs (a, b) of a distal radius and ulna nonunion in a Chihuahua. A 1.5 mm locking compression plate was used with two screws per fragment to stabilize the fracture after debridement of the nonunion and grafting with autogenous cancellous bone graft (c, d).

of potential pitfalls associated with them, including the inability to dictate screw orientation with some systems and the false sense of security perceived once the screwhead locks into the plate, as it does not guarantee adequate bone anchorage. Principles of fracture repair, including restoration of alignment while providing acceptable fragment apposition, must be respected regardless of the choice of construct. Considerations for ulnar fixation are made based on biomechanical factors such as location, comminution, and association with other lesions. If ulnar fixation is elected, we tend to prefer a laterally applied locking plate in proximal fractures and an intramedullary rod in more distal ones.

Toy-breed dogs represent a separate challenge due to their notorious predisposition to complications (Figure 14.8). Using small locking plates with high PBR and MIPO techniques could mitigate some of these complications by optimizing the fracture biology and mechanical properties of the construct.

References

1. Johnson, A.L., Houlton, J.E.F., and Vannini, R. (2005). *AO Principles of Fracture Management in the Dog and Cat*. Georg Thieme Verlag: Stuttgart Germany.
2. Piermattei, D.L., Flo, G.L., and DeCamp, C.E. (2006). Fractures: classification, diagnosis, and treatment. In: *Handbook of Small Animal Orthopedics and Fracture Repair*, vol. 1 (ed. L. Farthman), 25–159. Saunders Elsevier: St. Louis.
3. Rudd, R.G. and Whitehair, J.G. (1992). Fractures of the radius and ulna. *Vet. Clin. North Am. Small Anim. Pract*. 22: 135–148.
4. Bilgili, H., Kurum, B., and Captug, O. (2007). Treatment of radius-ulna and tibia fractures with circular external skeletal fixator in 19 dogs. *Pol. J. Vet. Sci*. 10: 217–231.
5. DeAngelis, M.P. (1975). Causes of delayed union and nonunion of fractures. *Vet. Clin. North Am*. 5: 251–258.
6. Field, J.R. (1997). Bone plate fixation: its relationship with implant induced osteoporosis. *Vet. Comp. Orthop. Traumatol*. 10 (6): 88–94.
7. Hunt, J.M., Aitken, M.L., Denny, H.R. et al. (1980). The complications of diaphyseal fractures in dogs:

a review of 100 cases. *J. Small Anim. Pract.* 21: 103–119.

8. Johnson, A.L. and Schaeffer, D.J. (2008). Evolution of the treatment of canine radial and tibial fractures with external fixators. *Vet. Comp. Orthop. Traumatol.* 21: 256–261.
9. Sumner-Smith, G. (1991). Delayed unions and nonunions. Diagnosis, pathophysiology, and treatment. *Vet. Clin. North Am. Small Anim. Pract.* 21: 745–760.
10. Haaland, P.J., Sjostrom, L., Devor, M. et al. (2009). Appendicular fracture repair in dogs using the locking compression plate system: 47 cases. *Vet. Comp. Orthop. Traumatol.* 22: 309–315.
11. Johnson, A.L., Kneller, S.K., and Weigel, R.M. (1989). Radial and tibial fracture repair with external skeletal fixation: effects of fracture type, reduction, and complications on healing. *Vet. Surg.* 18: 367–372.
12. Garofolo, Pozzi, S.a., A. (2013 Apr Apr). Effect of plating technique on periosteal vasculature of the radius in dogs: a cadaveric study. *Vet. Surg.* 42 (3): 255–261. doi: 10.1111/j.1532-950X.2013.01087.x Epub 2013 Feb 21.
13. Jain, R., Podworny, N., Hupel, T.M. et al. (1999 Mar-Apr). Influence of plate design on cortical bone perfusion and fracture healing in canine segmental tibial fractures. *J. Orthop. Trauma* 13 (3): 178–186.
14. Welch, J.A., Boudrieau, R.J., DeJardin, L.M., and Spodnick, G.J. (1997 Jan-Feb). The intraosseous blood supply of the canine radius: implications for healing of distal fractures in small dogs. *Vet. Surg.* 26 (1): 57–61.
15. Saikku-Backstrom, A., Raiha, J.E., Valimaa, T. et al. (2005). Repair of radial fractures in toy breed dogs with self-reinforced biodegradable bone plates, metal screws, and light-weight external Coaptation. *Vet. Surg.* 34 (1): 11–17.
16. Larsen, L.J., Roush, J.K., and McLaughlin, R.M. (1999). Bone plate fixation of distal radius and ulna fractures in small- and miniature-breed dogs. *J. Am. Anim. Hosp. Assoc.* 35 (3): 243–250.
17. Waters, D.J., Breur, G.J., and Toombs, J.P. (1993). Treatment of common forelimb fractures in miniature and toy-breed dogs. *J. Am. Anim. Hosp. Assoc.* 29: 442–448.
18. Perren, S.M. (2002 Nov). Evolution of the internal fixation of long bone fractures. The scientific basis of biological internal fixation: choosing a new balance between stability and biology. *J. Bone Joint Surg. Br.* 84 (8): 1093–1110.
19. Johnson, A.L., Seitz, S.E., Smith, C.W. et al. (1996). Closed reduction and type-II external fixation of comminuted fractures of the radius and tibia in dogs: 23 cases (1990–1994). *J. Am. Vet. Med. Assoc.* 209: 1445–1448.
20. Perren, S.M. (2002). The technology of minimally invasive percutaneous osteosynthesis (MIPO). *Injury* 33 (Suppl 1): VI–VII.
21. Guiot, L.P. and Dejardin, L.M. (2011). Prospective evaluation of minimally invasive plate osteosynthesis in 36 nonarticular tibial fractures in dogs and cats. *Vet. Surg.* 40: 171–182.
22. Anderson, G.M., Lewis, D.D., Radasch, R.M. et al. (2003). Circular external skeletal fixation stabilization of antebrachial and crural fractures in 25 dogs. *J. Am. Anim. Hosp. Assoc.* 39: 479–498.
23. Pozzi, A. and Lewis, D. (2009). Surgical approaches for minimally invasive plate osteosynthesis in dogs. *Vet. Comp. Orthop. Traumatol.* 22: 316–320.
24. Piermattei, D.L. and Johnson, K.A. (2004). *An Atlas: Surgical Approaches to the Bones and Joints of the Dog and Cat (Ed 4)*. Philadelphia, PA: Saunders.
25. Pozzi, A., Hudson, C.C., Gauthier, C.M., and Lewis, D.D. (2013 Jan). Retrospective comparison of minimally invasive plate osteosynthesis and open reduction and internal fixation of radius-ulna fractures in dogs. *Vet. Surg.* 42 (1): 19–27. doi: 10.1111/j.1532-950X.2012.01009.x Epub 2012 Nov 26.
26. Guiot, L.P., Guillou, R.P., and Dejardin, L.M. (2012). Minimally invasive plate Osteosynthesis for the treatment of antebrachial fractures in dogs; proceeding of the 21st ECVS annual scientific meeting. *Vet. Surg.* 41: E4.
27. Gautier, E. and Sommer, C. (2003). Guidelines for the clinical application of the LCP. *Injury* 34 (Suppl 2): B63–B76.

15 Femur Fractures

Ian Gordon Holsworth

15.1 Introduction

Fracture of the femur in companion animals is common, often involves high force impact and is complicated by the extensive muscular envelope that surrounds the bone. The combination of traumatic hemorrhage at the fracture site and along the muscular planes, swelling and edema of the associated soft tissues, contraction of the muscular surround, fracture site displacement, and a propensity for the hip and stifle joint to lose their rotational alignment makes successful fracture repair challenging. The restoration of linear and rotational alignment of the femur along with the need to have a stable repair construct has lent the femoral fracture to bone plate repair. The evolution of plate design and capabilities has seen the locking plate (LP) become a staple of femoral fracture repair over the past 15 years. The ability to affix the bone screws securely to the bone plate and the fracture segments has, in the author's opinion, improved the strength and durability of the fracture repair construct and decreased implant and therefore construct failure. The relative strength of the LP in comparison to the more traditional dynamic compression plate (DCP) with or without the addition of an intramedullary (IM) rod has also been investigated experimentally to determine the relative biomechanical qualities of the different construct types. A more recent trend in the orthopedic surgical field is away from the classic open reduction and internal fixation (ORIF) toward biological osteosynthesis and the development of minimally invasive plate osteosynthesis (MIPO) with a limited surgical approach and reduced iatrogenic trauma. This approach hopes to preserve bone vascularity, improve fracture consolidation, decrease infection rate and avoid the need for bone grafting and transforms the plate construct into an internal extramedullary splint. The MIPO treatment goal is the anatomic reconstruction of the articular area, if involved, and axis, rotation and length reestablishment for the metaphyseal-diaphyseal area. The placement of a plate that bridges the fracture site and is only affixed to the femur proximally and distally with a limited number of bone screws is the underlying technical guideline. The establishment of sufficient fracture site stability with a degree of relative instability with MIPO is in contrast to the more traditional anatomic reduction and rigid fixation by bone plates with the goal of the technique being absolute fracture stability.

Locking Plates in Veterinary Orthopedics, First Edition.
Edited by Matthew D. Barnhart and Karl C. Maritato.

The challenge of the MIPO technique is the decreased operative visualization of the fracture segments, the adjustment of the surgeon to less open visual cues to anatomic restoration and the need in many cases for intraoperative fluoroscopic examination. The term *minimally invasive percutaneous plate osteosynthesis (MIPPO)* is used to describe the use of small, multiple surgical skin incisions and the development of skin "windows" to access the bone surface. The plates are placed blindly up the bone shaft under the muscular layer to lie adjacent but not compressing the periosteum. In cases of concurrent articular fracture, the use of a transarticular approach and retrograde plate osteosynthesis (TARPO) is utilized to expose the articular surface by arthrotomy, reduce the articular fracture anatomically and implant the epiphysis area sufficiently to provide rigid stability to the articular fracture repair. The adjacent metaphyseal-diaphyseal zone is then stabilized under MIPO guidelines.

Internal fixators can be expected to maintain but not obtain fracture reduction, so care must be taken to ensure adequate fracture reduction before insertion of the locked screws. The challenge to the trauma surgeon of reestablishing the length, axis and rotation of displaced femoral fractures during minimally invasive techniques is an ongoing area of both intraoperative imaging and surgical technique refinement.

15.2 Anatomy

In the normal dolichocephalic and mesocephalic dog, the femoral shaft in the diaphyseal region has a slight caudal curve in the sagittal plane and a slight medial curve in the frontal/coronal plane at the distal diaphyseal-metaphyseal junction. The measurement of the anatomic and mechanical angles of the femur and pelvic limb has been performed and documented by several authors for several different dog breeds [1–4].

The relative location of the femoral head in comparison to the frontal plan of the femoral condyles is very important in terms of restoration of the femoral alignment of the femur during fracture repair. The measurement of this angle has been investigated with multiple imaging modalities and there is large variation between individuals [5–10].

The tendency of the femoral head and neck's sagittal axis to rotate into a significantly increased anteverted location in relationship to the distal femur postfracture must be recognized and addressed during the realignment phase of femoral fracture repair. Failure to do so can lead to permanent femoral deformity and the resultant stability and biomechanics of the hip joint may be compromised. If adversely affected to a significant degree there is a propensity for hip luxation and development of hip joint osteoarthritis.

The use of computer tomography and three dimensional modeling has further allowed assessment and quantification of the other morphometric parameters of the canine femur which has improved both our understanding of the bone geometry present and subsequently our efforts to restore the patients femoral alignment to prefracture conformation [11].

15.3 Biomechanics

Under load, the medial cortical wall of the femoral diaphysis is the compression aspect of the bone, the lateral aspect the tension aspect. The proximal femur has a complex biomechanical loading pattern due to the offset femoral head. The femoral neck is under a complex interplay of both compressive and tension forces during normal daily activity. Neutralization of these forces to allow progressive bone healing is the surgical goal. Fracture configuration, including the degree of comminution, will affect the choice of surgical implant and its placement location. Accepting the limitations and challenges of the individual fracture and devising an appropriate response is the surgical challenge. Placement of the bone plate on the lateral, tension aspect, is commonly performed although medial aspect plating, while far less common, can also be used if the fracture configuration favors it, LPs are used or there is significant lateral thigh skin abrasions or open trauma to the thigh.

15.4 Materials

The advent of LPs in their myriad of forms from a range of manufacturers gives individual surgeons options to choose. Experimental comparison between standard limited-contact dynamic compression plates (LC-DCP) and LP plates mechanically has not shown the LP to be superior biomechanically in most aspects of testing, but the LP also did not underperform in a consistently significant way [12–17]. Personal experience with many LP types has been very positive personally and they have become first choice and invaluable in the author's clinical practice. Individual surgeons are faced with choosing an implant type based on availability and personal preference. There are inherent differences in mechanical strength between different LP types, which are to be expected and accepted by the surgeon [18, 19].

The lack of plate compression to the bone appears to affect construct stiffness adversely in some biomechanical models with a suggestion that ideally the LP be placed at 2 mm or less from the bone surface [20]. To adhere to this guideline in the femur, contouring of the plate may be necessary in both the proximal and distal aspects of the bone shaft. The degree of LP contouring possible by the surgeon intra-operatively varies between designs. Overcontouring without protection of the threaded plate holes can lead to distortion of the plate hole threads with a resultant inability to correctly lock the threaded screwheads into the plate. The presence of combination compression or locking holes in some LP designs with half of the hole a dynamic compression design for use with standard screws and the other half conical and threaded allows the surgeon to chose the appropriate screw for the current repair.

The addition of an IM rod to the femoral bone and plate construct to increase construct stability and fatigue life is an approach that has been used widely with traditional and now locking plating systems to good effect [21]. Biomechanical comparison in a femoral fracture model of a LC-DCP-IM rod to a LP alone showed the LC-DCP-IM construct had higher stiffness and resistance to failure, lower interfragmentary motion and lower plate strain and stress. A pin of any size increases resistance to axial loads, but a pin size of 30% or more of intra-medullary diameter is required to increase bending stiffness. Plate length changes do affect stiffness, but the presence of an IM pin has more overall construct strength significance [22, 23]. When comparison of a combined LP intramedullary pin (LP-IM) construct is made to the LC-DCP-IM construct experimentally in canine femurs, there was no significant difference biomechanically [24].

The option of placing monocortical versus bicortical screws in the femoral LP is also one the surgeon must deliberate on. The presence of bicortical screws in cadaver testing has increased torsional stiffness compared to monocortical screw constructs. Monocortical screws are sometimes necessary in bone segments without a trans cortex at the screw site or in constructs where the bicortical locking screw interferes with the presence of an IM pin. The use of bicortical locking screws in the most proximal and distal bone plate hole along with varying numbers of monocortical screws has been investigated in cadaver femurs, and the addition of multiple monocortical screws increased construct stiffness in a linear relationship but did not influence load-to-failure. The presence of bicortical screws in the femur model tested did not confer any significant biomechanical advantage and appears to not be an essential step in experimental fracture construct builds [25]. When the mode of construct failure is compared, bicortical screw constructs failed by bone fracture under the applied loads, whereas monocortical screw constructs failed at the bone–screw interface.

15.5 Surgical Approach

Surgical access to the femur bone is from a lateral or medial approach. Both approaches have their place in fracture repair and both approaches have similar but distinct challenges.

The lateral approach is performed by incising the biceps femoris fascia adjacent to the vastus lateralis and reflecting the vastus cranially to expose the bone surface. In the proximal femur, this is complicated by the presence of the tensor fascia lata and gluteal muscles and distally by the soft tissues associated with the stifle joint. The medial approach to the femur is made by initially incising the fascial connection between the cranial and caudal sartorius muscles. This fascial connection is distinct in canines but non-existent in felines, requiring a muscle-splitting technique. Once the sartorius muscles are separated and retracted, the vastus medialis is identified and it can be separated from the neurovascular tract that runs caudal to its caudal margin. This must be performed carefully to avoid iatrogenic damage to these structures. Once the separation between the neurovascular tract and the muscle belly is complete and any perforating vasculature is isolated and ligated as necessary the vastus medialis muscle belly can be retracted cranially to expose the femoral bone surface. As the dissection proceeds proximally the femoral bone shaft, it becomes more difficult to isolate effectively and the musculature of the inguinal area impedes good access.

15.6 Application on the Femur

Classification of femoral fractures is separated into several broad but important categories. The most important early assessor is the presence of an open vs. closed fracture. Open fractures vary in their severity depending on the degree of bone exposure and concurrent soft tissue trauma. The urgency of surgical therapy is proportional to the degree of open bone exposure and concurrent soft tissue trauma. The fracture location on the bone is divided into proximal, shaft and distal. The proximal category includes intracapsular (epiphyseal, physeal, subcapital, and transcervical) and extracapsular (cervical, intertrochanteric, and subtrochanteric). The shaft fractures are described by the fracture orientation and segments (transverse, short oblique, long oblique, spiral, segmental, butterfly, and comminuted) (Figure 15.1). The distal fractures are described as supracondylar, condylar, or intercondylar.

15.7 Proximal

Application of LPs to the proximal femur is from a standard lateral approach with proximal extension to ensure complete exposure of the greater trochanter. Plating of subtrochanteric and proximal shaft fractures will often involve contouring the plate over the greater trochanter to its proximal extent to allow screw placement into the trochanter. The use of LPs in intracapsular fractures is not possible and in the case of extracapsular subtrochanteric fractures they are commonly used in conjunction with additional screw fixation to attempt stable fracture fixation. In addition to fracture reduction, the other major challenge is contouring the LP sufficiently to bring the plate surface in good proximity to the heavily contoured proximal femoral diaphysis.

15.8 Shaft

The placement of the LP in the femoral shaft area is most commonly performed laterally. Medial plate placement is possible but is

(a)

(b)

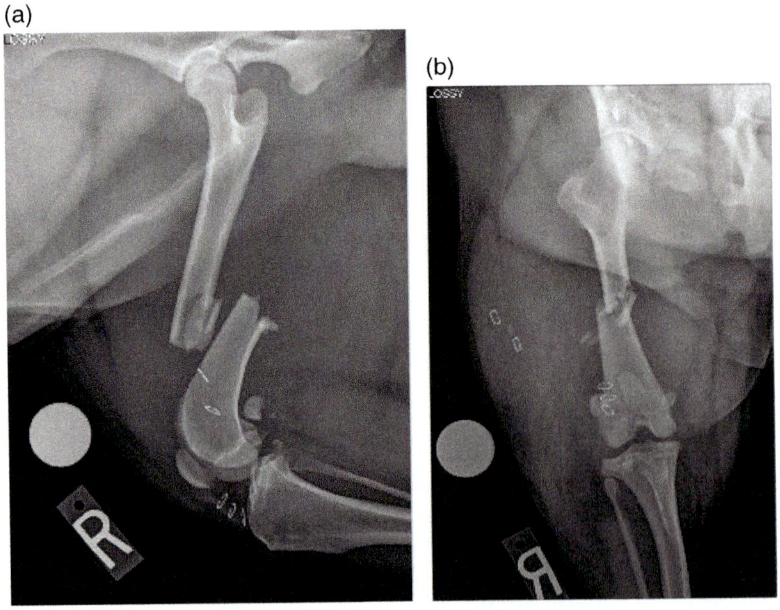

Figure 15.1 (a) and (b) Lateral and PA view of a right closed mid-diaphyseal transverse closed femoral shaft fracture with moderate caudal and proximal displacement of the distal femoral fracture segment. Skin staples indicate the presence of lateral aspect thigh concurrent soft tissue trauma repair.

normally reserved for distal shaft fractures. Traditionally ORIF technique has been employed for this process with fracture site reduction and plate-bone surface contouring being performed. Unfortunately this approach often requires considerable soft tissue dissection and femur exposure. The use of MIPPO technique is suited to mid femoral shaft fractures and can be employed by the experienced surgeon in some cases. The bone plate is introduced through a distal or proximal mini-approach to the femur and advanced over the lateral aspect of the femur below the biceps femoris and vastus lateralis. The plate is allowed to bridge the fracture site without exposure and then is secured proximally and distally to the unaffected bone surface once alignment of the femur is normalized. Fluoroscopic guidance during the procedure is not essential but very helpful and attention to proximal and distal joint alignment must be prioritized. It is helpful to recognize the femoral head may have rotated into an abnormally anteverted position post-fracture event, and this should be corrected prior to definitive implant placement. When employing a more minimal surgical approach to the femur, a decision of the concurrent placement of an IM rod must be made. The author typically inserts the rod retrograde to emerge from the femur in the inter-trochanteric area, and its direction is then reversed to allow it to seat into the distal femoral segment. Removal of the trocar tip if present on the distal end of the rod implant is advised to prevent inadvertent penetration through the articular surface of the distal femur and resultant stifle joint damage. Apart from the well-recognized biomechanical advantages the rod addition brings, it also is very helpful in many cases in restoring femoral length and overcoming fracture site collapse. Once placed, the intact proximal and distal femoral segments can be aligned more readily prior to LP placement. The length of plate, the choice of monocortical, bicortical, locking, or cortical compressive screws are all based on the individual patient and fracture configuration (Figure 15.2).

The surgical aim of a stable construct that will maintain femoral alignment and basic configuration while fracture healing progresses

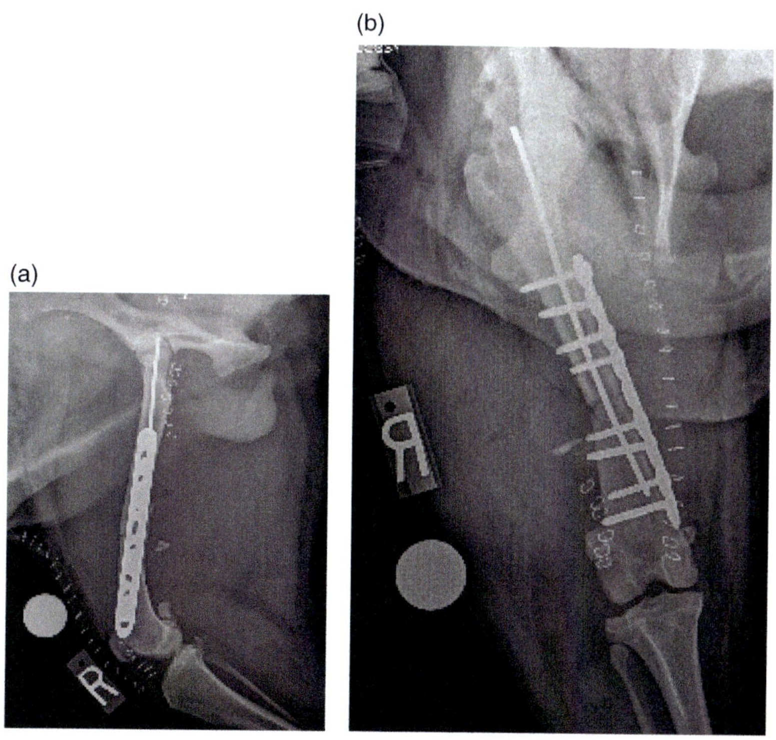

Figure 15.2 (a) and (b) Immediate postoperative films of femoral fracture repair construct. An IM pin in combination with a medially applied locking plate (LP) with mixed use of cortical and locking screws has been utilized.

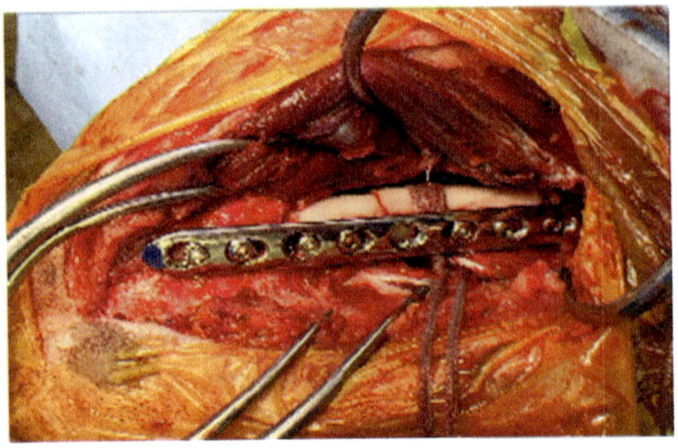

Figure 15.3 Intra-operative appearance of a medial femoral shaft approach with intra-operative use of a multistrand multifilament surgical suture to aid in fracture segment reduction prior to placement of a medial locking plate. The surgical suture can be maintained or removed following fracture repair construct completion according to surgeon preference.

must be prioritized. Minimizing soft tissue dissection and maximizing vascular supply to the area assists in achieving that aim. With the heavy thigh musculature often present in many dog breeds, the MIPPO technique allows the surgical dissection to be decreased from ORIF technique and surgical trauma is reduced. When performing a medial approach to the mid-femur in cases of lateral aspect trauma, a more classical ORIF approach will likely be necessary (Figure 15.3).

15.9 Distal

Distal femoral fractures are subclassified into two groups, those with an articular component and those that are extracapsular in relationship to the stifle. The latter group is far more common but often requires significant dissection around the stifle joint capsule and peri-articular structures to allow fracture isolation, reduction, and implant placement. If an articular fracture is present, the TARPO technique may be utilized to achieve a well-reduced, stable articular fracture repair with plate tie-in to the distal diaphysis. These fractures are more challenging, the degree of open arthrotomy and exposure of the joint surfaces is more significant, and placing the bone screws in safe and effective bone corridors to achieve stability without iatrogenic damage to joint structures is a challenge. Regardless of whether a medial or lateral approach is utilized it is important that the quadriceps complex, including the patella, is well aligned & stabilized post fracture fixation and that a stable and central patella results.

15.10 Postsurgical Care and Monitoring

The severity of concurrent soft tissue injury, the presence of other orthopedic trauma, the patient size and attitude, the owner's limitations, and the successful progression of healing are all factors that will dictate postsurgical recommendations. It is imperative that patient activity be well curtailed, regular revisits be performed to allow patient and fracture site reassessment, and relaxation of restrictions corresponds to evidence of good radiographic healing and appropriate limb use by the patient (Figure 15.4).

It is vital to the overall limb use that an assessment of proximal and distal joint function be made sequentially and maintenance of appropriate joint range-of-motion and limb flexibility be prioritized during the recovery period to avoid quadriceps contracture and loss of stifle and hip joint function.

15.11 Complications & Limitations

Implant complications are seen in approximately 10% of femoral fractures using locking compression plates (LP) and this rate appears constant regardless of patient and implant size [26, 27]. Decreased muscle mass, loss of adjacent joint ROM, quadriceps contracture, and persistent limb lameness may all occur and adversely affect the perceived success of the fracture repair. Minimizing complication rates is a complex interplay of surgical experience, skillset, patient selection, client education, preoperative patient preparation, surgery duration, implant choice, appropriate postoperative care, regular reevaluation of patient progress and client monitoring and support. Improvements in many of these areas are possible in most surgical scenarios and should be prioritized to improve patient care. Continued technique and implant evolution will hopefully continue to improve patient outcomes and decrease

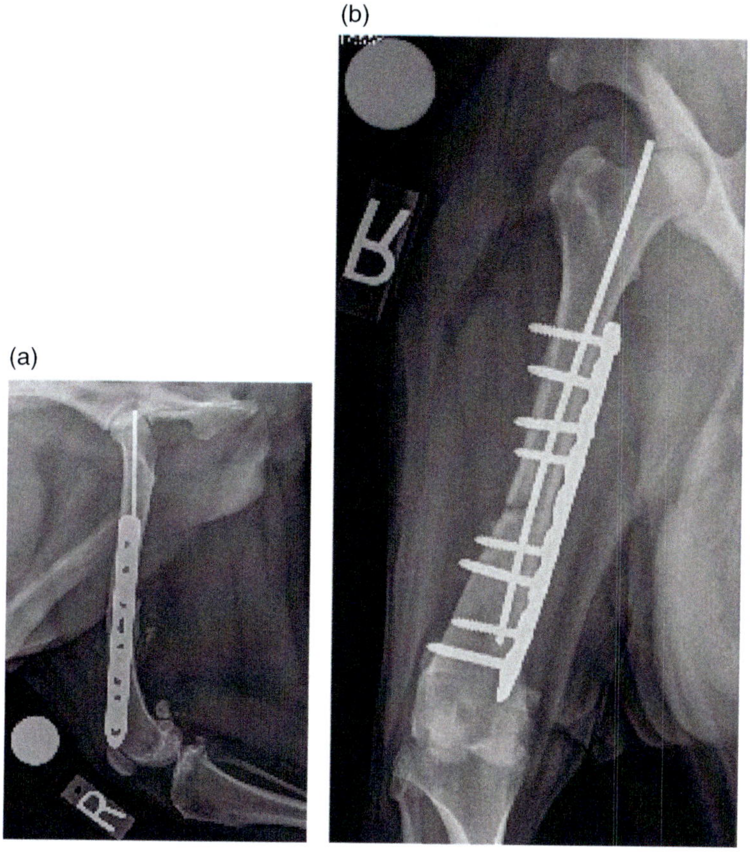

Figure 15.4 (a) and (b) Follow-up radiographs six weeks postsurgical repair. Fracture site appearance, implant location, and femoral alignment appear appropriate and unchanged from postsurgery (Figure 15.2a and b). Progressive bone deposition is apparent and of an appropriate degree.

individual surgeon's complication rates. The author's personal experience with LPs has been very positive in comparison with previous experiences with standard DCP plates. The ability to more securely capture bone segments and affix those fracture segments more securely to the plate with locking screws has decreased implant detachment and fracture construct failure in my opinion. The increased surgeon confidence in fracture repair construct that LPs brings is invaluable and reflects the advancement the LP introduction to clinical orthopedics has achieved.

References

1. Tomlinson, J., Fox, D., Cook, J.L. et al. (2007). Measurement of femoral angles in four dog breeds. *Vet. Surg.* 36 (6): 593–598.
2. Swiderski, J.K., Radecki, S.V., Park, R.D. et al. (2008). Comparison of radiographic and anatomic femoral varus angle measurements in normal dogs. *Vet. Surg.* 37 (1): 43–48.
3. Dismukes, D.I., Fox, D.B., Tomlinson, J.L. et al. (2008). Determination of pelvic limb alignment in the large-breed dog: a cadaveric radiographic study in the frontal plane. *Vet. Surg.* 37 (7): 674–682.
4. Palmer, R.H., Ikuta, C.L., and Cadmus, J.M. (2011). Comparison of femoral angulation measurement between radiographs and anatomic specimens across a broad range of varus conformations. *Vet. Surg.* 40 (8): 1023–1028.
5. Bardet, J.F., Rudy, R.L., and Hohn, R.B. (1983). Measurement of femoral torsion in dogs using a biplanar method. *Vet. Surg.* 12: 1–6.
6. Montavon, P.M., Hohn, R.B., Olmstead, M.L. et al. (1985). Inclination and anteversion angles of the femoral head and neck in the dog: evaluation of a standard method of measurement. *Vet. Surg.* 14 (4): 277–282.

7. Hauptman, J., Cardinet, G.H. 3rd, Morgan, J.P. et al. (1985). Angles of inclination and anteversion in hip dysplasia in the dog. *Am. J. Vet. Res.* 46 (10): 2033–2036.
8. Dudley, R.M., Kowaleski, M.P., Drost, W.T. et al. (2006). Radiographic and computed tomographic determination of femoral varus and torsion in the dog. *Vet. Radiol. Ultrasound* 47: 546–552.
9. Ginja, M.M., Gonzalo-Orden, J.M., Jesus, S.S. et al. (2007). Measurement of the femoral neck anteversion angle in the dog using computed tomography. *Vet. J.* 174 (2): 378–383. Epub 2006 Oct 2.
10. Kaiser, S., Cornely, D., Golder, W. et al. (2001). The correlation of canine patellar luxation and the anteversion angle as measured using magnetic resonance images. *Vet. Radiol. Ultrasound.* 42 (2): 113–118.
11. Savio, G., Baroni, T., Concheri, G. et al. (2016). Computation of femoral canine morphometric parameters in three-dimensional geometrical models. *Vet. Surg.* 45 (8): 987–995.
12. Stoffel, K., Dieter, U., Stachowiak, G. et al. (2003). Biomechanical testing of the LCP - how can stability in locked internal fixators be controlled? *Injury* 34 (Suppl 2): B11–B19.
13. Aguila, A.Z., Manos, J.M., Orlansky, A.S. et al. (2005). In vitro biomechanical comparison of limited contact dynamic compression plate and locking compression plate. *Vet. Comp. Orthop. Traumatol.* 18 (4): 220–226.
14. Niemeyer, P. and Südkamp, N.P. (2006). Principles and clinical application of the locking compression plate (LCP). *Acta Chir. Orthop. Traumatol. Cechoslov.* 73 (4): 221–228. Review.
15. DeTora, M. and Kraus, K. (2008). Mechanical testing of 3.5mm locking and non-locking bone plates. *Vet. Comp. Orthop. Traumatol.* 21 (4): 318–322.
16. Filipowicz, D., Lanz, O., McLaughlin, R. et al. (2009). A biomechanical comparison of 3.5 locking compression plate fixation to 3.5 limited contact dynamic compression plate fixation in a canine cadaveric distal humeral metaphyseal gap model. *Vet. Comp. Orthop. Traumatol.* 22 (4): 270–277.
17. Irubetagoyena, I., Verset, M., Palierne, S. et al. (2013). Ex vivo cyclic mechanical behaviour of 2.4mm locking plates compared with 2.4mm limited contact plates in a cadaveric diaphyseal gap model. *Vet. Comp. Orthop. Traumatol.* 26 (6): 479–488.
18. DeTora, M. and Kraus, K. (2008). Mechanical testing of 3.5mm locking and non-locking bone plates. *Vet. Comp. Orthop. Traumatol.* 21 (4): 318–322.
19. Malenfant, R.C. and Sod, G.A. (2014). In vitro biomechanical comparison of 3.5 string of pearl plate fixation to 3.5 locking compression plate fixation in a canine fracture gap model. *Vet. Surg.* 43 (4): 465–470.
20. Ahmad, M., Nanda, R., Bajwa, A.S. et al. (2007). Biomechanical testing of the locking compression plate: when does the distance between bone and implant significantly reduce construct stability? *Injury* 38 (3): 358–364.
21. Hulse, D., Hyman, W., Nori, M. et al. (1997). Reduction in plate strain by addition of an intramedullary pin. *Vet. Surg.* 26 (6): 451–459.
22. Matres-Lorenzo, L., Diop, A., Maurel, N. et al. (2016). Biomechanical comparison of locking compression plate and limited contact dynamic compression plate combined with an intramedullary rod in a canine femoral fracture-gap model. *Vet. Surg.* 45 (3): 319–326.
23. Pearson, T., Glyde, M., Hosgood, G. et al. (2015). The effect of intramedullary pin size and monocortical screw configuration on locking compression plate-rod constructs in an in vitro fracture gap model. *Vet. Comp. Orthop. Traumatol.* 28 (2): 95–103.
24. Goh, C.S., Santoni, B.G., Puttlitz, C.M. et al. (2009). Comparison of the mechanical behaviors of semicontoured, locking plate-rod fixation and anatomically contoured, conventional plate-rod fixation applied to experimentally induced gap fractures in canine femora. *Am. J. Vet. Res.* 70 (1): 23–29.
25. Field, E.J., Parsons, K., Etches, J.A. et al. (2016). Effect of monocortical and bicortical screw numbers on the properties of a locking plate-intramedullary rod configuration. An in vitro study on a canine femoral fracture gap model. *Vet. Comp. Orthop. Traumatol.* 29 (6): 459–465.
26. Haaland, P.J., Sjöström, L., Devor, M. et al. (2009). Appendicular fracture repair in dogs using the locking compression plate system: 47 cases. *Vet. Comp. Orthop. Traumatol.* 22 (4): 309–315.
27. Vallefuoco, R., Le Pommellet, H., Savin, A. et al. (2016). Complications of appendicular fracture repair in cats and small dogs using locking compression plates. *Vet. Comp. Orthop. Traumatol.* 29 (1): 46–52.

16 Tibia Fractures

Kei Hayashi

Fractures of the tibia are relatively common in dogs and cats, accounting for 10–20% of all fractures [1–3]. Tibia fractures often result from trauma, and the majority of tibia fractures are diaphyseal fractures. Immediate immobilization of the crus is recommended and surgical treatment is often indicated. A variety of repair methods can be applied for tibial fractures, and the selection of repair technique depends on multiple factors, including the type and location of the fracture, the age of the animal, the presence of associated soft tissue defects and infection (particularly in open fractures), economic considerations, and the surgeon's preference. The overall prognosis following fracture of the tibia and fibula is generally good when appropriate treatment is applied.

Locking plate (LP) systems can provide simple, reliable, and effective treatment of challenging tibial fractures, nonunions, and deformities. The application of locking plate implant systems may have several significant advantages over conventional repair options, particularly in the following four specific situations:

1. Diaphyseal fractures treated with a minimally invasive technique, often in a "bridging" plate function
2. Proximal or distal juxta-articular fractures with a short segment of bone available for implant application
3. Revision of fracture repair complications including nonunions
4. Tibial deformity (pes varus and pes valgus) treated with corrective osetotomy/ostectomy based on the center of rotation of angulation (CORA) methods

16.1 Relevant Anatomy

The tibia has several unique anatomic features amenable to applications of locking plate systems. For example, the medial aspect of the tibia has a nominal soft tissue envelope, and therefore minimally invasive plate application can be performed easily, especially when a locking plate is used in bridging fashion. However, due to the tibia's sigmoid shape, adequate contouring is often necessary to prevent postoperative limb deformity. Anatomical landmarks are relatively easy to palpate in the tibia, and identification of the joint space is crucial in LP application to prevent inadvertent insertion of screws into the joints, as the majority of LP systems employ fixed-angle designs

Locking Plates in Veterinary Orthopedics, First Edition.
Edited by Matthew D. Barnhart and Karl C. Maritato.

for screw placement. Wide variation in the length and shape of the tibia and fibula is seen among canine breeds. The anatomy of the tibia in cats is similar to that of dogs. The medullary cavity of the feline tibia appears to be more uniform in diameter than in dogs, but no other substantial differences have been noted.

The proximal half of the tibia is three-sided proximally (medial, lateral, and caudal surfaces), whereas the distal half is essentially cylindrical and the entire medial part of the distal extremity of the tibia forms the medial malleolus. The proximal tibial metaphysis is relatively flat medially but is concave both laterally and caudally. All these surfaces blend into the tibial diaphysis, which is uniform in diameter but slightly S-shaped. It curves from medial to lateral in the proximal one-half and then from lateral to medial in the distal one-half. The distal part of the tibia is flared slightly and forms the distal articular surface and the medial malleolus. The medial malleolus is the proximal attachment of the medial collateral ligament of the talocrural joint.

The cranial branch of the medial saphenous artery and vein and the saphenous nerve pass obliquely across the diaphysis of the tibia, and care must be taken not to injure this bundle during surgical approach to medial diaphysis of the tibia. Arteries (such as the tibial and popliteal arteries) and nerves (such as the peroneal and cutaneous nerves) run along the lateral and caudal aspects of the tibia and fibula; however, surgical lateral approaches are rarely required.

16.1.1 Practical Tips and Tricks

- Locating joint spaces (stifle and tarsal joints) is crucial in LP application in order to prevent inadvertent screw insertion into a joint.
  - Palpation of landmarks around stifle (e.g. tibial tuberosity, fibular head) and placement of 25G needles at the proximal extent of tibia will help locate stifle joint space.
  - Palpation of medial malleolus will help locate talocrural joint space. It should be noted that the malleoli extend distal to the articular surface, and care must be taken not to place implants into talocrural joint space. In the majority of dogs, a safe corridor for screw insertion lies approximately halfway between the maximum peak of the malleolus and the start of the flare of the malleolus in the metaphysis.
- The medial aspect of the tibia is well-suited for LP application, as it has minimal soft tissue envelop and is relatively flat.
- Wide variation in shape of the proximal tibia is seen among canine breeds. Examination radiographs of the contralateral tibia will help identify this variation, if needed.
- In general, LP systems do not require precise countering for fracture fixation. However, in the tibia, due to its S-shaped anatomy, appropriate plate contouring is necessary to prevent postoperative valgus malalignment. Presurgical contouring of a plate using a ventrodorsal radiograph of the normal tibia as a template can help reduce operative time and facilitate minimally invasive plate osteosynthesis application.
- The tibia's S-shape typically precludes placement of a large-diameter intramedullary (IM) pin, and a large straight pin can cause valgus malalignment. If an IM pin is used (as a temporary reduction device, or as in a plate-rod combination), a pin approximately 30–40% of the diameter of the medullary canal at the tibial isthmus is chosen.
- The distal part of the tibia is flared slightly, which may provide some extra bone stock for screw placement, particularly when T-plate or plate-rod combination is chosen.

16.2 Minimally Invasive Plate Osteosynthesis of Diaphyseal Fractures

Diaphyseal fractures account for 70–80% of all tibial fractures. Oblique and spiral fractures are the most common fracture patterns recognized in small-animal patients of all ages, whereas comminuted and open fractures are more common in mature animals. Minimally invasive plating techniques, particularly using a locking plate, have been introduced for repair of tibial fractures in an effort to improve bone healing [4–6]. This

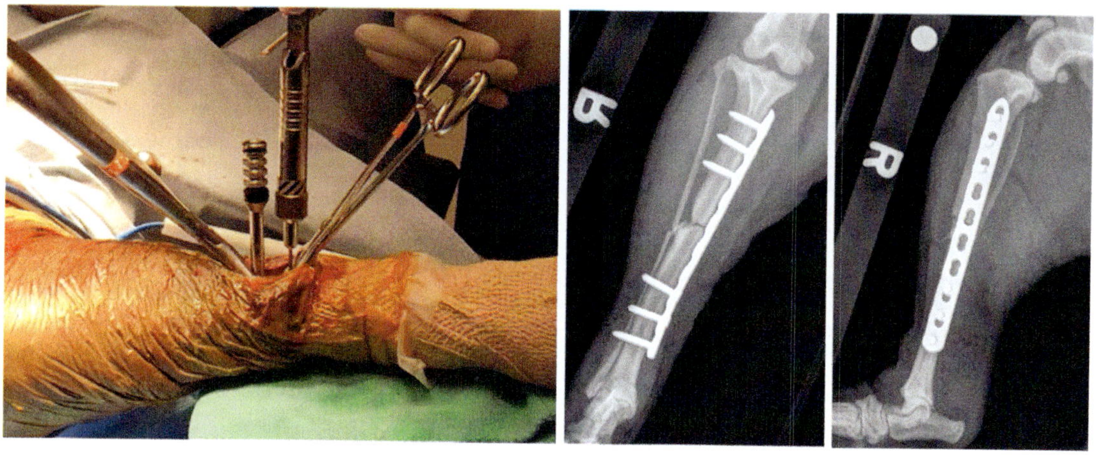

Figure 16.1 Minimally invasive plating techniques using a locking plate in a simple tibial fracture in a mature dog. This approach involves a small, medially located skin incision over the proximal and distal aspects of the tibia, remote from the fracture site. A soft tissue tunnel is created between the periosteal surface of the tibia and the overlying muscular fascia/vascular bundles, connecting the two incisions. A plate is then slid along the surface of the tibia, and screws are applied through the proximal and distal incisions. A locking plate usually functions as a bridging plate but can function as a compression plate, depending on fracture configuration, plate type, and application method.

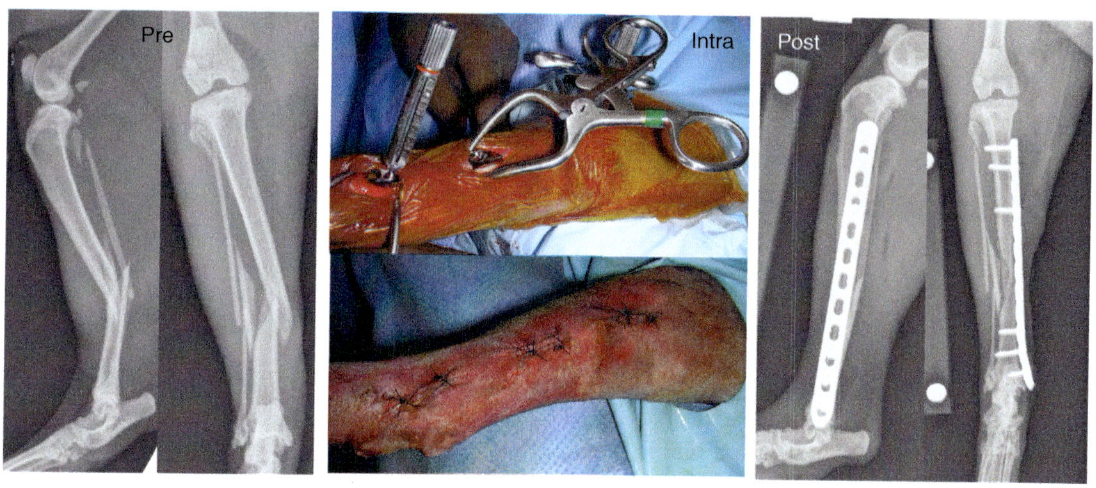

Figure 16.2 Minimally invasive plating techniques using a locking plate in a comminuted tibial fracture in a mature cat, applied in a bridging plate function. This approach involves a small, medially located skin incision over the proximal and distal aspects of the tibia. An additional small skin incision over the fracture site can be made to aid appropriate reduction and alignment. A carefully countered plate is then slid along the surface of the tibia, and screws are applied through the proximal and distal incisions. (Source: Courtesy of Dr. Amy Kapatkin.)

approach, also called *minimally invasive plate osteosynthesis (MIPO)*, involves a small, medially located skin incision over the proximal and distal aspects of the tibia, remote from the fracture site (Figures 16.1–16.3) [4, 7]. A soft tissue tunnel is created between the periosteal surface of the tibia and the overlying muscular fascia connecting the two incisions (Figures 16.1 and 16.2). A plate is then slid along the surface of the tibia, and screws are applied through the proximal and distal incisions. An IM pin can be combined with MIPO application (Figure 16.3). The technique has clinical efficacy and greatly improves postoperative patient comfort, but there is no documented difference in healing times between MIPO and open plating techniques [6, 8].

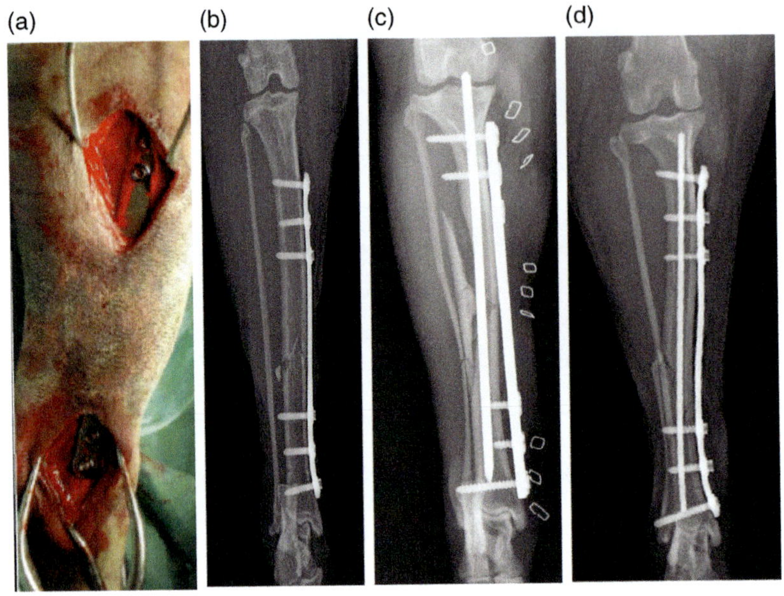

Figure 16.3 Intramedullary (IM) pin and locking plate combination. Minimally invasive plating techniques can be combined with IM pin to facilitate fracture reduction, reduce the necessity of precise plate countering, and extend fatigue life of implants. Through small skin incisions (a), a countered locking plate alone (b), an IM pin and an uncountered locking plate (c), or an IM pin and a countered locking plate can be applied in tibial fractures (d). (Source: Courtesy of Dr. Brian Beal.)

16.2.1 Practical Tips and Tricks for Tibia MIPO

- Functional limb alignment needs to be restored by carefully examining the joints above and below, particularly for comminuted fractures. Rotational and valgus/varus malalignment will result in limb dysfunction.
- Careful palpation of anatomical landmarks may help restore cranio-caudal alignment; the cranial border of the tibial crest is fairly parallel to the axis of the mid-distal tibia.
- In plate-rod combinations, a normograde IM pin can be placed with a minimal approach to the stifle/proximal tibia. This will achieve general restoration of alignment, length, and reduction of the fractured tibia. Then, through two small proximal and distal skin incisions, the locking plate is pushed under the soft tissue and neuro-vascular bundles, immediately over the bone. Two or three locking screws are placed through both incisions, away from the fracture site.

16.3 Proximal and Distal Fractures with a Short Fracture Segment

Proximal and distal fractures present a unique challenge for repair because the segment can be very short, and the amount of bone available for implant application is significantly limited. Plating may be applicable, depending on the size of the patient and the fracture pattern. Specially designed plates (such as the T-plate) are advantageous if three (or more) screws can be inserted into the short segment. Circular (ring) or hybrid external skeletal fixators are an excellent choice for fractures with a short segment; however, they can be technically demanding, postoperative care is intensive, complications are common, and postoperative patient comfort can be a problem. The application of locking plates may allow simpler fracture management in the proximal/distal tibia, as two locking screws in the short segment may provide adequate stability (Figures 16.4 and 16.5) [4, 9].

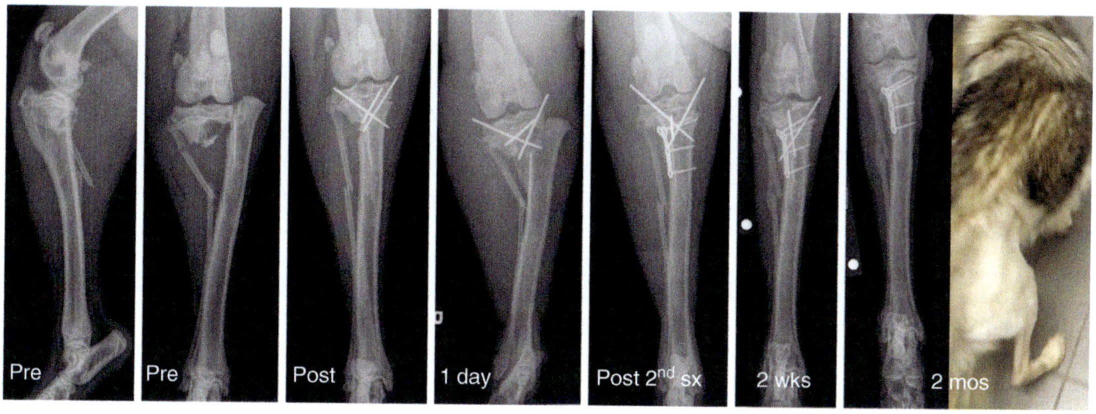

Figure 16.4 A locking T-plate applied in a "buttress" fashion after failure of pin fixation in a physeal comminuted fracture in a four-month-old large-breed puppy. The plate was applied to a very short segment of proximal metaphysis without violating physis, on the side of the comminution in order to function as a buttress plate. The patient demonstrated an excellent limb function at two months after plate fixation.

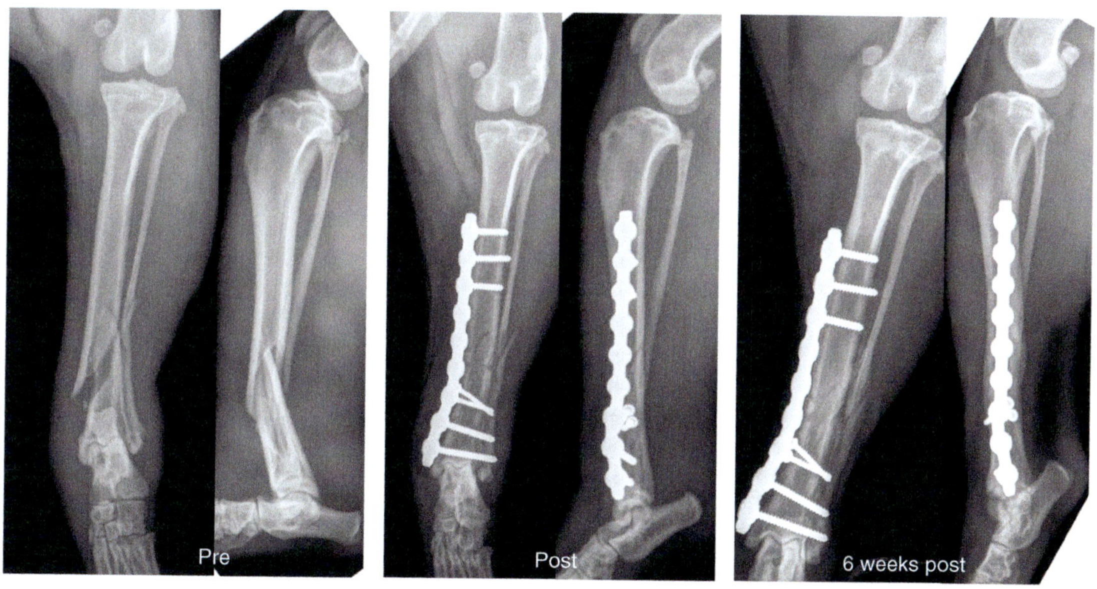

Figure 16.5 Distal diaphyseal/metaphyseal fractures of the tibia and fibula repaired with two lag screws and a "neutralization" plate in a mature dog. Note there are only two locking screws in the short distal segment, but postoperative radiographs show stable bone-implant construct and adequate bone healing at six weeks postsurgery.

16.3.1 Practical Tips and Tricks

- In cases with proximal Salter-Harris type fractures, locating growth plate (as well as joint space) is crucial. This can be done by intra-operative direct visual inspection and/or size/distance measurement on preoperative radiographs. Extremely small bone stock in metaphyseal segments often requires locking T-plate application.
- Plate contouring is necessary for both proximal and distal fractures.
- It should be noted that the malleoli extend distal to the articular surface, and care must be taken not to place implants into talotibial joint space.

- After contouring a locking plate, the screw angles will be altered; therefore, care must be taken not to insert a screw into the joint, particularly when fixed-angle locking plates are used.
- While a few veterinary LP systems allow for polyaxial screw insertion, and thus permit angling of the screws away from the joint space, the majority of LP systems employ a fixed-angle mechanism. To avoid screw insertion into the joint in these systems, you can (i) use regular cortical screws at a desired angle (before locking screw placement), (ii) use short mono-cortical locking screws, or (iii) adjust contouring.

16.4 Revision of Fracture Complications

Complications associated with repair of fractures of the tibia are similar to those reported for other long-bone fracture repairs and include infection, implant failure, delayed union, nonunion, and malunion. Nonunion occurred in approximately 4% of tibial diaphyseal fractures in a study of 195 dogs and cats [2].

A variety of cases series and case reports describe outcomes following plate fixation in the repair of tibial fractures. A case report documenting the use of a locking plate applied to the medial aspect of the tibia of a large dog with a comminuted diaphyseal fracture and multiple limb injury included a description of a major complication with plate failure (bending) and resultant valgus deformity [9]. Malalignment or angular or rotational limb deformity is a serious complication that may be associated with inappropriate fixation technique, as seen in medial bone plate fixation with under contouring, or with implant failure, particularly in medial plating for comminuted fractures that have no lateral cortical support (Figure 16.6) [9–11]. Revision surgery with more rigid fixation is often necessary to correct postoperative malalignment (Figure 16.6) [9].

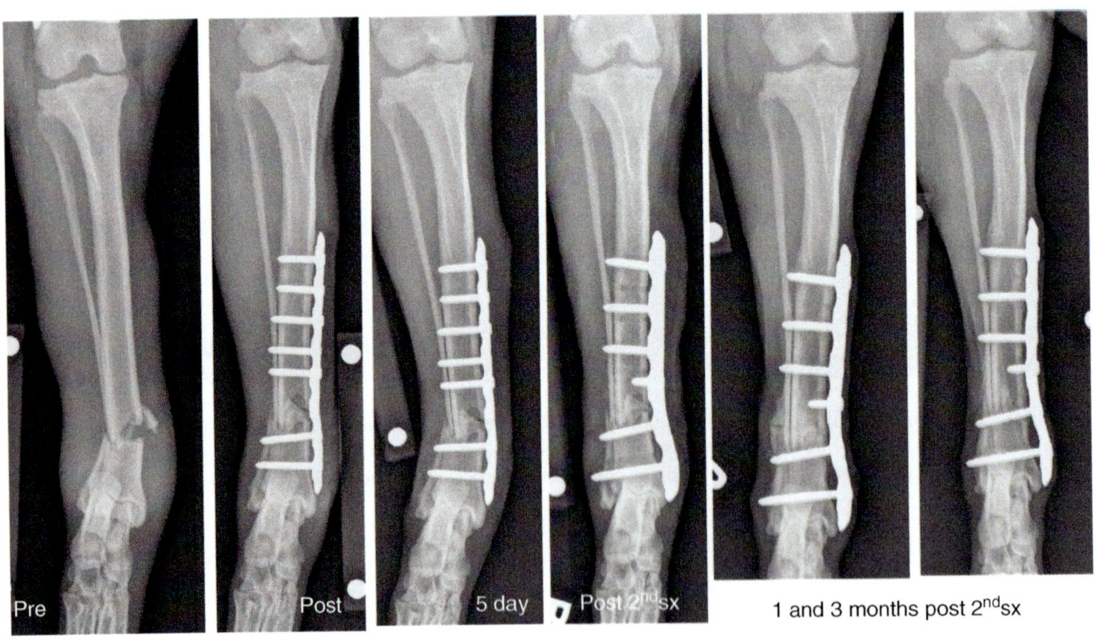

Figure 16.6 Revision of implant failure of an undersized and undercountered locking plate applied to the medial aspect of the tibia with a comminuted distal diaphyseal fracture in a mature dog. Plate failure (bending) and resultant valgus deformity were revised with a much larger, better-countered locking plate. Postoperative radiographs show stable bone-implant construct and progressive bone healing with maintenance of excellent limb alignment.

16.4.1 Practical Tips and Tricks

- Undercounting of the medial plate will result in valgus deformity and severe dysfunction of the limb. Revision with locking plate systems may be necessary to restore bone-screw security and rigid construct stability, as existing screw holes may have been compromised.
- Implant failure (such as plate bending) will result in valgus deformity and severe dysfunction of the limb. Revision with locking plate systems may be necessary to restore bone–screw security and rigid construct stability, as existing screw holes have been compromised and damaged.
- Plate breakage at a screw hole over/near the fracture site may be caused by a phenomenon called stress concentration. Revision by a large locking plate in a braiding plate fashion may be necessary to restore rigid construct stability.

The cause of nonunion and malunion in the tibia is usually inappropriate fixation and resultant inadequate stability, as is commonly seen with external coaptation, IM pin fixation, and external skeletal fixators. In some cases, bone healing is complicated by infection and osteomyelitis (Figures 16.7 and 16.8). Closed reduction and external skeletal fixator repair of comminuted fractures of the tibia generally result in a good outcome; however, reported complications include nonunion, malunion, and infection/osteomyelitis associated with the wire/pin tract (Figure 16.8) [12–14]. Locking plate systems can be effectively applied for revision surgery for complications associated with repair of tibial fractures (Figures 16.6–16.8).

16.4.2 Practical Tips and Tricks

- Chronic infection and pin tract morbidity can be associated with external skeletal fixators, cerclage wires, and loosened screws. In these situations, these devises need to be removed, and the bone must be stabilized if it has not yet healed. Internal fixation with locking plate system may be an ideal choice since they provide excellent stability, and locking screws can be placed distant from the infection sites. Fresh autogenous cancellous bone graft is always recommended.

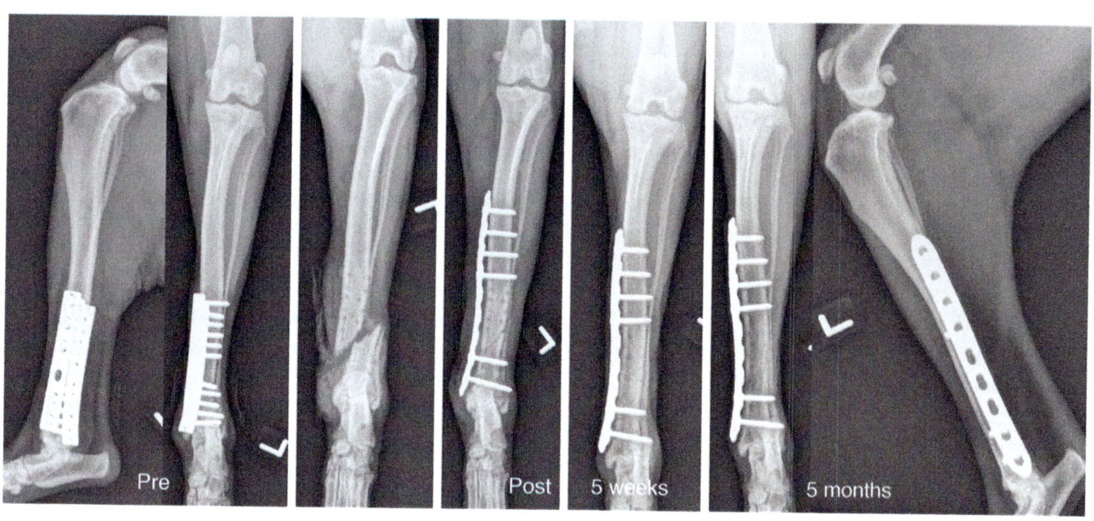

Figure 16.7 Revision of nonunion and chronic infection of distal tibia in a mature dog. Chronic draining from double plate site was originally treated with plate removal, which resulted in an immediate refracture. A countered locking plate was applied to the medial aspect of the tibia and the infection was treated with systemic antibiotics based on culture/sensitivity tests for over eight weeks. Postoperative radiographs show adequate bone healing and resolution of infection.

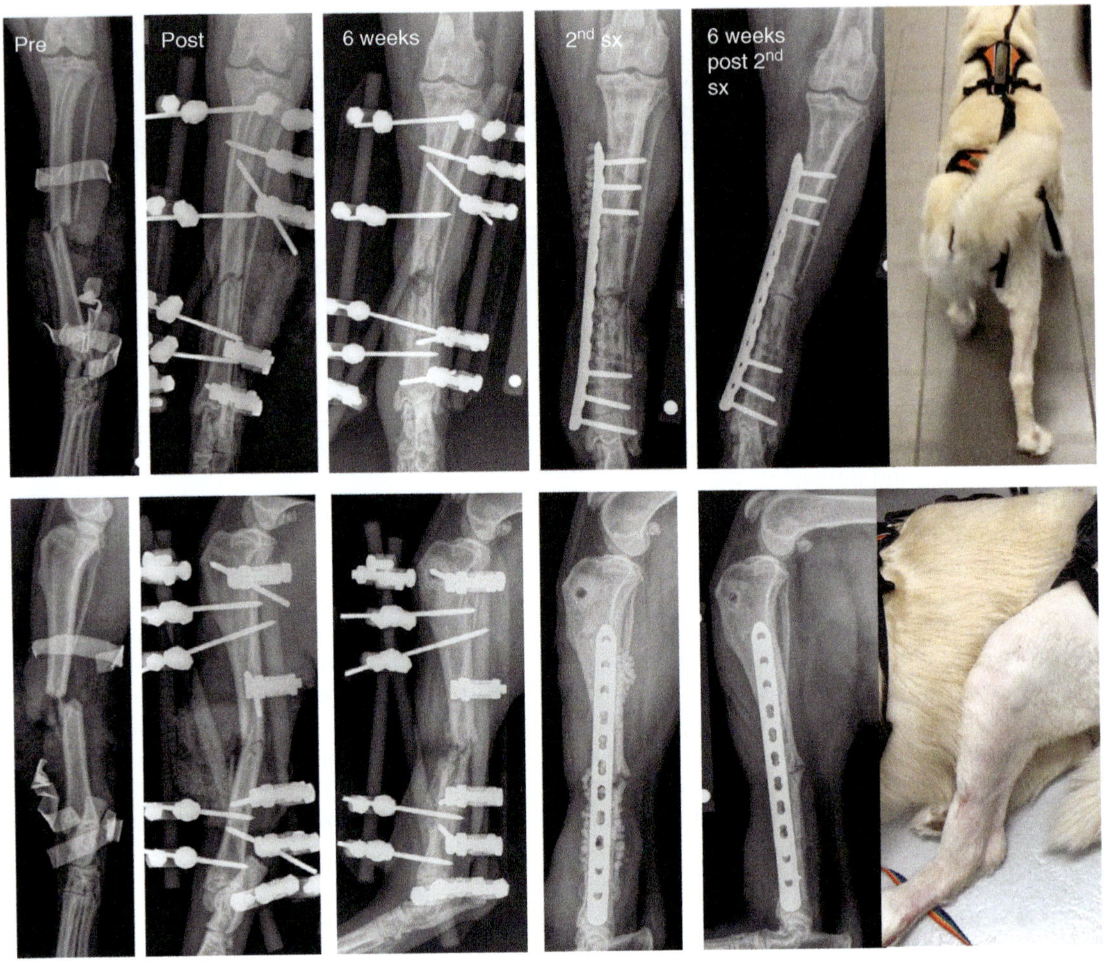

Figure 16.8 Revision of delayed union and osteomyelitis of tibia in a mature dog. Open fracture of the tibia with significant soft tissue loss was originally treated with external skeletal fixators and vacuum-assisted closure system, which resulted in chronic osteomyelitis, malalignment, and delayed union at six weeks after the injury. A large locking plate was applied to the medial aspect of the tibia with antibiotics impregnated absorbable beads around the infection sites. Postoperative radiographs show progressive bone healing and resolution of infection at six weeks after the plating, and the patient demonstrated excellent limb function.

- Local and regional antibiotic delivery can be considered with antibiotic-impregnated absorbable beads, nonabsorbable beads or pluronic gel, or by frequent local antibiotic injections when internal fixation is used.

16.5 Surgical Correction of Tibial Deformity

Deformity of the tibia can occur without trauma/fracture; these conditions are considered congenital and developmental. Pes valgus has been recognized in large-breed dogs (Figure 16.9), and pes varus has been recognized in Dachshunds (Figure 16.10) [15–19]. In these reported cases, there was no history of trauma and the condition was often bilateral; therefore, a hereditary cause was suspected [19, 20]. Pes valgus and pes varus are often associated with abnormal limb alignment and stifle pathology, including patellar luxation [21, 22]. Pes valgus and pes varus that cause clinical signs of lameness may require surgical correction. Surgical treatment for these deformities involves corrective osteotomy/ostectomy and realignment of the limb.

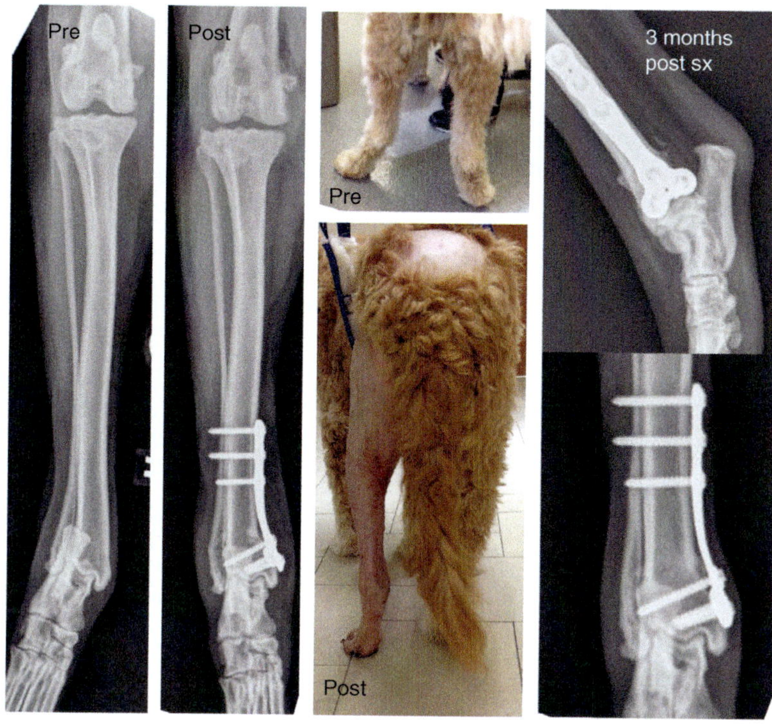

Figure 16.9 Pes valgus treated with corrective closing wedge ostectomy in a 1.5-year-old large-breed dog. The short distal segment was fixed with a countered locking T-plate, resulting in immediate improvement in limb alignment. Postoperative radiographs showed stable bone-implant construct and adequate healing of the ostectomy at three months postsurgery. (Source: Courtesy of Dr. Adrienne Bentley.)

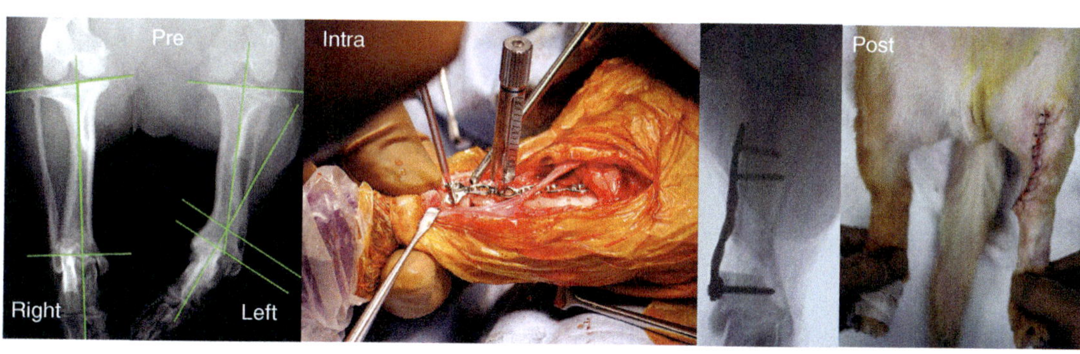

Figure 16.10 Pes varus treated with corrective opening wedge osteotomy in a mature Miniature Dachshund. The distal short segment was fixed with a countered locking T-plate, and autogenous cortico-cancellous bone graft was applied to the gap, resulting in immediate improvement in limb alignment. (Source: Courtesy of Drs. Satoshi Kobayashi and Hirokazu Mori.)

Successful surgical correction for pes valgus has been reported using plate and plate-rod combinations [15, 16]. Pes varus is most commonly recognized in Dachshunds, and surgical treatment with open-wedge corrective osteotomy has been reported using linear external skeletal fixators, hybrid external skeletal fixators, plate fixation, and plate-rod fixation [18, 19, 22]. To aid planning of the corrective osteotomy and to improve the outcome of surgical correction, standardized radiographic techniques and measurement methods of various parameters in dogs have been investigated [23]. Corrective osteotomy and ostectomy based on the CORA methods is recommended; however, surgery is highly challenging because the CORA is typically very distal, so the amount of bone available for implant application is limited. Use of locking plates may allow simpler management of tibial deformities, as two to three locking screws in the distal segment may provide adequate stability (Figures 16.9 and 16.10) [4, 7–9].

16.5.1 Practical Tips and Tricks

- Determining the clinical relevance of a tibial deformity can be a challenge, since they do not always cause pain or lameness, and it can be bilateral. Additionally, breed standards for "normal" tibial anatomy have not been fully documented, and currently there are no guidelines for surgical indication.
- Careful planning is crucial in corrective osteotomy/ostectomy. A CT scan will greatly aid in defining the deformity and will help with planning correction. Additionally, planning and practicing corrective surgery by creating a model from the CT scan using a 3D printer has become an increasingly practical option.
- Use of fluoroscopy (C-arm) is helpful for avoiding the articular structures distally and maximizing screw purchase.
- It should be noted that bone segments after osteotomy are extremely small in Miniature Dachshunds. Locking T-plate application has numerous advantages over previously reported methods.

References

1. Boone, E.G., Johnson, A.L., and Hohn, R.B. (1986). Distal tibial fractures in dogs and cats. *J. Am. Vet. Med. Assoc.* 188: 36.
2. Boone, E.G., Johnson, A.L., Montavon, P. et al. (1986). Fractures of the tibial diaphysis in dogs and cats. *J. Am. Vet. Med. Assoc.* 188: 41.
3. Unger, M., Montavon, P.M., and Heim, U.F.A. (1990). Classification of fractures of long bones in the dog and cat: introduction and clinical application. *Vet. Comp. Orthop. Traumatol.* 3: 41.
4. Pozzi, A. and Lewis, D. (2009). Surgical approaches for minimally invasive plate osteosynthesis in dogs. *Vet. Comp. Orthop. Traumatol.* 22: 316.
5. Sarrau, S., Meige, F., and Autefage, A. (2007). Treatment of femoral and tibial fractures in puppies by elastic plate osteosynthesis: a review of 17 cases. *Vet. Comp. Orthop. Traumatol.* 20: 51.
6. Schmökel, H.G., Stein, S., Radke, H. et al. (2007). Treatment of tibial fractures with plates using minimally invasive percutaneous osteosynthesis in dogs and cats. *J. Small Anim. Pract.* 48: 157.
7. Guiot, L.P. and Déjardin, L.M. (2011). Prospective evaluation of minimally invasive plate osteosynthesis in 36 nonarticular tibial fractures in dogs and cats. *Vet. Surg.* 40: 171–182.
8. Boero Baroncelli, A., Peirone, B., Winter, M.D. et al. (2012). Retrospective comparison between minimally invasive plate osteosynthesis and open plating for tibial fractures in dogs. *Vet. Comp. Orthop. Traumatol.* 25: 410–417.
9. Schwandt, C.S. and Montavon, P.M. (2005). Locking compression plate fixation of radial and tibial fractures in a young dog. *Vet. Comp. Orthop. Traumatol.* 18: 194.
10. Dudley, M., Johnson, A.L., and Olmstead, M. (1997). Open reduction and bone plate stabilization, compared with closed reduction and external fixation, for treatment of comminuted tibial fractures: 47 cases (1980–1995) in dogs. *J. Am. Vet. Med. Assoc.* 211: 1008.
11. Piermattei, D.L., Flo, G.L., and DeCamp, C.E. (2006). Fractures of the tibia and fibula. In: *Flo's Handbook of Small Animal Orthopedics and Fracture Repair*, 4 (ed. P. Brinker), 633. Philadelphia: Saunders.
12. Anderson, G.M., Lewis, D.D., Radasch, R.M. et al. (2003). Circular external skeletal fixation stabilization of antebrachial and crural fractures in 25 dogs. *J. Am. Anim. Hosp. Assoc.* 39: 479.
13. Johnson, A.L., Seitz, S.E., Smith, C.W. et al. (1996). Closed reduction and type-II external fixation of comminuted fractures of the radius and tibia in dogs: 23 cases (1990–1994). *J. Am. Vet. Med. Assoc.* 209: 1445.
14. Kraus, K.H., Wotton, H.M., and Boudrieau, R.J. (1998). Type-II external fixation, using new clamps and positive-profile threaded pins, for treatment of fractures of the radius and tibia in dogs. *J. Am. Vet. Med. Assoc.* 212: 1267.
15. Altunatmaz, K., Ozsoy, S., and Guzel, O. (2007). Bilateral pes valgus in an Anatolian sheepdog. *Vet. Comp. Orthop. Traumatol.* 20: 241.
16. Burton, N.J. and Owen, M.R. (2007). Limb alignment of pes valgus in a giant breed dog by plate-rod fixation. *Vet. Comp. Orthop. Traumatol.* 20: 236.
17. Jevens, D.J. and DeCamp, C.E. (1993). Bilateral distal fibular growth abnormalities in a dog. *J. Am. Vet. Med. Assoc.* 202: 421.

18. Johnson, S.G., Hulse, D.A., Vangundy, T.E. et al. (1989). Corrective osteotomy for pes varus in the dachshund. *Vet. Surg.* 18: 373.
19. Radasch, R.M., Lewis, D.F., McDonald, D.E. et al. (2008). Pes varus correction in dachshunds using a hybrid external fixator. *Vet. Surg.* 37: 71.
20. Yoneji, K., Yoneji, W., Okamura, T. et al (2007). Incidence and inheritable character of Dachshund tibial dysplasia in Japan. Presented at: 34th Veterinary Orthopedic Society, Sun Valley, ID, March 4–10, p 89.
21. Yoneji, K., Higuchi, M., Kawata, M. (2006). Corrective osteotomy for tibial dysplasia in Dachshund. Presented at: 2nd World Veterinary Congress, Keystone, CO, February 25–March 4, p. 215.
22. Petazzoni, M., Nicetto, T., Vezzoni, A. et al. (2012). Treatment of pes varus using locking plate fixation in seven dachshund dogs. *Vet. Comp. Orthop. Traumatol.* 25: 231–238.
23. Dismukes, D.I., Tomlinson, J.L., and Fox, D.B. (2008). Radiographic measurement of canine tibial angles in the sagittal plane. *Vet. Surg.* 37: 300.

Section IV

Trauma Applications: Clinical Case Examples

IV-B Axial Skeletal Fractures

17 Pelvic Fractures

Shawn C. Kennedy

Pelvic fractures in the dog and cat represent approximately 20–30% of all fractures and are usually associated with severe trauma [1, 2]. Surgical therapy is focused on important structural fractures, such as fractures causing significant pelvic canal collapse, fractures disrupting load transmission from the limb to the spine, and disruption of the continuity of the articular surface of the acetabulum with subsequent instability. The presence of significant pain and neurologic dysfunction are also indications for repair. Generally, pelvic fractures are repaired if involving the ilial body, acetabulum, and/or sacroiliac joints. Locking plates are particularly well-suited for treatment of comminuted ilial body fractures, acetabular fractures associated with ilial body fracture, supracotyloid fractures, young patients with "soft" bone, and patients with poor mineral bone density.

The pelvis is a continuous osseous box composed of an ilium, ischium, pubis, and acetabulum on each side. Fractures generally displace if three or more bones are involved or if the sacroiliac joint(s) is involved; in immature patients, two fractures can be present because of the elasticity of the bone. Not all ilial body fractures are simple transverse or oblique fractures, in which reduction and compression is an excellent way to repair the fracture quickly. Frequently, a surgeon will be presented with a supracotyloid fracture (small distal ilial fracture cranial to the acetabulum) or with a small fragment of the cranial aspect of the ilial wing available for screw purchase. Fortunately, comminuted ilial fractures are not common (approximately 16%) because open repair and anatomic reconstruction is difficult [3]. Locking plate technology allows for a more biologic repair compared to traditional anatomic reduction and compression with dynamic compression plating (DCP) systems (Table 17.1).

Lateral plate fixation is the most commonly used approach, although the tension side of the ilial body is located ventrally [4]. However, access to the ventral surface of the ilium is difficult clinically, and application of a locking plates to the tension side of a bone is less critical than for conventional plates. A ventrolateral approach provides the most thorough access to all aspects of the ilium (dorsal, ventral, and lateral) and the most optimal visualization through a gluteal roll-up. It also provides access to the bone via muscle separation and subperiosteal elevation rather than muscle transection. The middle gluteal can be elevated and rolled up or down, depending on the aspect of the

Locking Plates in Veterinary Orthopedics, First Edition.
Edited by Matthew D. Barnhart and Karl C. Maritato.

Table 17.1 Comparison of veterinary locking systems in regards to properties important to pelvic fracture repair.

	Locking or nonlocking screws	Axial compression	Variable or fixed-angle screws	Three-dimensional contour
Synthes LCP[a]	Both same hole	Yes	Fixed	Yes, reconstruction only
Orthomed SOP[b]	Locking only	No	Fixed	Yes
Veterinary instrumentation	Both	Variable	Fixed	Yes, reconstruction only
Securos PAX[c]	Locking only	No	Variable	Variable
Kyon ALPS[d]	Both same hole	Yes	Variable for regular screws and fixed for locking screws	Yes
Traumavet Fixin	Locking only	No	Fixed	No

[a] Locking compression plate.
[b] String of pearls.
[c] Polyaxial.
[d] Advanced locking plate system.

ilium needed (ventral, lateral, or dorsal aspects). Although branches of the cranial gluteal vein, artery, and nerve can be retracted or transected if needed, care should be taken to preserve the lateral circumflex femoral vessels immediately cranial to the acetabulum. The sciatic nerve lies immediately dorsomedial to the ilium and traverses the ilium at the ischiatic notch and must not be injured during reduction and stabilization. Reduction of the caudal fragment is best with reduction forceps and/or through the use of the plate placed in the caudal segment. A precontoured plate (based on opposite side anatomy or cadaver) will significantly improve reduction of medially displaced caudal fragments as well as realignment of the weight-bearing axis of the pelvis. The usage of a Verbrugge clamp or a plate-reduction clamp applied to the cranial aspect of the plate/ilium allows reduction.

Although simple transverse fractures are easily compressed and locking plate technology is not critical for this type of repair, the unique morphology of the ilium allows for early screw loosening and subsequent pelvic canal narrowing. In cats, screw loosening occurred less often with locking plates or doubling the locking plate application compared to DCP [5]. Hybrid locking systems, which accommodate nonlocking screws with oval dynamic compression style screw holes, may be ideal for transverse fractures because they combine the benefits of the compression reduction of a DCP, and the screw-loosening prevention of a locking plate. If using the combination of locking and nonlocking screws in the ilium, it is important to apply the nonlocking screws in the caudal fragment first, prior to the locking screws, as the locking screws will hold the plate in a fixed position relative to the bone. After using the plate to help reduction of the fracture, the cranial compression screw is applied next prior to the subsequent locking screws, allowing for the advantage of the bone holding strength of the locking screws. However, only hybrid-style locking plates allow concurrent compression and locking screws within the same plate, limiting the benefits of the compression to those types of plating systems.

When applying a locking plate to an acetabular fracture, proper apposition and alignment of articular surfaces is as critical as with nonlocking plates. Segmental ilial body fractures involving the acetabulum will likely cause gross displacement of the free segment(s), resulting in narrowing of the pelvic canal and disruption of skeletal continuity between the spinal column and the pelvic limb and osteoarthritis of the acetabulum. Reconstruction plates have been a valuable implant that allows repair of concurrent ilium and acetabular fractures, as the plate allows three planes of contour compared to two planes of the conventional DCP. There are some locking plate systems (polyaxial [PAX] and string of pearls [SOP], for example) that allow this type of contouring as well; however, when twisting and bending a locking plate, the screw holes can become deformed, resulting in a failed locking mechanism. Different systems have techniques designed to limit this negative consequence. Certain locking systems have been utilized to aid in similar fixation as a traditional reconstruction plate when combining ilial and acetabular fracture repair. One study did not show a significant advantage when using locking plate technology in a simple transverse acetabular model compared to a traditional plate in respect to joint congruity, displacement of fracture gap, construct stiffness, or ultimate load to failure. However, the locking plate used unicortical screws, adding a large advantage to the locking plate [6].

Given the degree of difficulty contouring acetabular plates, there is a substantial advantage of being able to use a unicortical screw near the acetabulum to avoid acetabular penetration with a bicortical screw. Also, because precise contouring of the plate is unnecessary, it can be applied more easily once the fracture is anatomically reduced without loss of reduction. Polyaxial locking plates have an advantage over fixed-angle locking plates around the acetabulum because the degrees of freedom in these plates makes the task of exposing an acetabular fracture less burdensome. PAX plates have up to 10° of freedom, interchangeable screws between 2.0–2.4 mm and 2.7–3.5 mm systems, and the ability to remove screws and adjust angulation as needed. Therefore, in this location, the placement of the plate around the acetabulum can be improved as less soft tissue dissection is necessary. Unfortunately, since acetabular fractures are articular, absolute stability is best. The relative stability of locking plates makes their use in simple acetabular fractures not the best choice.

Supracotyloid fractures, given the small fragments of bone available, are a great option for the relative stability given by the locking plates, as well as the ability to use fewer screws per segment of bone. Reconstruction plates can be added side by side to add more purchase to small bone segments. T-type plates are also valuable in this location to aid in bone purchase.

References

1. Lanz, O.I. (2002). Lumbosacral and pelvic injuries. *Vet. Clin. North Am. Small Anim. Pract.* 32: 949–962.
2. Hill, F.W.G. (1977). A survey of bone fractures in the cat. *J. Small Anim. Pract.* 18: 457–463.
3. Breshears, L.A., Fitch, R.B., Wallace, L.J. et al. (2004). The radiographic evaluation of repaired canine ilial fractures (69 cases). *Vet. Comp. Orthop. Traumatol.* 17: 64–72.
4. Vangundy, T.E., Hulse, D.A., Nelson, J.K. et al. (1988). Mechanical evaluation of two canine iliac fracture fixation systems. *Vet. Surg.* 17: 321–327.
5. Schmierer, P.A., Kircher, P.R., Hartnack, S. et al. (2015)). Screw loosening and Pelvic Canal narrowing after lateral plating of Feling Ilial fractures with locking and nonlocking plates. *Vet. Surg.* 44: 900–904.
6. Amato, N.A., Richards, A., Knight, T.A. et al. (2008). Ex vivo biomechanical comparison of the 2.4 mm uniLOCK reconstruction plate using 2.4 mm locking versus standard screws for fixation of acetabular osteotomy in dogs. *Vet. Surg.* 37: 741–748.

18 Maxillofacial and Mandibular Fractures

Boaz Arzi and Frank J.M. Verstraete

18.1 Anatomical Considerations

The mandibular and maxillofacial region is a complex area that poses challenges when planning the placement of internal fixation devices. In the mandibular, maxillary, and incisive bones, the teeth occupy a large portion of the bone preventing placement of screws without causing dental damage. Furthermore, the maxillary and the mandibular bones also contain important blood vessels and nerves, further limiting placement of internal fixation [1]. For example, the infraorbital foramen of the maxilla, through which the infraorbital neurovascular bundle emerges, lies dorsal to the third premolar tooth. The mandibular canal contains the inferior alveolar neurovascular bundle and rostrally the buccal surface of the mandible has the middle and caudal mental foramina through which the corresponding mental nerves and blood vessels emerge [1]. In addition, the relative position of the mandibular canal and the infraorbital foramen may differ, based on the size of the dog and skull configuration. These important aspects are the cornerstones of planning where to place plates and screws in order to avoid iatrogenic damage while still maintaining effective and biomechanically stable internal fixation. In the mandibular and maxillofacial region, plate exposure through the oral mucosa and endodontal damage to teeth and the mandibular canal, are potential complications when a plate is positioned near the alveolar margins [2, 3]. Furthermore, collateral damage to important anatomic structures such as major neurovascular bundles should also be avoided.

18.2 Biomechanics

Internal fixation failure is an important complication that can occur when the mechanical load is excessive in proportion to the implant, wrong implant selection and when bone quality is poor [2, 3]. Historically, for mandibular fracture fixation and reconstruction, miniplate systems were applied near the alveolar margin in an attempt to counter mandibular bone stresses in accordance with the tension band principle [3, 13]. Application of the tension band principle is based on the assumption that anatomic reconstructions are strongest when fixation devices are loaded in tension. Placement of a small plate along the lines of tensile stress (i.e. Champy lines) would be used to neutralize

Locking Plates in Veterinary Orthopedics, First Edition.
Edited by Matthew D. Barnhart and Karl C. Maritato.

applied functional forces [3, 13]. However, recent biomechanical studies have demonstrated that a plate near the alveolar margin is not needed, as adequate internal fixation can be achieved using a single mandibular locking reconstruction plate placed at mid-mandibular height [2]. Furthermore, miniplates applied on the alveolar margin are associated with unavoidable damage to the roots of the teeth and tend to become exposed to the oral cavity [2, 3].

Our clinical experience and research over the past several years using locking reconstruction plates for mandibular fracture and critical-sized defects repair has revealed that a single plate placed in a buccal position (just ventral to the tooth roots and dorsal to the mandibular canal) can adequately resist mechanical load without clinical or radiographic evidence of collateral damage to blood vessels, nerves, or tooth roots or plate exposure through the mucosa [4, 5].

The thin bones of the maxillofacial complex provide a lightweight but strong frame filled with the air spaces of the nasal cavity and paranasal sinuses [6, 7]. The maxillofacial frame is strengthened by the support of the buttresses that maintain the appropriate position of the maxilla in relation to the base of the skull and the mandibles [6, 7]. Implant selection should take these biomechanical factors into consideration. We use nonlocking miniplates for the maxillofacial region as they are easier to contour to match the complex tridimensional morphology and are not subjected to the sustained loads that mandibles are.

18.3 Materials

18.3.1 Locking Reconstruction Plates for the Mandible

The authors use 2.4–3.0 mm titanium locking plates (Synthes® Maxillofacial, Paoli, PA) for mandibular fracture fixation or reconstruction of critical-size defects in medium to large breed dogs [2, 4, 8]. Veterinary adaptation plates are available and can be cut as needed. A single plate is secured on each side of the fracture or defect with at least three 3 mm bicortical, locking screws of appropriate length in which two screw-threads are exposed on the lingual aspect. For small-breed dogs and cats, the authors use a single locking titanium 2.0 mm miniplate (Synthes Maxillofacial, Paoli, PA) that is adapted to the desired anatomical contour of the mandible and, at a minimum, two bicortical 2.0 mm locking screws are used on each side of the fracture or defect [5].

18.3.2 Nonlocking Titanium Miniplates for the Maxillofacial Bones

For the maxillofacial bones, the authors use a variety of low-profile titanium 2.0 mm nonlocking miniplates (Synthes Maxillofacial 2.0 mm Mandible Trauma, Paoli, PA) [6]. These plates can also be cut and contoured, using specially designed miniplate bending cutters and pliers. For controlled drilling, a 4 or 6 mm self-stopping drill bit or regular-length drill bit can be used to create a 1.5 mm core hole for the 2.0 mm screw thread diameter. The length of the screws placed can be determined by using computed tomography measurements of the bone thickness or a depth-gauge. At least two nonlocking, self-tapping 2.0 mm titanium screws should be placed on either side of the fracture.

18.4 Surgical Approach

The surgical approach for placing internal fixation into the mandibular and maxillofacial bones should be done in the least traumatic, yet effective, method of exposure [1]. As the region is very rich in major blood vessels, nerves, and salivary glands and ducts, care must be taken to avoid damaging these structures. However, if the region underwent trauma, the normal anatomy may be distorted. Exposure of the mandibular and maxillofacial bones frequently requires subperiosteal elevation of the muscles that adhere to the underlying bone.

There are three options to approach the mandibular and the maxillofacial bones: intraoral approach, extraoral approach, and a combination of the two. A step-by-step description of extra- and intraoral approaches for the bones of the region is not within the scope of this chapter; it has been described elsewhere [1]. Intraoral approaches can be used for fractures of the mandible, maxilla, and incisive bone. The typical intraoral incision lines are made within the alveolar mucosa 3–4 mm away from the mucogingival junction. Most commonly, an extraoral approach is used for placing internal fixation, as it allows better exposure of the fracture or bones to be plated. Regardless of the method used, an approach through a traumatic wound should be avoided. A limited approach should be avoided, as it will force the surgeon to exert excessive pressure when manipulating the wound, which will further injure the area and not provide adequate access to place plates and screws.

18.5 Application on the Mandible

18.5.1 Trauma

For fractures involving the mandibular body or caudal mandible, locking reconstruction plates or locking miniplates can be used to stabilize the fracture fragments and achieve the desired occlusion and return to normal function (Figure 18.1a and b) [7]. Typically, pharyngotomy intubation is required to assess and achieve the desired postoperative occlusion [9]. An extraoral approach to the mandible/s is performed with the dog in dorsal recumbency. A single plate is contoured to match the anatomy of the mandible and secured to the bone using three 2.4 or 3.0 mm screws in each fragment of the fracture. In small dogs, a single locking miniplate should be used and ideally three 2.0 mm locking screws should be placed in each fragment. The authors have occasionally used two locking screws in the caudal bone segment in small dogs and cats due to space limitation.

18.5.2 Segmental Mandibular Reconstruction

A combined surgical and regenerative strategy resulting in rapid return to normal function can be achieved using a single titanium locking reconstruction plate and locking screws that are contoured to match the normal anatomy of the mandible [4]. The reconstruction is aided by rapid bone regeneration using recombinant human bone morphogenetic protein (rhBMP-2) resulting in restoration of the biomechanics of the mandibles. Immediate mandibular reconstruction following mandibulectomy was previously published [4]. In general, a combined extra- and intraoral approaches are utilized [1]. Once the ostectomy area is measured and marked, a single titanium locking plate is contoured prior to the ostectomy in order to capture the normal anatomy of the ventrolateral mandible. The plate is then secured, just below the roots of the teeth and above the mandibular canal, to the bone with 3.0 mm titanium locking screws (i.e. at least three screws in each segment). Then, the plate and screws are removed and the segmental mandibulectomy is initiated extraorally and completed intraorally while following the principles of oncologic surgery with regards to

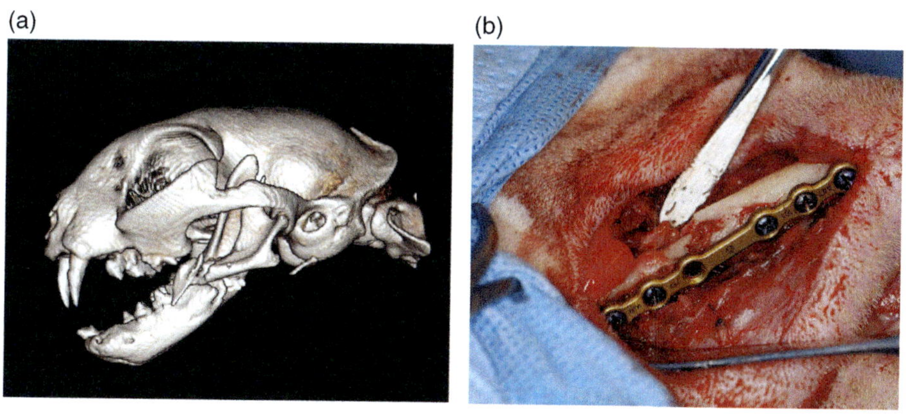

Figure 18.1 Repair of traumatic left mandibular fracture in a cat. (a) The tri-dimensional CT image demonstrates the comminuted fracture of the left mandible. (b) Repair using a 2.0 mm locking titanium miniplate and 2.0 mm titanium screws.

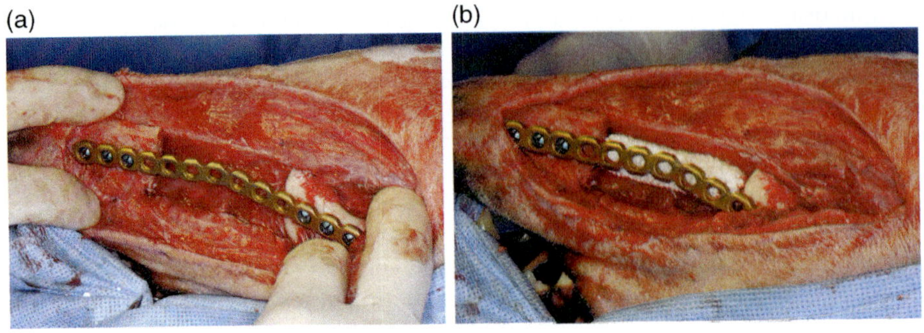

Figure 18.2 Immediate segmental mandibular reconstruction in a dog. (a) Following segmental mandibulectomy, a 2.4–3.0 mm titanium locking reconstruction plate is secured to the mandible using 3.0 mm locking titanium screws based on previously drilled holes. (b) A compression-resistant matrix infused with rhBMP-2 is placed at the defect site in order to regenerate bone at the defect site.

surgical margins. After intraoral closure, the plate is secured to the mandible via the extraoral approach (Figure 18.2a). A compression-resistant matrix (CRM) impregnated with rhBMP-2 is implanted into the defect to fit snugly (Figure 18.2b) and secured circumferentially with 4–0 poliglecaprone 25 sutures to prevent migration post-implantation. The surrounding soft tissues are sutured around the plate and CRM to provide a soft tissue envelope.

18.5.3 Rostral Mandibular Reconstruction

A regenerative approach to rostral mandibular reconstruction was developed by our group to correct the instability and malocclusion that follow extensive bilateral rostral mandibulectomy in dogs [8]. Rostral mandibles are challenging to reconstruct due their complex geometry. The use of three-dimensional (3D) printing, as described later, is highly beneficial for surgical planning. The reconstructive surgery should take place three to four weeks after rostral mandibulectomy has been performed and the soft tissues have healed appropriately [10]. In order to achieve the desired postoperative occlusion, pharyngotomy intubation is performed [9]. With the dog in dorsal recumbency, an extraoral approach to both mandibles is performed via a single midline incision. Using blunt dissection, the mandibles are exposed and the locking reconstruction plate is contoured and adapted to the bone. If a 3D-printed model is used, the plate can be contoured prior to surgery to save surgical time and better prepare for the reconstructive surgery. The plate is secured with at least three 3.0 mm locking screws in each mandible. The rhBMP-2 infused CRM is implanted in the defect to fit snugly and secured circumferentially with 4–0 poliglecaprone 25 sutures. The surrounding soft tissues are sutured around the plate and scaffold to provide a soft tissue envelope. The subcutaneous tissues and skin are closed routinely.

18.5.4 Defect Nonunion Mandibular Fracture Reconstruction

When a mandibular fracture nonunion occurs, it typically results in malocclusion [5]. According to the Weber-Cěch classification: a "defect nonunion" occurs when a critical-size section of the bone is lost as a result of trauma, periodontal disease, or surgery [11, 12]. A defect nonunion occurs most commonly in small-breed dogs and/or as a result of failure from inadequate fracture repair (Figure 18.3a). As described for segmental and rostral mandibular reconstruction, a regenerative approach is also ideal for treatment of defect nonunions. In cases where tooth proximity creates concern over root damage from screw placement, the teeth at risk are extracted three to four weeks prior to the reconstructive surgery. This permits bone regeneration at the empty tooth alveloi, which will allow an adequate purchase to the screws. The surgery is performed with the dog intubated via pharyngotomy to ensure the desired postoperative occlusion [5, 9]. The canine teeth are

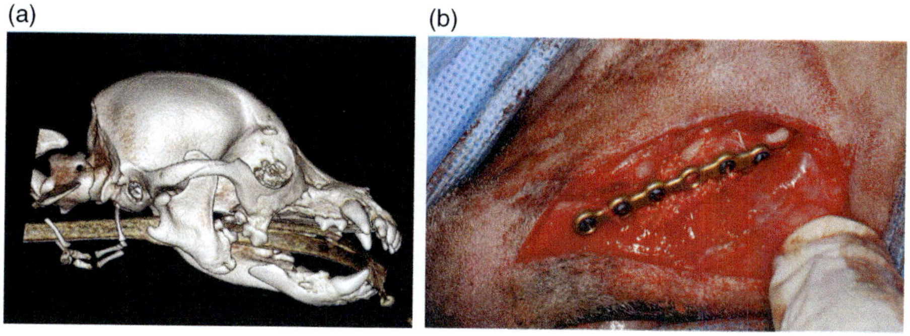

Figure 18.3 Reconstruction of defect nonunion mandibular fracture in a dog. (a) The tridimensional CT image demonstrates the defect nonunion of the right mandible. (b) Repair using 2.0 mm locking titanium miniplate and 2.0 mm titanium screws using a rhBMP-2 infused compression resistant matrix.

wired together using 28-gauge wire, bringing the mandibles and maxillas into the desired occlusion. An extraoral approach to the mandible is used and a single locking titanium 2.0 mm miniplate is adapted to the desired anatomical contour of the mandible in a lateral position while avoiding tooth root damage (Figure 18.3b). The fracture edges are debrided and the plate is secured to the bone with at least three locking titanium screws in each segment of the fracture. Because of the anatomic limitations in the caudal mandibles of very small dogs and cats, the authors may use two locking screws when necessary. Appropriately sized CRM impregnated with rhBMP-2 is implanted as described previously. The surrounding soft tissues are sutured around the plate and sponge to provide a soft tissue envelope. The subcutaneous tissue and skin are closed routinely.

18.6 Application on the Maxillofacial Bones

The authors use internal fixation by means of titanium nonlocking miniplates as a valuable surgical modality for the treatment of severe maxillofacial trauma in dogs. The use of miniplates allows for restoration of the normal anatomy, quick return to normal function, and excellent cosmesis [6, 7, 13]. Nonlocking plate and screws are used because the plates are easier to contour to adapt to the complex maxillofacial anatomy (Figure 18.4a–d). In addition, bending locking plates are likely to result in deformation of the delicate screw holes. Extraoral and/or intraoral approaches can be used based on the preferred accessibility to the fractured site [1, 6]. Periosteal elevators can be used to elevate depressed comminuted fracture segments in order to achieve normal anatomic contour. If a small bone fragment is found to be nonvital or devoid of blood supply, it should be discarded.

The miniplate selection is based on the size of the fractures and must be contoured to match the desired anatomical site. The plates are secured to the bone with at least two nonlocking, self-tapping titanium screws in each segment of the fracture. The sequence of plate placement is done with *simplification of the fracture* in mind, such that unstable fragments are secured to the surrounding stable bone. In addition, important surgical objectives are to restore nasofrontal vault, orbit, and dental occlusion. Following lavage, the subcutaneous tissue and skin are reconstructed and closed routinely. A Stent bandage can be placed and secured with sutures to prevent postoperative emphysema and swelling [6].

18.7 Three-Dimensional Printing for Preoperative Planning

For complex repair and reconstruction situations such as mandibular reconstruction of critical-size defects, severe maxillofacial trauma, or defects where aberrant anatomy is present, the use of 3D printed models provides important technical benefits. Apart from providing a better understanding of the complex anatomy, the 3D printed model is very useful for planning the osteotomy lines and for precontouring plates to

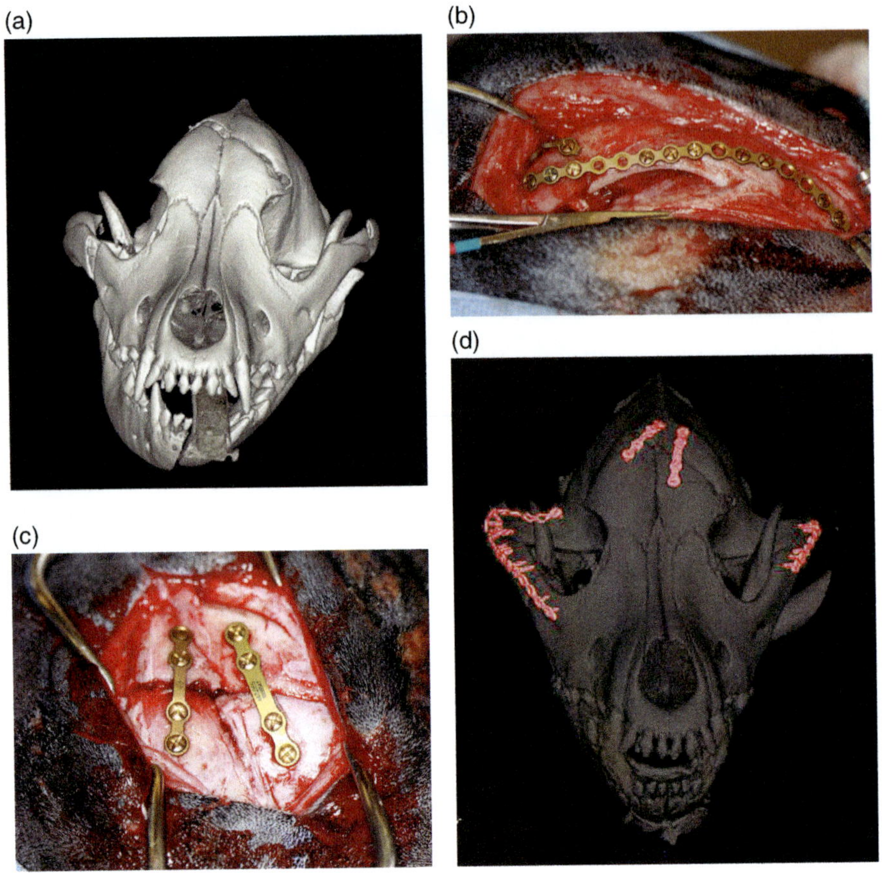

Figure 18.4 Severe maxillofacial fractures repair in a dog. (a) The tridimensional CT image demonstrates multiple maxillofacial fractures. (b) Repair using several 2.0 mm nonlocking titanium miniplates and 2.0 mm titanium nonlocking screws at the zygomatic arch and the temporal bone component. (c) Repair of the frontal sinus. (d) Postoperative CT demonstrating the reconstructed maxillofacial bones.

match the contour of the bone (i.e. before mandibulectomy and reconstruction). Three-dimensional printing is particularly beneficial when a segment of the mandible is missing because a mirror image of the intact contralateral mandible can be used to create an intact mandible model to which the plate can be anatomically contoured in advance of surgery.

References

1. Verstraete, F.J.M., Arzi, B., and Bezuidenhout, A.J. (2012). Surgical approaches for mandibular and maxillofacial trauma repair. In: *Oral and Maxillofacial Surgery in Dogs and Cats*, 1 (ed. F.J.M. Verstraete and M.J. Lommer), 259–264. Edinburgh: Elsevier.
2. Arzi, B., Stover, S.M., Garcia, T.C. et al. (2016). Biomechanical evaluation of two plating configurations for critical-sized defects of the mandible in dogs. *Am. J. Vet. Res.* 77 (5): 445–451.
3. Boudrieau, R.J. (2015). Initial experience with rhBMP-2 delivered in a compressive resistant matrix for mandibular reconstruction in 5 dogs. *Vet. Surg.* 44 (4): 443–458.
4. Arzi, B., Verstraete, F.J.M., Huey, D.J. et al. (2015). Regenerating mandibular bone using rhBMP-2: part 1 - immediate reconstruction of segmental mandibulectomies. *Vet. Surg.* 44 (4): 403–409.
5. Verstraete, F.J.M., Arzi, B., Huey, D.J. et al. (2015). Regenerating mandibular bone using rhBMP--2: part 2 - treatment of chronic, defect non-union fractures. *Vet. Surg.* 44 (4): 410–416.
6. Arzi, B. and Verstraete, F.J.M. (2015). Internal fixation of severe maxillofacial fractures in dogs. *Vet. Surg.* 44 (4): 437–442.

7. Boudrieau, R.J. (2012). Maxillofacial fracture repair using miniplates and screws. In: *Oral and Maxillofacial Surgery in Dogs and Cats*, 1 (ed. F.J.M. Verstraete and M.J. Lommer), 293–308. Edinburgh: Elsevier.
8. Arzi, B., Cissell, D.D., Pollard, R.E. et al. (2015). Regenerative approach to bilateral rostral mandibular reconstruction in a case series of dogs. *Front Vet. Sci.* 30 (2): 4. doi: 10.3389/fvets.2015.00004.
9. Lantz, G.C. (2012). Pharyngotomy and pharyngostomy. In: *Oral and Maxillofacial Surgery in Dogs and Cats*, 1 (ed. F.J.M. Verstraete and M.J. Lommer), 543–546. Edinburgh: Elsevier.
10. Lantz, G.C. (2012). Mandibulectomy techniques. In: *Oral and Maxillofacial Surgery in Dogs and Cats*, 1 (ed. F.J.M. Verstraete and M.J. Lommer), 467–480. Edinburgh: Elsevier.
11. Marretta, S.M. (2012). Maxillofacial fracture complications. In: *Oral and Maxillofacial Surgery in Dogs and Cats*, 1 (ed. F.J. Verstraete and M.J. Lommer), 333–342. Edinburgh: Elsevier.
12. Sumner-Smith, G. (2002). Non-union of fractures. In: *Bone in Clinical Orthopedics*, 2 (ed. G. Sumner-Smith and G.E. Fackelman), 349–358. Stuttgart.
13. Boudrieau, R.J. (2004). Miniplate reconstruction of severely comminuted maxillary fractures in two dogs. *Vet. Surg.* 33 (2): 154–163.

19 Spinal Fractures and Luxations

Bianca F. Hettlich

Vertebral column trauma often results in unstable injuries such as fractures and/or luxations. The most commonly injured area requiring surgical stabilization is the thoracolumbar spine, particularly the thoracolumbar (TL) and lumbosacral (LS) junctions. Vertebral luxation without fracture usually occurs in a ventral direction, resulting in damage to intervertebral disks and ligaments. Luxation may also occur laterally with concurrent articular facet fractures. Hyperflexion coupled with compression often results in vertebral body and endplate fractures with cranioventral displacement of the caudal fracture fragment.

Whether surgical stabilization is indicated depends on several factors such as patient age and weight, neurologic status, progression of neurologic deficits, pain caused by the injury, and degree of spinal instability. The latter can be difficult to discern radiographically. To provide a more objective evaluation, the surgeon can classify the injury according to the three-compartment classification. This method divides the vertebra into dorsal, middle, and ventral compartments and proposes that significant instability is present if two or three compartments are affected (Figure 19.1).

Rigid fixation methods described for the spine include a variety of techniques, including pins or screws and polymethylmethacrylate (PMMA), vertebral body plates, and external skeletal fixation. The most substantial anchorage of implants is achieved by placement into the vertebral bodies. For this, a dorsolateral to ventromedial trajectory is required unless implants can be placed directly laterally on the vertebral body. While fixation with pins and PMMA provides a high degree of versatility and freedom in placement of pins, this technique introduces a large amount of foreign material (PMMA) into the paraspinous musculature, making closure difficult. Once in place, adjustments to the construct can only be made by removing the PMMA. Furthermore, curing of PMMA causes an exothermic reaction that may damage surrounding tissues. By contrast, plate fixation eliminates these disadvantages and can provide strong, low-profile stabilization.

Compared to standard plates, locking plates do not require close bone contact, which makes perfect plate contouring unnecessary. Due to their angle-stable screw mechanism, locking plates can be applied with monocortical screws without significant loss of stiffness, as

Locking Plates in Veterinary Orthopedics, First Edition.
Edited by Matthew D. Barnhart and Karl C. Maritato.

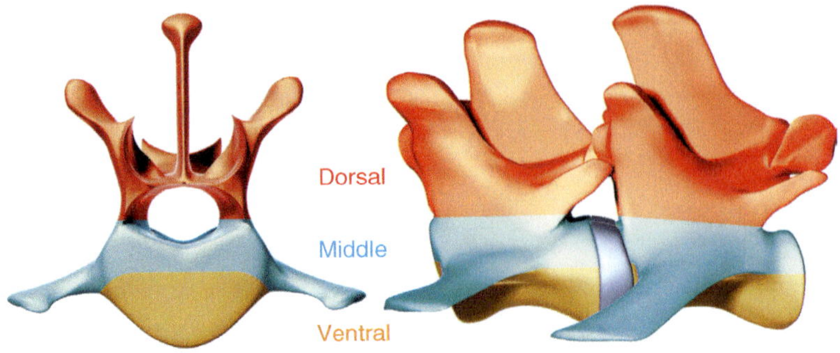

Figure 19.1 Illustration of the three-compartment classification depicting the ventral, middle, and dorsal compartment of canine vertebrae. (Source: Created by Tim Vojt.)

demonstrated in long-bone models. Both these qualities make locking plates very attractive for use in the vertebral column where contouring can be difficult and bicortical implants may pose risks to neurovascular structures. While locking plates can be applied to all parts of the spine, anatomic features and alignment can make their usage challenging. In these cases, despite the benefits of locking plates, alternative fixation methods (i.e. fixations with pins and PMMA, standard plates, polyaxial locking plates) should be considered, which allow easier adjustments in implant insertion location and angle. Examples include areas with physiologic changes in alignment such as the TL junction and malalignment due to deformities or nonreducible fractures.

Scientific literature on the use of locking plates in the canine and feline TL vertebral column is scarce. Clinical application of various locking plates has been described mainly for cervical vertebral stabilization, while *in vivo* comparison studies between locking plates and other fixation methods in the TL spine have not been reported. Description of locking compression plate (LCP) and string of pearls (SOP) use for TL vertebral column injuries is limited to a few cases [1–3]. While clinical publications on the use of titanium alloy plate systems in the TL spine are lacking, plates such as Advanced Locking Plate System (ALPS), UniLock, Polyaxial (PAX) Advanced Locking System, titanium reconstruction locking plates, and the recently introduced titanium SOP plate would have the advantage of improved MRI compatibility as titanium produces less artifact when compared to stainless steel.

Only one veterinary study has evaluated the *in vitro* biomechanical properties of a locking plates in comparison to pin-PMMA fixation in the canine cadaveric lumbar spine [4]. Bilateral bicortical pin/PMMA fixation with a total of four pins was compared to unilateral monocortical LCP fixation with a total of four screws. Results of this cadaveric study showed that pin/PMMA fixation was significantly stiffer and stronger and that for most testing directions, unilateral monocortical LCP fixation was only as strong as the intact spine. The authors of this study therefore recommend that LCP is only used in this particular configuration for inherently stable spinal injuries. There are no studies evaluating the biomechanical properties of LCP fixation in other configurations (i.e. unilateral with more screws, bilateral, bicortical screws), nor is there published biomechanical testing of other types locking plates in the TL spine.

Recently introduced PAX systems have been evaluated *in vitro* and *in vivo* for human and veterinary appendicular fractures. Unlike fixed-angle locking implants, these plate systems allow insertion of screws at varying angles. Depending on the system, screws are locked via different mechanisms such as expanding bushings, locking caps, or by cutting of the screw-head into the plate-hole metal. The ability to angle screws during spinal fracture repairs could offer considerable advantages, including greater flexibility of implant placement and an enhanced ability to avoid nervous tissues. However, their use has not been described for TL fractures in humans and there are no published reports on the use of these plates in veterinary TL surgery.

19.1 Preoperative Planning

Orthogonal radiographs are used to provide an overview of the injury. Since relying on radiographs alone can cause a surgeon to miss vertebral column injuries and compression within the spinal canal, CT or MRI are indicated for complete evaluation. Preoperative CT is also helpful in assessing patient specific anatomy and planning plate and screw location. Once the extent of the injury has been documented, degree of suspected instability is determined and the fixation construct chosen. Commonly used sizes for locking plates are 2.0 or 2.4 mm for small dogs and cats, 2.7 mm for medium, and 3.5 mm for large-breed dogs.

Preplanning screw location with the chosen locking plate type and size is extremely important, as the angle-fixed screw position can easily interfere with the intervertebral disk spaces. Due to screw hole spacing within the plates, only two screws can usually be placed per vertebral body.

The ideal implant stiffness required for appropriate vertebral column immobilization in cats and dogs is not known. The surgeon will have to make decisions on implant stiffness requirements based on each individual patient. Apart from size and shape of the affected vertebrae, a major factor will be degree of instability of the injury. With relatively stable injuries, unilateral plate fixation with two screws in adjacent vertebral bodies may be sufficient. With unstable injuries, unilateral locking plate fixation should span two vertebrae cranial and caudal to the lesion to assure sufficient points of fixation, or bilateral plate fixation should be used. This is expected to improve upon the reported biomechanical disadvantage of unilateral LCP fixation over bilateral pin/PMMA fixation in a cadaveric canine lumbar spine injury model [4].

It has been demonstrated that fixation with multiple monocortical locking screws has similar stiffness to bicortical fixation using nonlocking plates and cortical screws. While this is an important benefit of locking plates, it has only been assessed biomechanically in long bones, where cortical bone is more substantial compared to vertebral body bone, and multiple screws can be placed per segment to achieve the desired cortical purchase points. By contrast, vertebral cortices tend to be thin with soft medullary bone. Monocortical screw fixation is very attractive along the vertebral column, but it has not been sufficiently assessed biomechanically in the TL spine in cats or dogs. The surgeon will have to consider the possible implications of reduced stiffness with a monocortical fixation in addition to the planned fixation points cranial and caudal to the injury. If easily modified and achieved without violation of the vertebral canal or injury to adjacent ventrolateral perispinous vascular structures, bicortical screw purchase should be considered.

19.2 Approaches to the Vertebral Column

Depending on the surgeon's preference, the TL spine can be approached via a dorsal, dorsolateral, or lateral approach. The position of the animal is adjusted for the specific approach: ventral recumbency for dorsal, slightly lateralized for the other approaches. For unilateral plate application, the dorsolateral and lateral approach allows for improved access to the vertebral bodies and decreased soft issue interference during drilling and placement of screws. For bilateral plate fixation, a dorsal approach is chosen to provide access to both sides of the vertebral column.

Vacuum bags or other holding devices and tape are used to maintain the desired position of the animal on the operating table. It is important to account for the change in vertebral position in case of oblique lateral patient position when applying implants at specific angles. With the animal in a straight ventral recumbent position, desired vertical or horizontal insertion angles can be more easily determined.

During the approach to the affected TL segment, care must be taken to avoid iatrogenic injury by aggressive manipulation. The approach extends ventrally to expose the rib heads of the thoracic or the base of the transverse processes of the lumbar spine.

19.3 Reduction

Utilizing reduction forceps on spinous processes, careful traction and manipulation is performed to reduce vertebral subluxation and reestablish alignment. Comminuted vertebral body fractures or older injuries can be very difficult to manipulate, and emphasis may shift from realignment to establishing stability, which can impact the ability to apply plates for fixation.

Temporary reduction can sometimes be maintained with transarticular K-wires, which can be placed individually through each articular process or translaminar from one process through the dorsal lamina into the other. Kyphotic malalignment may not be reduced entirely this way, and further use of reduction forceps may be necessary.

19.4 Locking Plate Application

While they can be used along the entire vertebral column, application of locking plates is easier along the lumbar spine due to the lack of rib heads and the relatively flat lateral surface of the vertebrae. Implant insertion angle and corridors have been described [5]; however, patient-specific planning using preoperative CT images is recommended.

Once the area of injury has been approached and the lateral vertebral bones freed of soft tissue to allow visualization of landmarks, the intervertebral foramina are identified with their neurovascular bundle. Depending on plate location and contact with the bone, the bundle can be carefully freed and the plate placed underneath. However, unless plate position causes compression of the bundle, dissection is avoided and plates are placed over the bundles. Small-gauge hypodermic needles can be used to identify the cranial and caudal borders of the intervertebral disks to aid precise plate positioning and assure that screw placement will be in the desired location. Contouring of locking plates is limited, as it is not necessary for implant stability and changes orientation of the screw trajectories. If contouring is desired, it must be done with full recognition of the change in direction of the screw trajectories. Bending should also occur between screw holes, not over them, to avoid damaging the threaded portion of the locking mechanism.

19.5 Lumbar Spine

For vertebral body implants placed from dorsolateral, the recommended implant insertion angle for the lumbar spine is around 60° from vertical. It is easier to achieve this angle when using plates compared to pin/PMMA fixation, as soft tissue interference around fixation pins and cement is eliminated. However, when using a standard dorsal approach, soft tissues may still impair placement of the drill guide and drilling, tapping, and screw insertion. Screw insertion landmarks are the base of the pedicle and transverse process. An additional reported landmark is the accessory process; however, implant insertion must be sufficiently ventral to this process to avoid entering the vertebral canal. Along the lumbar spine, the plate naturally wants to lay relatively flat against the lateral laminar and pedicular bone. A small keyhole pediculectomy or mini-hemilaminectomy can be performed to probe or visualize the floor of the vertebral canal to further aid proper screw insertion points and trajectory.

19.6 Placement of a 3.5 mm LCP

The application of a LCP in a canine lumbar spine model is demonstrated in Figure 19.2.

Relatively stable injuries can be treated with unilateral fixation using a four- or five-hole 3.5 mm LCP. Fixation strength can be increased by spanning two vertebrae cranially and caudal and by applying bilateral plates. The threaded part of the combi hole in the LCP is situated toward the center of the plate. With the four-hole 3.5 mm LCP, this can be disadvantageous because it forces the locking screws to be placed very close together in the center of the plate, often interfering with the intervertebral disk space. In this case, changing to a five-hole plate usually allows two-screw fixation per vertebral body without violating the disk. While this leaves an empty screw hole over the disk space, it is unlikely to weaken the repair. Sometimes, a slightly longer plate may be chosen to improve screw hole location, leaving an empty hole toward the end of the plate. Due to the limited lateral bending of the spine, an overhanging plate across part of the next vertebra is unlikely to cause clinical problems.

The 3.5 mm LCP can be held in position using the threaded plate holder (longer) or threaded drill guide (shorter) placed in one of the holes away from the first screw to be placed. This allows easy adjustment of plate position but does not secure the plate well in its position and requires an assistant to hold the plate.

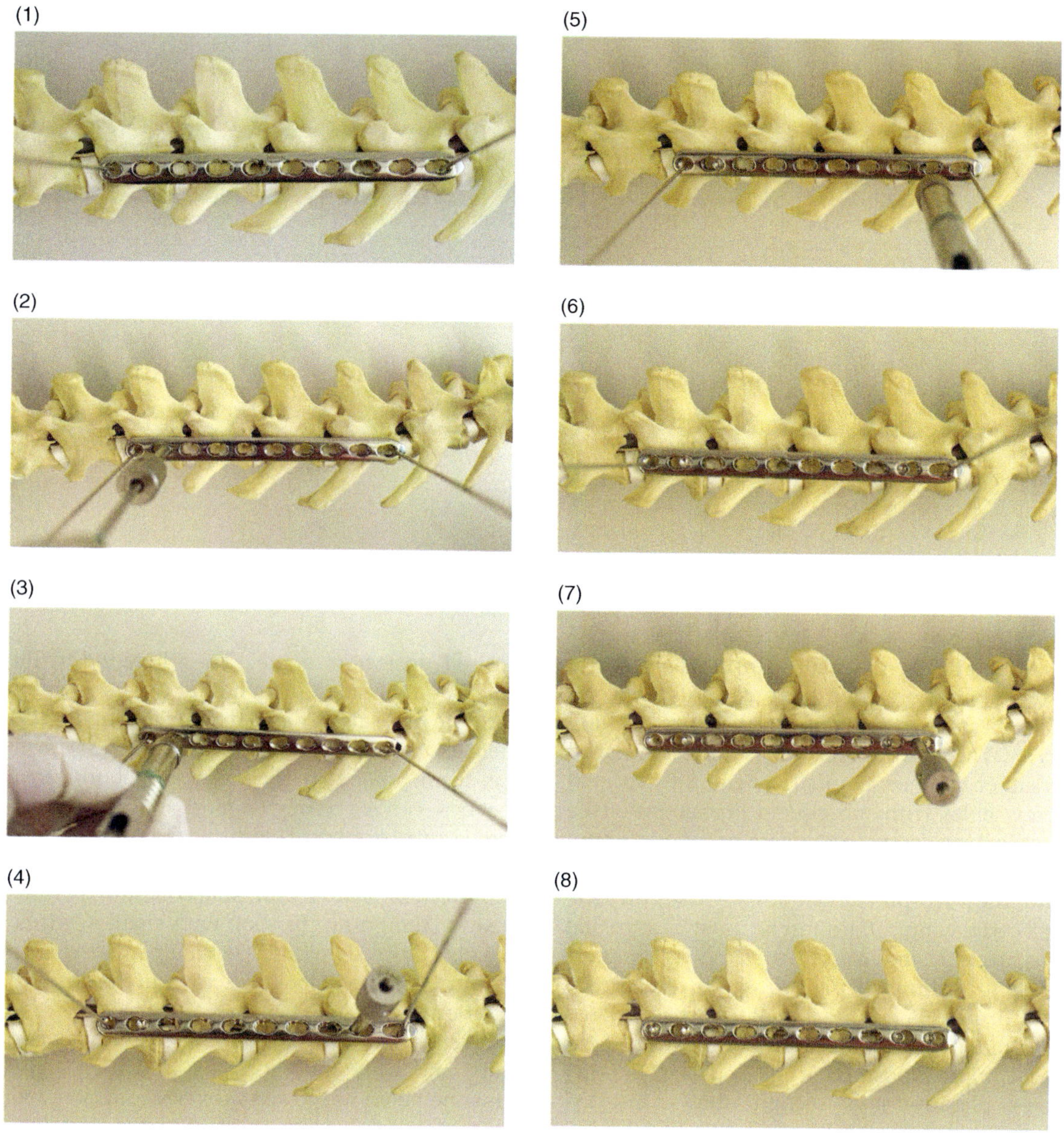

Figure 19.2 Placement of a 10-hole 3.5 mm LCP in a canine lumbar spine model spanning L1 (left of image) to L5 (right of image). (1) The plate is placed on the lateral aspect of the lumbar spine in a canine bone model spanning L2 to L5. The plate is not contoured and is placed just below the articular and at the base of the transverse processes. Two small Kirschner wires (K-wires) are used to hold the plate in position temporarily. They are placed in the outermost holes as far toward the ends as possible. (2) A threaded drill guide is placed into the second most cranial combi hole. This guide is used to tilt the plate to the desired angle before a 2.8 mm drill bit is used to drill the hole. (3) The depth gauge is used to carefully probe the walls of the bone tunnel for possible breaches. (4) The cranial screw is now in place and the drill guide is placed into the threaded part of the combi-hole next to the most caudal hole. (5) After drilling, the depth gauge is used again to assess drill tunnel integrity prior to placing the locking screw. (6) The caudal screw has been placed. The K-wires can now be removed since the plate is locked into position. (7) The most cranial and caudal screws can now be placed. Note that the hole made by the K-wire in the caudal hole is located in the dynamic compression part of the hole and that the locking screw will be placed in the treaded part of the hole. In the cranial hole, the drill tunnel will incorporate the K-wire hole. (8) Two screws each are now placed in the most cranial and caudal vertebrae. The remaining screws can be placed into holes, which will not interfere with the intervertebral disks. (9) Final implant construct. Note the four unfilled screw holes (*) located over or too close to intervertebral disk spaces. Only one screw per vertebrae could be applied in the centrally located vertebrae for the size of spine in this model. (10) View from dorsal showing the position of the uncontoured 10 hole 3.5 mm LCP plate on the lateral aspect of the vertebral column.

(10)

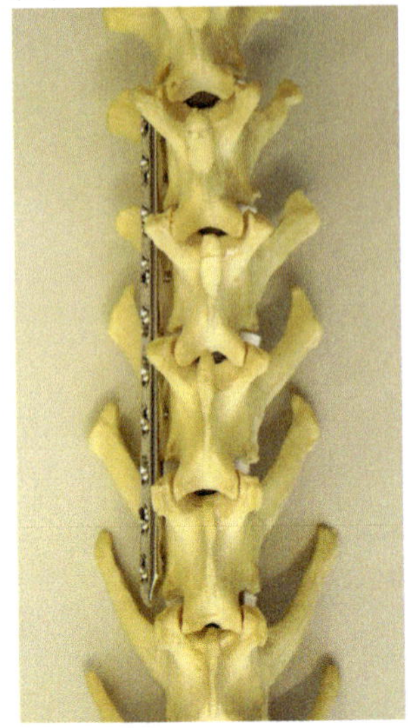

(9)

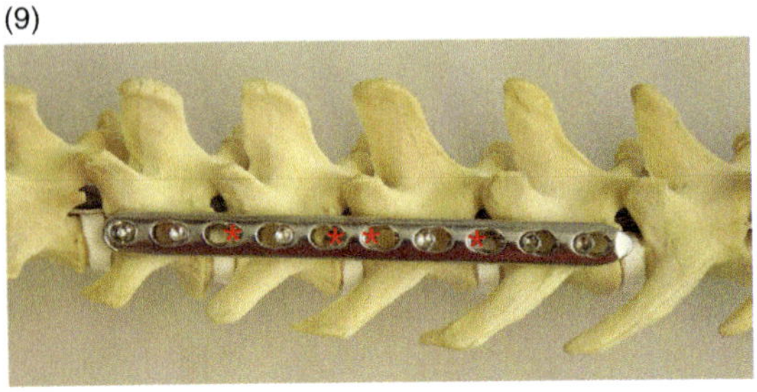

Figure 19.2 (Continued)

Alternatively, the plate can be temporarily fixed in position using the push-pull device to allow easier placement of the first locking screw. The push-pull device is typically placed in either the most cranially or caudally located screw holes with subsequent placement of the first locking screw in the vertebral body opposite the push-pull. Since temporary fixation with the push-pull device already fixes the LCP at a certain angle, the surgeon must be sure that this angle is similar to the desired screw angle prior to drilling. If plate position after push-pull fixation is not ideal, it should be adjusted to avoid inappropriate placement of the screws. Once implant position is checked after the first screw placement, the second screw is inserted in the same vertebral body as the push-pull. The push-pull can then be removed and the remaining two screws can be placed.

Another method to maintain the LCP in position but still allow tilting of the plate for proper drill hole angulation is the use of small K-wires for temporary fixation. For this, two 1–1.5 mm K-wires are placed at the cranial and caudal extend of the plate, holding it at the desired level along the vertebral column. K-wires are placed away from the center of the plate, in the dynamic compression part of the combi hole. When drilling the hole for the first locking screw, the plate can still be tilted to achieve the desired insertion angle. The threaded drill guide or a threaded plate holder can be used to hold the plate at the desired angle during placement of the first screw. Once a locking screw has been placed in each vertebral body, the K-wires can be removed and the remaining screws are placed. The cortical bone defects made by the K-wires are small enough to not compromise stability of subsequently placed screws. Temporary fixation with small K-wires can also be used on other locking plates to facilitate application of locking screws in the desired position.

If screws are purposefully placed monocortically and only the cis-cortex is drilled, care must be taken not to select overly long screws. This may lead to contact of the advancing screws with the trans-cortex, lifting of the plate away from the spine and/or stripping of the cis-cortical bone. Depending on location of the drill hole in the cis-cortex, screws may be accidentally diverted during advancement within the vertebral bone by the inner cortex of the canal. While such a diversion is good, as it hopefully avoids vertebral canal violation, it shifts the screw trajectory and may cause shifting of the plate position or cross threading/ malposition of the locking screw.

If screws are placed bicortically, both cortices must be drilled and the length of the drill tunnel should be measured. The depth gauge can also be used as a probe to carefully palpate the integrity of the drill tunnel for possible breaches into the vertebral canal. On principle, locking screws with a self-tapping end should be of sufficient length to have the entire cutting tip extend beyond the trans-cortex. This goal must be weighed against the possible risk of damage to perispinous vasculature.

Depending on the type of implant, screws can be power inserted or hand inserted. Use of a torque limiting device is recommended for Synthes locking screws. Considering the confines of the surgical area, thin cortex, and potentially interfering inner cortical bone, hand insertion of screws may be preferable.

19.7 Thoracic Spine

Plate application in the thoracic spine is more challenging due to the differences in vertebral anatomy and presence of ribs. On principle, vertebral body plates can be applied through a lateral intrathoracic approach. More commonly, dorsolateral plate application with disarticulation of the rib heads or drilling of a notch to accommodate the plate is performed. Implant insertion angles are different in the thoracic compared to the lumbar spine, with trajectories becoming steeper in the more cranial thoracic vertebrae. At T13 insertion angles are around 45° from vertical and reduce to 20–25° at T10. This is due to the changes in vertebral body shape from broad oval in the lumbar spine to tall and almost hourglass shape in the thoracic spine. Identification of the disk space borders can again be achieved using small needles, and K-wires can aid in temporary positioning of the plate prior to locking screw placement.

Due to the natural kyphotic curvature of the TL spine, it can be difficult to apply long locking plates across multiple vertebrae. When plates with fixed-angle screws are used, screw location at the cranial and caudal extend of the plate might not be centered, requiring adjustments of plate positioning that may compromise vertebral canal safety or sufficient bone purchase. Some locking plates can be bent to fit the natural curvature of the spine (i.e. SOP, locking reconstruction plate); however, any contouring of the plate must be done with care to assure that screw trajectory is still going in the desired direction.

19.8 Placement of a 3.5 mm SOP Plate

Placement of a 3.5 mm SOP plate in the canine TL spine is depicted in Figure 19.3.

SOP plates, applied along the dorsolateral surface, are often used in the caudal thoracic/cranial lumbar spine. Since they can be bent in three planes with 6° of freedom, the kyphotic curvature can be mimicked and screw holes can be twisted to accommodate differences in screw insertion angle between the cranial and caudally located screws. Based on preoperative CT and radiographs, the plate can be precontoured, which will greatly decrease intraoperative time for adjustments. Inserting the screws into the plate during planning will aid assuring their desired trajectory since specific angles can be determined.

As with LCP and other locking plates, a maximum of two screws can usually be placed per vertebral body. To achieve the appropriate number of cortical fixation points, it is common to span two vertebrae on each side of the injury. Even with this, unilateral SOP plating may not be sufficient for unstable injuries. Since normal cortical screws are used, failure mode of SOP implants is through shearing just below the screwhead. To strengthen fixation and avoid implant failure, bilateral SOP plate fixation should be considered and is recommended.

19.9 Problem Solving with Locking Plates

Malalignment and poor reducibility of the vertebral column due to injury may require placement of screws in locations and at angles that prohibit usage of a locking plate. Alignment can sometimes be adjusted to fit the selected implant; however, this must be done with great care and without additional iatrogenic injury. Flexibility to change to a different implant type is an important component of pre- and intraoperative decision-making.

Interference of anatomic structures such as ribs can impair ideal application of locking

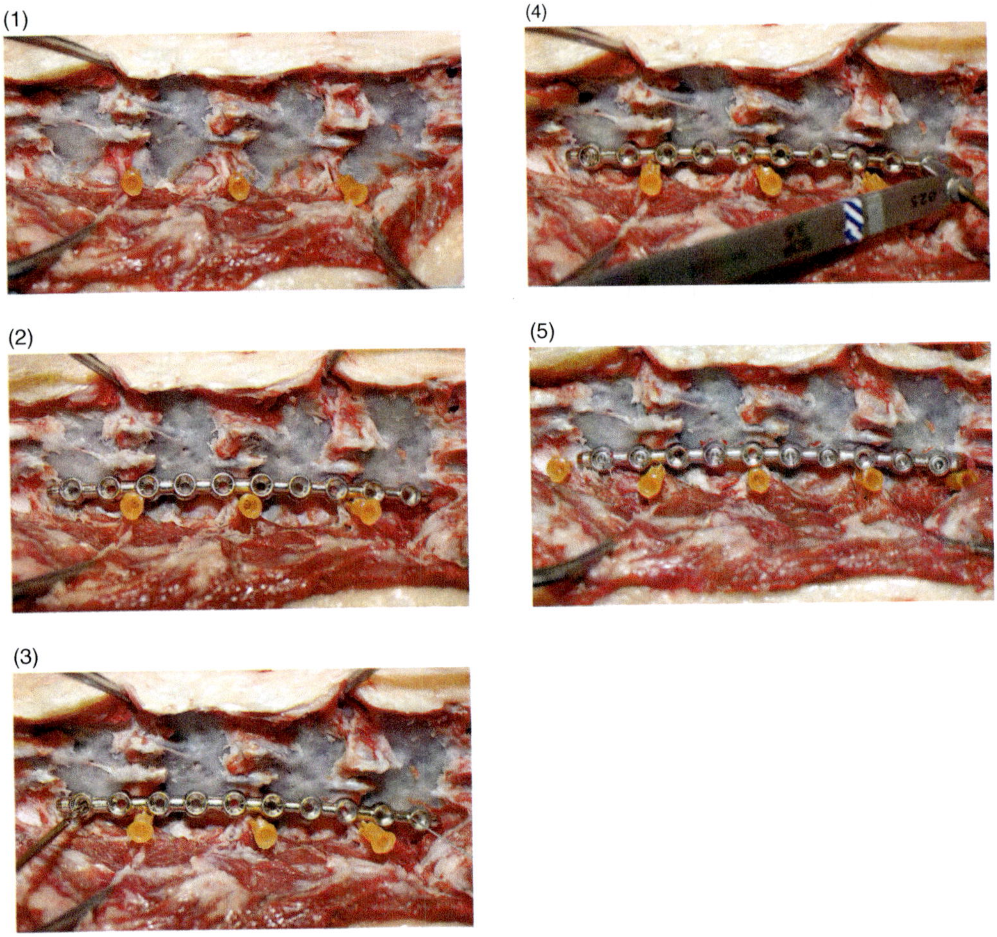

Figure 19.3 Placement of a 10-hole 3.5 mm SOP plate in the canine thoracolumbar (TL) spine spanning T13 (left of image) through L3 (right of image). (1) Hypodermic needles identify the intervertebral disk spaces. Note the neurovascular bundles, which have been carefully prepared. (2) The plate has been contoured to fit the natural kyphotic curvature of the spine in this region. Placement of the plate will be immediately below the articular processes at the base of the transverse processes. (3) Drilling of the first screw hole in the most cranial aspect of the plate. In this case, temporary plate fixation was aided by placing a small K-wire in the caudal most hole. The K-wire still allows changes in plate position and angulation. The first hole was drilled without a drill guide with focus on the desired angle of the screw within the vertebral body. With correct position and angle, this first screw will place the plate in the correct position for subsequent screws. (4) The K-wire was removed and the most caudal screw is placed. Since the plate position is now locked in place regarding the angulation, the SOP drill guide can now be used to assure proper screw position within the plate. (5) The SOP plate has been applied with seven screws. Note that three plate holes are left without a screw, as these would have been placed too close or in the intervertebral disk space.

plates. Rib heads can be disarticulated to allow plate positioning and either be reattached with heavy suture or wire or left disarticulated. Rib heads can also be partially removed by rongeurs or drill. If the base of the transverse process is interfering with ideal placement, it can be notched or partially removed.

After placement of the first locking screw, the plate is locked in position apart from some rotary movement around the first point of fixation. This locked position determines the trajectory for the remaining screws within the vertebral bodies. Prior to placing more screws, it is important to carefully assess the position of the remaining screw holes. It may become apparent that plate position or angle of screws has shifted and that screw trajectories with this position will not engage bone properly, are positioned to close to the vertebral canal or will enter the intervertebral disk.

While standard plates allow some degree of freedom with the angle of screw placement in relation to the plate, screws for many locking plates are fixed-angle. This means that a poor screw trajectory once the plate is locked cannot be adjusted by angling a locking screw. It might be necessary to remove the first screw, adjust the plate, and redrill. Considering the limited bone stock of the vertebral bodies, this should be avoided as much as possible by assuring the best possible position and angulation of the first screw. In most locking plates, it is possible to combine locking and nonlocking screws within the same plate, such as in the combi hole of the LCP. The use of polyaxial locking plates may alleviate some of the restrictions on the use of regular locking plates as these allow some angulation of screws within the screw holes.

The important application principle should be followed, when combining locking and nonlocking screws. In such case, the nonlocking screws are applied first in an area where appropriate plate/bone contact can be achieved to create compression of the plate to the bone. After this, the locking screws can be applied. In reverse order, the locking screws would prevent compression of bone against the plate by the nonlocking screws. When locking plates are chosen for spinal fixation, the need for placement of nonlocking screws typically arises when plate positioning is not ideal and screws must enter the vertebral bone at a different trajectory than allowed by the locking screw path. Most often, in these scenarios, the plate is already applied with several locking screws in place. For long bone fractures, one should loosen the locking screws at this point, apply the nonlocking screws, then retighten the locking screws. Along the uneven spine, this may not be ideal, as the nonlocking screws may shift the plate enough out of position to prevent proper locking of the locking screws. Going against the principle rules of application, in some cases, nonlocking screws may need to be applied after their locking counterparts, without loosening the construct again.

Failure of locking plates depends on the implant used. Many locking plates are very strong and unlikely to fail along the plate. Common modes of failure in the spine are screw pullout of the bone or fracture and shearing of screws between the plate and bone. The risk of screw breakage is higher with regular cortical screws, which have a weak point between the screwhead and shaft, compared to locking screws, which tend to have a larger core diameter than the regular screws.

19.10 Postoperative Assessment

Orthogonal spinal radiographs are obtained to assess vertebral column alignment and implant position. Radiographs have a poor accuracy to determine position of bicortical implants in relation to the vertebral canal. While locking plates can be applied using monocortical screws, accidental violation of screws into the vertebral canal is still possible, depending on the location of the plate. Computed tomography is an outstanding tool to assess implant placement in relation to the vertebral canal and can be used with excellent accuracy despite metal artefact.

References

1. Downes, C.J., Gemmill, T.J., Gibbons, S.E. et al. (2009). Hemilaminectomy and vertebral stabilisation for the treatment of thoracolumbar disc protrusion in 28 dogs. *J. Small Anim. Pract.* 50: 525–535.
2. Kumar, B.N. and Nagaraja, B.N. (2015). Stabilization of vertebral fractures by locking plate fixation in dogs. *Indian J. Vet. Surg.* 36: 129–131.
3. McKee, W.M. and Downes, C.J. (2008). Vertebral stabilisation and selective decompression for the management of triple thoracolumbar disc protrusions. *J. Small Anim. Pract.* 49: 536–539.
4. Sturges, B.K., Kapatkin, A.S., Garcia, T.C. et al. (2016). Biomechanical comparison of locking compression plate versus positive profile pins and Polymethylmethacrylate for stabilization of the canine lumbar vertebrae. *Vet. Surg.* 45: 309–318.
5. Watine, S., Cabassu, J.P., Catheland, S. et al. (2006). Computed tomography study of implantation corridors in canine vertebrae. *J. Small Anim. Pract.* 47: 651–657.

Section V

Nontrauma Applications: Clinical Case Examples

V-A Corrective Osteotomies

20 Tibial Plateau Leveling Osteotomy for Cranial Cruciate Ligament Rupture

Mary Sarah Bergh

20.1 Introduction

Cranial cruciate ligament (CCL) disease is a common cause of pelvic limb lameness in dogs worldwide and surgery is often recommended to allow a faster and more complete return to function [1]. While numerous surgical procedures have been described to treat stifle pain and instability that occur secondary to CCL deficiency, the tibial plateau leveling osteotomy (TPLO) has been one of the most commonly performed orthopedic procedures worldwide and is the only surgical procedure that has been shown to allow a return to normal clinical function [2–5]. Initially developed and reported by Slocum and Slocum in 1993, the TPLO eliminates cranial tibial subluxation through a rotational cylindrical osteotomy in the proximal tibia that decreases the tibial plateau angle (TPA), thereby eliminating cranial tibial thrust. The osteotomy is stabilized with a bone plate [6]. Initially, only the Slocum TPLO plate was used for the TPLO due to patent restrictions, but once the patent expired, numerous bone plates were applied to and designed specifically to be used to stabilize the TPLO. Of these, both locking and nonlocking constructs have become widely available for dogs and cats of all sizes.

20.2 Locking TPLO Plate Design

While the shape, specific design features, and the locking mechanism differ between manufacturers, locking TPLO plates share the commonality of allowing the screw to lock into both the bone plate and the bone. (Figure 20.1) As such, direct contact to the bone is not necessary for construct stability. Some locking TPLO plate designs are precontoured to match the shape of the proximomedial tibia. This feature not only minimizes the offset of the plate from the bone and subsequent working length of the screws but can also decrease surgical time.

Fixed-angle locking screw holes dictate the direction that the screw can be placed. The angle of these screws is often directed to avoid the joint surface and converge in the region of maximal bone stock. The Synthes bone plate (DePuy Synthes Vet, West Chester, PA), for example, directs the proximal screw 3° distally

Locking Plates in Veterinary Orthopedics, First Edition.
Edited by Matthew D. Barnhart and Karl C. Maritato.

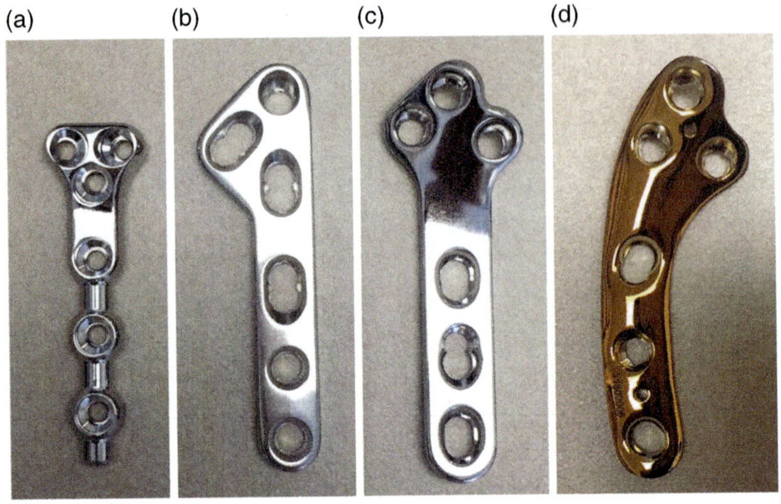

Figure 20.1 Examples of commercially available locking tibial plateau leveling osteotomy (TPLO) plate designs. (a) String of pearls TPLO plate (Orthomed, Huddersfield, West Yorkshire); (b) Unity cruciate plate (New Generation Devices, Glen Rock, NJ); (c) Synthes locking TPLO plate (DePuy Synthes Vet, West Chester, PA); (d) TPLO Curve™ plate (Biomedtrix, Whippany, NJ). The proximal portions of plates c and d are precontoured to fit the shape of the proximomedial tibia.

and 5° caudally, the cranial screw 3° caudally, and the caudal screw is directed 3° cranially. This convergent placement of locking screws provides superior anchorage to bone, as compared to locking screws placed in parallel orientation and nonlocking screws, because more bone must be displaced for screw stripping to occur [7].

Several TPLO plate designs allow a combination of both locking and standard screw fixation. This hybrid fixation allows for axial compression if the nonlocking screw is placed in load fashion in a DCP hole. Such interfragmentary compression results in direct bone healing across the osteotomy (Figure 20.2). The Biomedtrix TPLO Curve™ plate (Biomedtrix, Whippany, NJ) achieves compression across the osteotomy site in a novel fashion: an angled compression hole rotates the plate to compress the osteotomy cranially, and an axial compression slot compresses the osteotomy distally (Figure 20.3). Other plate designs, such as the string of pearls TPLO plate (Orthomed, Huddersfield, West Yorkshire), allow pure locking fixation that would provide bridging fixation unless interfragmentary compression is applied with other means.

The Synthes TPLO plate design allows both locking screw and conventional screw fixation in all holes of the proximal portion of the plate and either one or two holes in the distal portion of the plate. When both screw types are used, the standard screws should be secured prior to the placement of the locking screws. While the author routinely uses locking screws in the proximal portion of the plate and standard screws in the distal portion, locking screws may be used in the distal portion for very large dogs, for dogs that have subjectively poor bone quality, or if stripping of the cis-cortex of one of the standard screws occurs during insertion (Figure 20.4). A standard screw may be used in the proximal portion of the plate if the locking screw strips the drill hole or if redirection of the screw is desired to avoid crossing the osteotomy or articular surface.

20.3 Clinical Benefits of Locking TPLO Plates

The standard technique for the TPLO utilizes a medial approach to the proximal tibia for execution of the osteotomy and bone plate application on the proximomedial metaphysis and diaphysis. Anatomically, this location can be challenging to accurately contour a plate due to the complex three-dimensional shape of the tibia

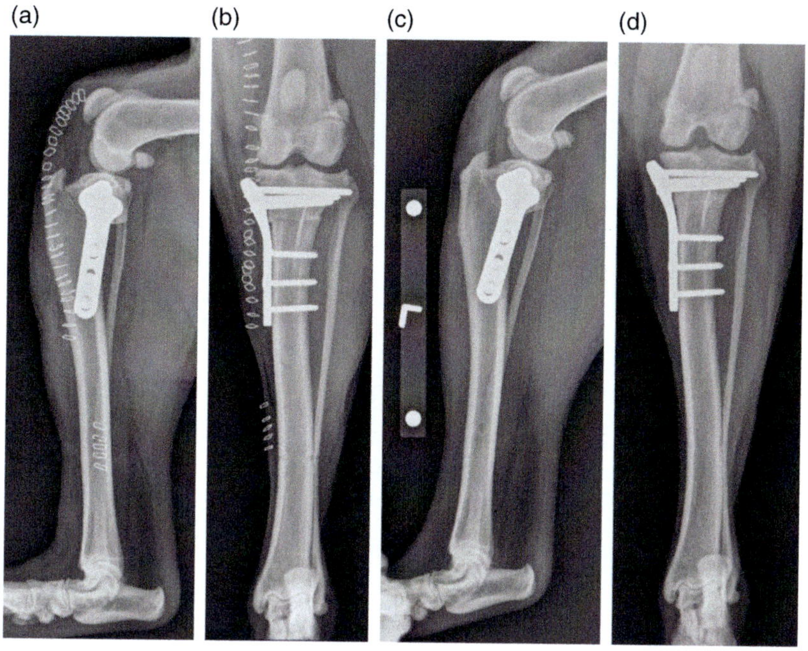

Figure 20.2 Immediate postoperative (a and b) and eight-week follow-up radiographs (c and d) from a tibial plateau leveling osteotomy (TPLO) performed on a 36 kg female spayed Labrador retriever using a Synthes 3.5 mm locking TPLO plate with hybrid locking fixation. Locking screws were used in the proximal portion of the plate and conventional cortical screws were used to achieve axial compression in the distal portion of the plate. Uncomplicated direct bone healing occurred across the osteotomy site.

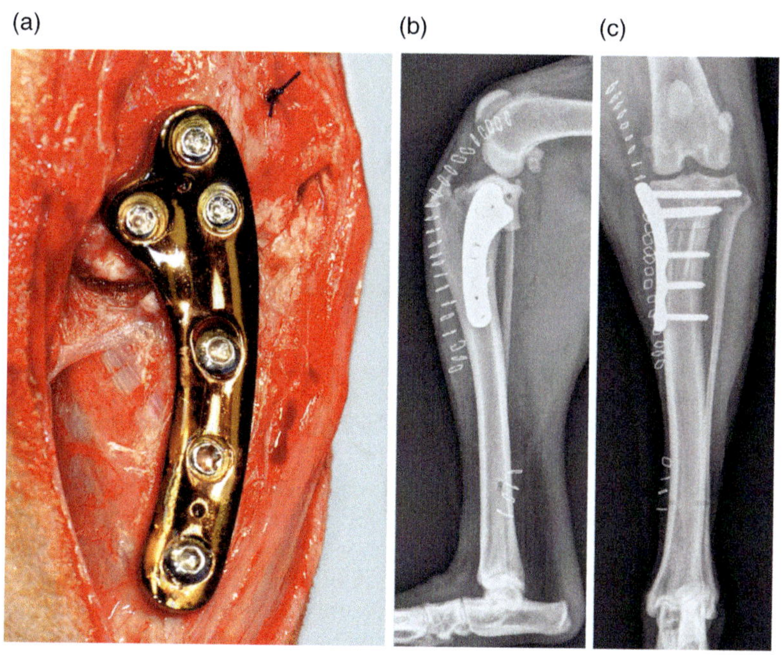

Figure 20.3 Intraoperative photograph (a) and immediate postoperative radiographs (b and c) of a TPLO stabilized with TPLO Curve™ plate. This plate has two compression holes to allow compression across both the cranial and distal aspects of the osteotomy and is coated with a silver-based plasma antimicrobial coating.

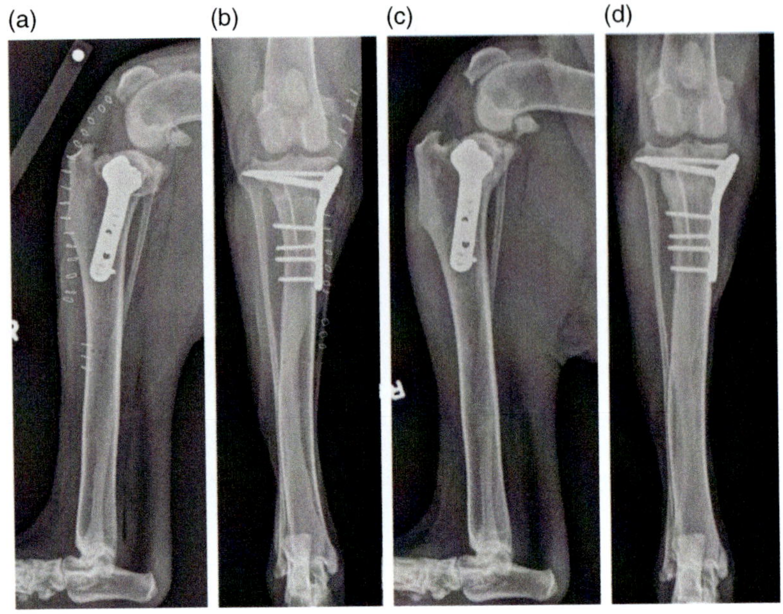

Figure 20.4 Immediate postoperative (a and b) and 12-week follow-up radiographs (c and d) from a TPLO performed on a 68.2 kg female spayed Mastiff using a single Synthes 3.5 mm broad TPLO plate. Four locking screws were used in the proximal segment and one locking screw (screw #7) was used with three conventional cortex screws in the distal segment. Uncomplicated healing and excellent clinical function was achieved.

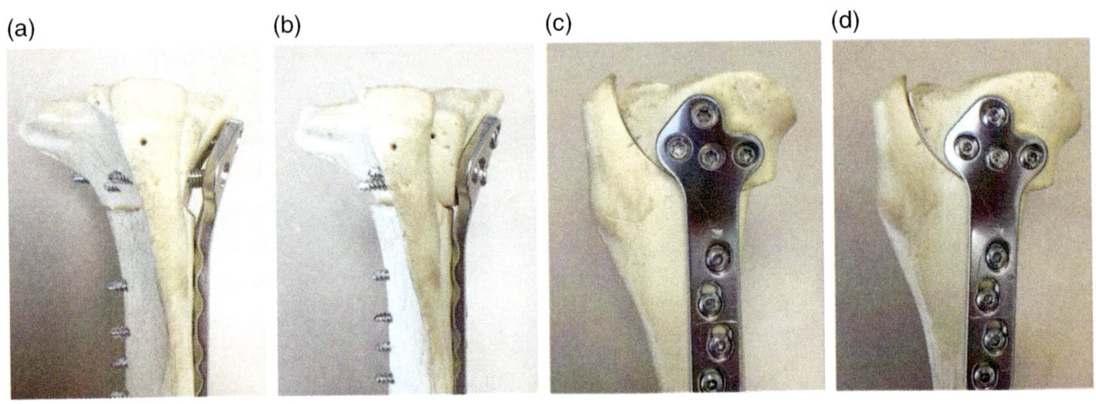

Figure 20.5 Bone models showing TPLO stabilized with locking screws (a and c) and conventional screws (b and d) placed through the same drill holes in the proximal segment. Axial and torsional alignment of the bone, osteotomy rotation, and compression across the osteotomy are only maintained with the locking construct.

and the variable – and often substantial – amount of medial buttress present in animals with CCL disease. Failure to precisely contour standard bone plates to the shape of the tibia can have a significant impact on reduction of the osteotomy as the conventional screws are tightened, leading to translation of the plateau segment, loss of osteotomy rotation, and the introduction of torsional or angular deformities in the tibia – all of which can negatively affect clinical function [8, 9] (Figure 20.5). Locking plate fixation does not require contact of the bone to the plate for stability; therefore, osteotomy rotation and reduction can be maintained during screw tightening. Some fixed-angle locking screws have a larger core diameter than conventional screws, to withstand the larger cantilever loading forces under these conditions.

In addition to maintenance of the desired TPA intraoperatively, locking TPLO plates allow less change in the TPA in the postoperative period, as compared to conventional bone plates [10, 11]. When a gap is present at the osteotomy site, biomechanical studies have shown that the Synthes locking TPLO plate has significantly greater construct stiffness as compared to two types of conventional TPLO plate constructs [12].

20.4 Complications of Locking TPLO Plates

Locking plates may reduce the complication rates of TPLO due to a reduction in surgical time, less loss of reduction of the osteotomy and plateau segment, more rigid constructs with decreased implant breakage, and lower infection rates [13–15]. The reduction in postoperative infection with locking TPLO plates may be due to enhanced construct stability, shorter surgical times, or better preservation of blood supply to the surgical region. The TPLO Curve™ plate has a HyProtect™ silver-based plasma antimicrobial coating that provides a continuous release of silver ions that inhibit bacteria growth and biofilm formation for over three months after implantation, which may further decrease postoperative infection rates.

While locking-angle stable screws increase construct strength, this feature can be problematic on occasion. If the bone plate requires bending to accommodate a large medial buttress, it will direct the screws toward the joint surface. Joint penetration may occur in these cases. If the bone plate is contoured around medial buttress, prior to drilling, the mediolateral trajectory of the drill bit can be estimated by evaluating the angle of the threaded drill guide as it locks into the plate hole and comparing it to palpable anatomical landmarks. If the angle suggests that the joint may be penetrated, the plate may be positioned more distally, or a conventional nonlocking cortex screw can be placed and aimed parallel to or angulated away from the joint. After drilling the hole, it is helpful to carefully palpate the drill hole with the depth gauge to ensure that violation of the joint has not occurred.

The aforementioned advantage of the converging angle of locking screws in the Synthes plate design can be problematic if fixation failure occurs. In contrast to conventional screw fixation, where fixation failure usually occurs by screw toggling within the plate hole and subsequently backing out of the bone, fixation failure of locking plates usually occurs by bone slicing. When this occurs, the screws remain in the same orientation relative to the bone plate and cut through the metaphyseal bone, resulting in a large region of damaged bone (Figure 20.6). This large segment of metaphyseal bone loss can complicate revision, as it reduces bone stock for adequate stabilization of the osteotomy.

Specialized threaded drill guides assist screw direction to match with the threads in the screw hole for several plate designs. Cross threading of the drill guide or malpositioning of the screw in the hole will result in cross-threading of the threads in the head of the screw in the plate hole. While this has been shown to decrease construct strength experimentally, to the author's knowledge, clinical problems have not been attributed to this in TPLO.

20.5 Specific Clinical Applications of Locking TPLO Plates

Locking TPLO plates can offer a direct clinical advantage to patients of all sizes by maintaining the desired TPA and limb alignment both intraoperatively and postoperatively. Increased construct strength of locking fixation allows a single broad plate to be used to stabilize very large and giant breed dogs without the need for a secondary bone plate (Figure 20.4). This results in a reduction of surgical time and cost to the client. A clinical study has evaluated the use of locking TPLO plates in dogs weighing greater than 50 kg and found them to be both effective and associated with a decreased postoperative infection rate [16].

The TPLO can be combined with other surgical procedures such as the correction of patellar luxation or angular deformities of the tibia. The increased construct strength of locking TPLO plates in buttress fashion makes them especially useful in these cases, because there is often a gap at the osteotomy site and the plate construct acts as a bridge (Figure 20.7). As discussed earlier, locking plate fixation is superior to conventional plating in this application.

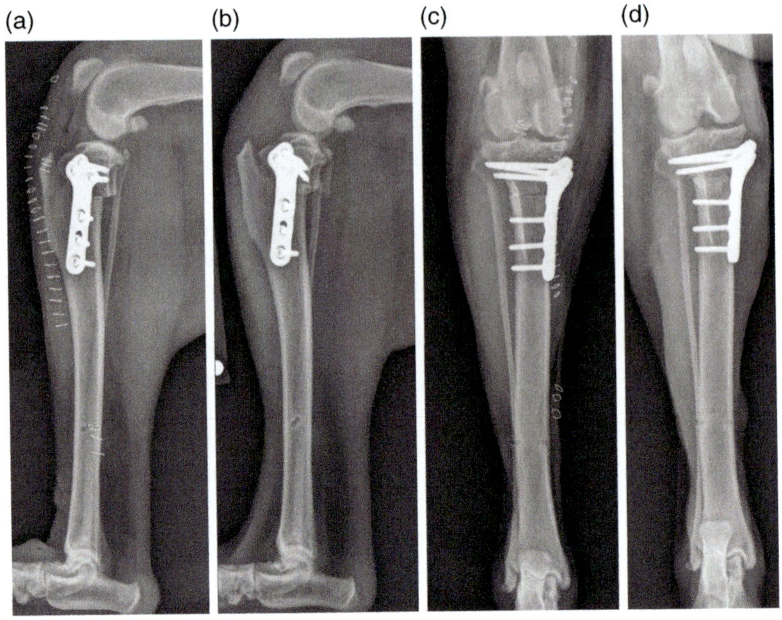

Figure 20.6 Immediate postoperative (a, c) and three-week postoperative (b, d) radiographs taken following TPLO in a seven-year-old dog. Fixation failure of the locking TPLO construct occurred due to slicing of the implants through the bone. Note the relatively unchanged position of the proximal screws, the lateral and caudal collapse of the plateau segment, and the fracture of the proximal fibula.

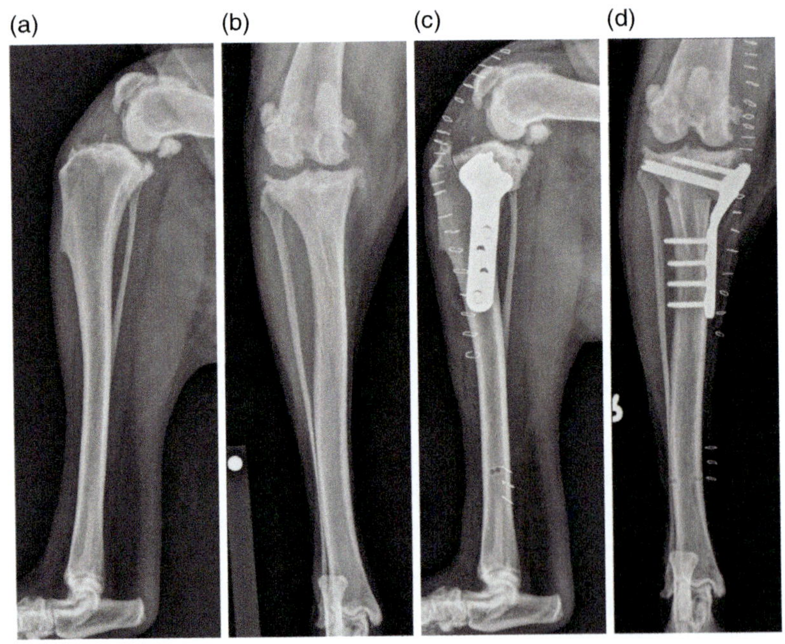

Figure 20.7 Mediolateral (a) and craniocaudal (b) tibial radiographs of a 45.5 kg 5.5-year-old male castrated Labrador retriever with cranial cruciate ligament (CCL) rupture and grade II/IV medial patellar luxation. Postoperative radiographs (c and d) show correction of both conditions; the TPLO is stabilized with hybrid locking fixation.

20.6 Conclusion

The TPLO is one of the most commonly performed veterinary orthopedic surgical procedures. The evidence suggests that optimal placement of the TPLO plate and screws, accurate rotation, and maintenance of the plateau in the desired position are critical to a successful outcome following the procedure. The relatively recent use of locking TPLO plate constructs has provided substantial clinical and biomechanical advantages over conventional plating techniques in achieving these goals. While locking screws and plates may be more expensive than conventional screws, locked plating constructs lead to improved construct strength and maintenance of osteotomy position and limb alignment, which positively affect outcome. Moreover, using locking plate constructs may reduce the possibility of costly complications.

References

1. Wucherer, K.L., Conzemius, M.G., Evans, R. et al. (2013). Short-term and long-term outcomes for overweight dogs with cranial cruciate ligament rupture treated surgically or nonsurgically. *J. Am. Vet. Med. Assoc.* 242 (10): 1364–1372.
2. Bergh, M.S., Sullivan, C., Ferrell, C.L. et al. (2014). Systematic review of surgical treatments for cranial cruciate ligament disease in dogs. *J. Am. Anim. Hosp. Assoc.* 50 (5): 315–321.
3. Duerr, F.M., Martin, K.W., Rishniw, M. et al. (2014). Treatment of canine cranial cruciate ligament disease. A survey of ACVS diplomates and primary care veterinarians. *Vet. Comp. Orthop. Traumatol.* 27 (6): 478–483.
4. Gordon-Evans, W.J., Griffon, D.J., Bubb, C. et al. (2013). Comparison of lateral fabellar suture and tibial plateau leveling osteotomy techniques for treatment of dogs with cranial cruciate ligament disease. *J. Am. Vet. Med. Assoc.* 243 (5): 675–680.
5. Krotscheck, U., Nelson, S.A., Todhunter, R.J. et al. (2016). Long term functional outcome of tibial tuberosity advancement vs. tibial plateau leveling osteotomy and extracapsular repair in a heterogeneous population of dogs. *Vet. Surg.* 45 (2): 261–268.
6. Slocum, B. and Slocum, T.D. (1993). Tibial plateau leveling osteotomy for repair of cranial cruciate ligament rupture in the canine. *Vet. Clin. North Am. Small Anim. Pract.* 23: 777–795.
7. Perren, S.M. (2002). Evolution of the internal fixation of long bone fractures. *J. Bone Joint Surg. Br.* 84-B: 1093–1110.
8. Leitner, M., Pearce, S.G., Windolf, M. et al. (2008). Comparison of locking and conventional screws for maintenance of tibial plateau positioning and biomechanical stability after locking tibial plateau leveling osteotomy plate fixation. *Vet. Surg.* 37: 357–365.
9. Wheeler, J.L., Cross, A.R., and Gingrich, W. (2003). In vitro effects of osteotomy angle and osteotomy reduction on tibial angulation and roation during the tibial plateau-leveling osteotomy procedure. *Vet. Surg.* 32 (4): 371–377.
10. Conkling, A.L., Fagin, B., and Daye, R.M. (2010). Comparison of tibial plateau angle changes after tibial plateau leveling osteotomy fixation with conventional or locking screw technology. *Vet. Surg.* 39: 475–481.
11. Krotscheck, U., Thompson, M.S., Ryan, K.K. et al. (2012). Comparison of TPA, bone healing, and intra-articular screw placement using conventional nonlocked application of surgeon-contoured versus locked application of precontoured TPLO plates in dogs. *Vet. Surg.* 41: 931–937.
12. Kloc, P.A., Kowaleski, M.P., Litsky, A.S. et al. (2009). Biomechanical comparison of two alternative tibial plateau leveling osteotomy plates with the original standard in an axially loaded gap model: an in vitro study. *Vet. Surg.* 38: 40–48.
13. Barnes, D.C., Trinterud, T., Owen, M.R. et al. (2016). Short-term outcome and complications of TPLO using anatomically contoured locking compression plates in small/ medium-breed dogs with "excessive" tibial plateau angle. *J. Sm. Animal. Prac.* 57: 305–310.
14. Kowaleski, M.P., Boudrieau, R.J., Beale, B.S. et al. (2013). Radiographic outcome and complications of tibial plateau leveling osteotomy stabilized with an anatomically contoured locking bone plate. *Vet. Surg.* 42: 847–852.
15. Gordon, S., Moens, N.M., Runciman, J. et al. (2010). The effect of the combination of locking screws and non-locking screws on the torsional properties of a locking-plate construct. *Vet. Comp. Orthop. Traumatol.* 23: 7–13.
16. Solano, M.A., Danielski, A., Kovach, K. et al. (2015). Locking plate and screw fixation after tibial plateau leveling osteotomy reduces postoperative infection rate in dogs over 50kg. *Vet. Surg.* 44: 59–64.

21 Double Pelvic Osteotomy for Hip Dysplasia

Matthew D. Barnhart

The triple pelvic osteotomy (TPO) was first described as a surgical treatment for juvenile canine hip dysplasia in 1969, and its efficacy has been well proven in numerous publications since. The original stair-step osteotomy procedure has undergone a number of iterations over time to ultimately become the current technique that involves pubic, ischial, and ilial osteotomies stabilized by a dedicated TPO plate and an ischial interfragmentary wire. While this TPO is effective at producing acetabular ventroversion and thereby reducing hip subluxation by improving femoral head coverage and articular surface contact, it has reported complication rates of 35–70% [1–3].

Screw loosening is the most common TPO complication, with reported rates of 30–62.5%, which is likely due to a combination factors including the low density of juvenile bone, minimal load sharing between osteotomy ends, and the high amount of motion generated at the ilial osteotomy site [2–5]. While screw loosening can be an incidental finding on routine postoperative radiographs, the potential for catastrophic loss of internal fixation and need for additional surgery is a real concern. Contradictory information exists regarding whether principles aimed at preventing screw loosening, including the use of cancellous screws, trans-sacral screw placement and ischial wiring, offer any benefit at all [2]. Other reported remedies for screw loosening include retightening of screws via open or fluoroscopic assisted approaches, ilial hemicerclage wire placement, and application of a ventral ilial plate [6, 7]. Clearly, any technique or implant that could reduce or prevent screw loosening would be very valuable in this application.

Arguably, there are few other veterinary surgical techniques that have been as positively impacted and improved by the introduction of locking implants as has the TPO. The use of locking TPO plates has dramatically reduced the reported overall complications rates to 5–7% and nearly eliminated screws loosening as a complication [8, 9]. Between two reports in which 371 screws were used in pre-angled seven-hole locking TPO plates (New Generation Devices, Glen Rock NJ), only a single loosened screw was documented (Rose). Noteworthy is that a combination of locking and nonlocking screws was used in the cases. The lack of loosening of the nonlocking screws can likely be attributed to the single beam construct formed by the locking components, which eliminates motion between the plate, screws, and bone. An

Locking Plates in Veterinary Orthopedics, First Edition.
Edited by Matthew D. Barnhart and Karl C. Maritato.

in vitro report also found that screw loosening was significantly reduced by the use of locking TPO plates [10]. Perhaps as importantly, locking TPO plates have truly made the double pelvic osteotomy (DPO) a viable alternative with distinct advantages over its predecessor.

In 2006, P.H. Haudiquet and J.F. Guillon presented the results from an *in vitro* study evaluating the feasibility of achieving sufficient acetabular ventroversion when only the ilium and pubic bones are osteotomized [11] (Figure 21.1). The goal of sparing the ischium was to simplify the TPO and maintain a more biomechanically stable construct that could reduce postoperative complications and morbidity. Segmental rotation was in fact possible because the intact ischium deformed through bending of the open pubic symphysis. Ironically, this same "soft plastic" juvenile bone, which is necessary to achieve rotation, is also what contributes to the aforementioned screw-loosening complications.

The ability of the DPO to improve coxofemoral joint congruity with a lower complication rate than that of TPOs has been described. A restoration of a normal joint congruity of 50–72% of femoral head coverage by the acetabulum following DPO was reported by Vezzoni et al. This has been postulated to be advantageous over the TPO, which tends to result in excessive femoral head coverage [12]. While using a locking plate when performing a TPO does significantly reduce implant associated complications, a DPO still offers a number of advantages comparatively (Table 21.1). To date, no clinical studies have directly compared DPOs and TPOs. Anecdotally, this author and other surgeons feel that DPO dogs appear to be significantly more comfortable and mobile after surgery compared to TPO patients. As such, many surgeons now feel there is no compelling reason to continue to perform the TPO, and in our practice, it has been replaced by the DPO. However, consideration should be given to some important technical differences between the two procedures.

Without question, forced rotational deformation of the intact ischial table is physically more challenging than maneuvering an osteotomized ischium. Holding the caudal segment of the pelvis in rotation while applying the DPO plate can be difficult. However, even with the ischium intact, the caudal osteotomized segment can still be "stacked" on top of the cranial segment, which makes applying the caudal portion of the DPO plate much easier. In cases where stacking is not possible, the author has found inserting a freer periosteal elevator between the two

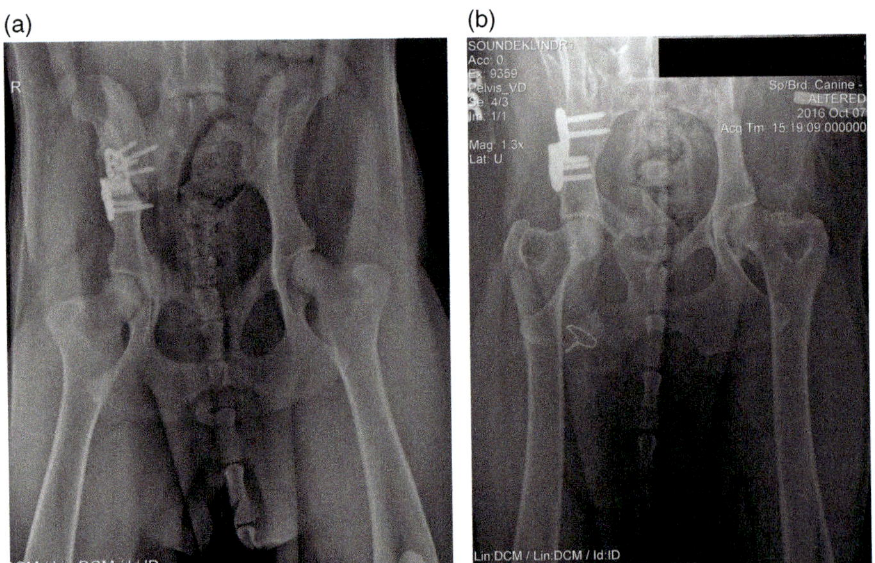

Figure 21.1 **(a, b)** Approximately six-week postoperative double pelvic osteotomy (DPO) and triple pelvic osteotomy (TPO) radiographs. Note lack of a ischial osteotomy and hemicerclage wire with the DPO.

Table 21.1 Double pelvic osteotomy (DPO) vs. triple pelvic osteotomy (TPO): Pros and cons.

DPO pros	TPO pros	DPO cons	TPO cons
No ischial osteotomy No ischial wire	Easier to rotate ilium More accurate rotation result (?)	Challenging to rotate Less accurate rotation result (?)	3 vs. 2 osteotomies Slower recovery (?)
Cantilever support by intact ischium		More expensive locking implant	More stress on ilial segment
Less screw loosening[a]			Screw loosening[b]
Preservation of pelvic geometry			Pelvic canal narrowing occurs
Restoration of normal joint congruity (50–72% coverage)			Excessive femoral head coverage (≥90%)

[a] Locking implants.
[b] Nonlocking implants.

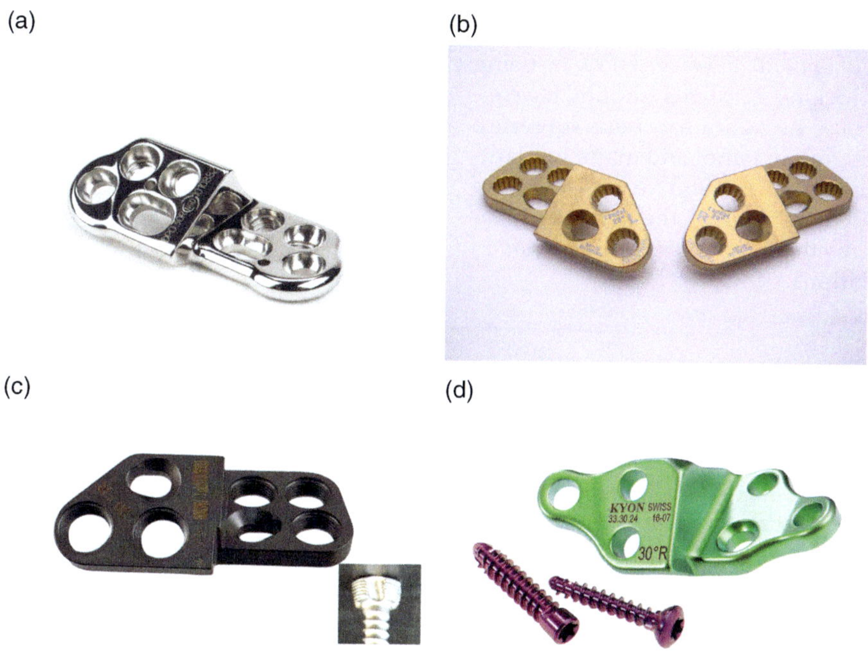

Figure 21.2 Some examples of locking DPO plates: (a) New Generation Device's DPO plate, (b) PAX DPO plate, (c) Freedom Lock DPO plate, and (d) ALPS DPO plate.

fragments can be used to elevate the caudal fragment, allowing proper placement of the plate. Additionally, the author favors a locking DPO plate that has a compression hole in addition to the locking holes (Figure 21.2). This allows the surgeon to place a cortical screw in compression to help bring the plate flush to the bone and assist with rotation. While this can be achieved in plates with only locking holes by placing a cortical screw initially in place of a locking screw (and then replacing it with a locking screw), the surgeon is limited by how much this screw can be angled in such holes. Compression of the plate against the bone is critical in order to achieve the full desired rotation and can be further assisted by placing bone reduction forceps against the plate and ilium. The author also prefers a polyaxial locking screw insertion option (PAX DPO plate, Securos, Fiskdale MA, Freedom Lock DPO plate, Everost, Sturbridge MA) since a fixed-angle requirement can be challenging in this area and may require more aggressive surgical dissection to expose dorsal aspect of the cranial segment (Figure 21.2).

Additionally, unlike with TPOs, the actual amount of acetabular ventroversion achieved via DPO is typically 5° less than the applied plate angle [13]. Both *in vitro* and clinical studies have demonstrated that a maximum rotation of 20° is ideal and that there is no difference in Norberg angles nor femoral head coverage when increasing from 20–30° of rotation [14, 15]. As such, a 25° DPO plate should be used in order to achieve a 20° rotation.

Whether or not a TPO or DPO is being performed, locking implants should be considered the new necessity for these surgeries. Proven reductions in minor and major implant-associated complications and favorable *in vitro* and clinical data prove the unquestionable advantages this implant technology has in these applications.

References

1. Plante, J., Dupuis, J., Beuregard, G. et al. (1997). Long-term results of conservative treatment, excision arthroplasty, and triple pelvic osteotomy for treatment of hips dysplasia in the immature dog. *Vet. Comp. Orthop. Tramatol.* 10: 101–110.
2. Hosgood, G. and Lewis, D.D. (1993). Retrospective evaluation of fixation complications of 49 pelvic osteotomies in 36 dogs. *J. Small Anim. Pract.* 34: 123–130.
3. Remedios, A.M. and Fries, C.L. (1993). Implant complications in 20 triple pelvic osteotomies. *Vet. Comp. Orthop. Tramatol.* 6: 202–207.
4. Doornink, M.T., Nieves, M.A., and Evans, R. (2006). Evaluation of ilial screw loosening after triple pelvic osteotomy in dogs: 227 cases (1991–1999). *J. Am. Vet. Med. Assoc.* 229: 535–541.
5. Koch, D.A., Hazewinkel, H.A., Nap, R.C. et al. (1993). Radiographic evaluation and comparison of plate fixation after triple pelvic osteotomy in 32 dogs with hip dysplasia. *Vet. Comp. Orthop. Traumatol.* 34: 123–130.
6. Fitch, R.B., Kerwin, S., Hosgood, G. et al. (2002). Treatment for mechanically failed triple pelvic osteotomies in four dogs–part II. *Vet. Comp. Orthop. Tramatol.* 15: 172–176.
7. Bogoni, P. and Rovesit, G.L. (2005). Early detection and treatment of screw loosening in triple pelvic osteotomy. *Vet. Surg.* 34: 190–195.
8 Rose, S.A., Peck, J.N., Tano, C.A. et al. (2012b). Effect of a locking triple pelvic osteotomy plate on screw loosening in 26 dogs. *Vet. Surg.* 14: 156–162.
9. Rose, S.A., Bruecker, K.A., Peterson, S.W. et al. (2012a). Use of locking plate and screws for triple pelvic osteotomy. *Vet. Surg.* 41: 114–120.
10. Case, J.B., Wilson, D.M., Knudsen, J.M. et al. (2012). Comparison of the mechanical behaviors of locked and nonlocked plate/screw fixation applied to experimentally induced rotational osteotomies in canine ilia. *Vet. Surg.* 41: 103–113.
11. Haudiquet, P.H., Guillon, J.F. Radiographic evaluation of double pelvic osteotomy versus triple pelvic osteotomy in the dog: an in vitro experimental study. Proceedings of the 13th ESVOT Congress; 10–14 September 2006; Munich, Germany. pgs. 85–86.
12 Vezzoni, A., Boiocchi, S., Vezzoni, L. et al. (2010). Double pelvic osteotomy for treatment of hips dysplasia in dogs. *Vet. Comp. Orthop. Tramatol.* 23 (6): 444–452.
13. Punke, J.P., Fix, D.B., Tomlinson, J.L. et al. (2011). Acetabular ventroversion with double pelvic osteotomy versus triple pelvic osteotomy: a cadaveric study in dogs. *Vet. Surg.* 40: 555–562.
14. Dejardin, L.M., Perry, R.L., and Arnoszky, S.P. (1998). The effect of triple pelvic osteotomy on the articular contact area of the hip joint in dysplastic dogs: an *in vitro* experimental study. *Vet. Surg.* 27: 194–202.
15. Tomlinson, J.L. and Cook, J.L. (2002). Effects of degree of acetabular rotation after triple pelvic osteotomy on the position of the femoral head in relationship to the acetabulum. *Vet. Surg.* 31: 398–403.

22 Distal Femoral Osteotomy for Patella Luxation

Ian Gordon Holsworth and Kirk L. Wendelburg

22.1 Introduction

Corrective osteotomies of the distal femur as part of the surgical technique for addressing congenital patellar luxation have become commonplace for some veterinary orthopedists over the past 10 years. Distal femoral corrective osteotomy (DFCO) has been reported as a successful surgical method for the treatment of the excessive distal femoral angulation that can play a role in patellar luxation. While several methods exist for performing a DFCO, they can be divided into closing or opening wedge osteotomies/ectomies. The use of tibial plateau leveling osteotomy (TPLO) jigs, intramedullary pins, interlocking nails, various plating systems, and Ilizarov fixators, have been reported in the past as techniques to help control, manipulate, and stabilize the osteotomies.

The realization that valgus and varus deformities of the distal femur may contribute to quadriceps complex malalignment and predispose the patella to luxation has changed our understanding of patellar instability and forced the development of presurgical imaging and assessment of femoral anatomy. Many individual variations in the technique of distal femoral (corrective) osteotomy (DFO or DFCO) are present. The major differences lying in presurgical planning, intraoperative use of bone jigs, osteotomy technique, correction of femoral torsion if present, medial, or lateral or combined bone plate application site and choice of implant. The use of locking plates and screws is common with the DFO procedure with several options available to the orthopedic surgeon.

22.2 Anatomy

The normal canine femoral diaphysis has a slight caudal curve in the mid-sagittal/median plane and a slight medial curve in the coronal/frontal plane. While the normal reference range of anatomic angles have been investigated, documented, and published [1], some less documented variation exists, particularly in the chondrodystrophic breeds. It has been postulated that with increased degrees of distal curvature, the tracking of the patellar mechanism is affected and luxation due to malignment across the stifle joint may result. Distal torsion of the femur is also recognized as influencing femoral condyle alignment and patellar stability.

Locking Plates in Veterinary Orthopedics, First Edition.
Edited by Matthew D. Barnhart and Karl C. Maritato.

The attachment location of the straight patellar ligament (i.e. patellar tendon) on the proximal tibial tuberosity of the tibial crest also plays a significant role in quadriceps-patellar complex alignment. The term *tibial torsion* is applied to varying degrees of abnormal tibial conformation with the end result being variations in the medial or lateral location of the tibial tuberosity.

In patellar luxation, patients the surgeon should attempt to assess the location and degree of skeletal malalignment pre and intraoperatively to allow adjustment of the anatomical malalignment into a normal range. The presurgical imaging techniques that have been utilized for this purpose include both radiography and computed tomography. Debate exists concerning which of these techniques is best suited for surgical assessment, how the patient should be positioned for these studies, and what degree of abnormal angulation justifies a corrective osteotomy. Publications investigating the different techniques are available for review by the individual surgeon [1–10].

22.3 Surgical Approach

Surgical access to the femur is from a lateral or medial approach. Both approaches have their place in both fracture repair and corrective osteotomies, and both approaches have similar but distinct challenges.

The lateral approach is performed by incising the biceps femoris fascia adjacent to the vastus lateralis m. and reflecting the vastus lateralis m. cranially to expose the bone surface. In the proximal femur, this is complicated by the presence of the tensor fascia lata and gluteal muscles and distally by the soft tissues associated with the stifle joint. The exposure is normally continued distally adjacent to the caudal line of the vastus lateralis m. with incision into the joint capsule to open the joint and allow medial luxation of the patella. The aim of the approach is to expose the complete condylar surfaces and mid to distal femur in the cranial aspect. Incision and retraction of the joint capsule cranially is necessary to achieve this aim.

The medial approach to the femur is made by initially incising the fascial connection between the cranial and caudal sartorius muscles. This fascial connection is distinct in canines but nonexistent in felines, requiring a muscle-splitting technique. Once the sartorius muscles are separated and retracted, the vastus medialis m. is identified and it can be separated from the neurovascular tract that runs caudal to its caudal margin. This must be performed carefully to avoid iatrogenic damage to these structures. Once the separation between the neurovascular tract and the muscle belly is complete and any perforating vasculature is isolated and ligated as necessary, the vastus medialis muscle belly can be retracted cranially to expose the femoral bone surface. As the dissection proceeds proximally the femoral bone shaft becomes more difficult to isolate effectively and the musculature of the inguinal area impedes good access. Placing deep retractors between the vastus medialis m. and the tendon of the pectineus m. will allow good visualization of the medial and cranio-medial wall of the femur. If a medial arthrotomy has been performed, the joint capsule incision is continued proximally and laterally to release the patellar complex and allow complete lateral luxation of the patella.

Prior to femoral osteotomy a decision on whether a trochleoplasty is to be performed should be made and completed. Awareness of the depth of the trochlear bone cuts for both a block and wedge-recession trochleoplasty is important as an excessively deep trochleoplasty may cause issue with distal bone segment bone screws being placed during the implantation phase.

22.4 Ostectomy Technique

22.4.1 Technique 1: Medial or Lateral Femoral Plating with Jig Assistance by IG Holsworth

Once the chosen femoral and stifle approach is completed and the cranial surface of both the intra-articular and mid to distal femoral shaft is exposed, the intraoperative ostectomy planning can begin (Figure 22.1).

In most cases of distal femoral varus or valgus, the center of rotation and angulation (CORA) is directly proximal to the joint capsule attachment on the cranial aspect of the femur. This can be assessed presurgically on planning

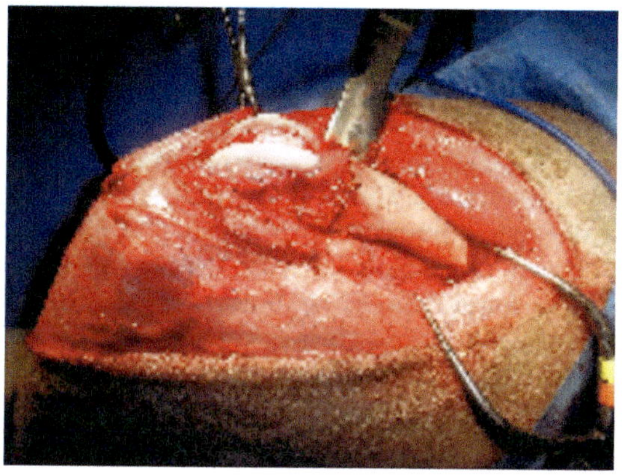

Figure 22.1 Intraoperative exposure of the cranio-lateral aspect of the distal left femur with open arthrotomy and previously performed recession wedge trochleoplasty.

imaging, and every effort should be made to perform the corrective osteotomy as close to this location as possible (Figure 22.2a and b).

Another factor that must be considered prior to definitive choice of the osteotomy line(s) is the configuration of the locking bone plate that will be implanted. It is wise to place the intended bone plate on the medial or lateral wall of the femur in an approximation of final location to confirm appropriate spanning of the osteotomy site.

An additional consideration that must be entertained is the location of the jig's bone pins. The distal pin should be placed, in most cases, directly proximal to the cartilage surface in the cranial midline of the distal femur. The final osteotomy location should consider the first

(a) (b)

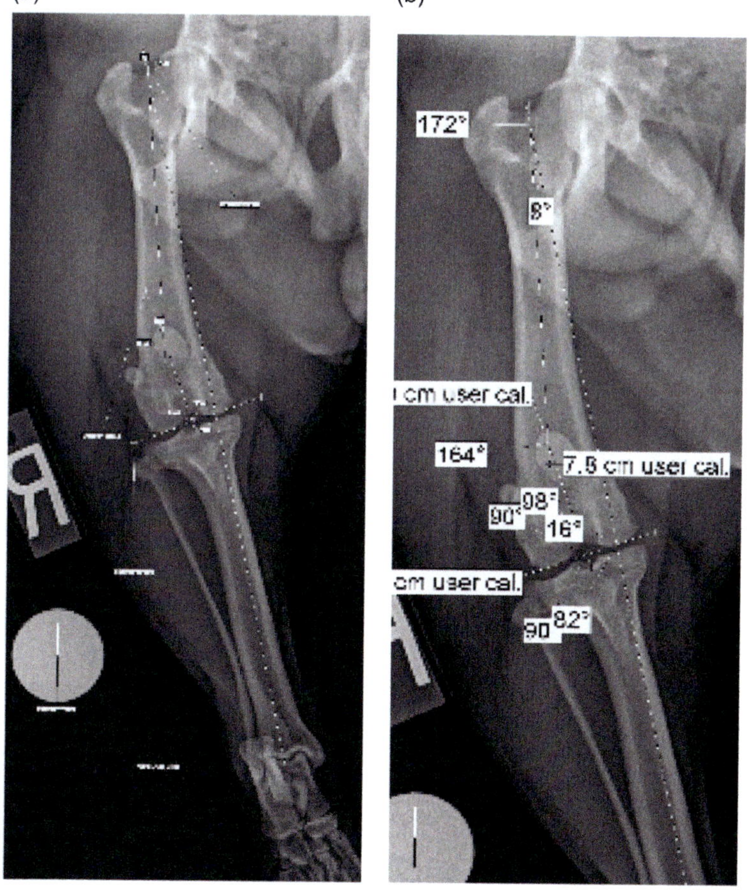

Figure 22.2 (a and b) Full right limb posterior–anterior alignment radiograph (a) and isolated femoral shaft with 16° measured femoral varus. The center of rotation and angulation (CORA) in the frontal plane is seen close to the proximal pole of the patella.

distal screw location and alignment below the osteotomy so that drilling of the screw hole does not interfere or contact the jig pin. In the majority of implants, the screw will engage the bone distal to that jig pin. The other issue that must be addressed before jig placement is the proximal jig pin location. It is also imperative that the proximal jig pin be placed in the midline of the cranial femur at a site where the implant spans that pin so that the first proximal plate screw is proximal to the jig pin. Failure to do this can lead to fracture through the jig pin site, as it is not protected by the bone plate if placed too far proximally. Once the jig and plate locations have been determined, the osteotomy location can be finalized and the cranial bone surface is scored to reflect the wedge ostectomy lines (Figure 22.3a and b).

It is also helpful to lightly score the cranial surface of the bone in the midline sagittal plane to allow accurate realignment during ostectomy reduction, and if a torsional adjustment is made, the degree of rotation can be subjectively assessed more accurately.

In the case of an opening wedge DFO, a single bone cut is made; in the case of a closing wedge osteotomy, a second osteotomy is made to remove a triangular ostectomy segment that has been predetermined in size and orientation to correct the abnormal anatomic lateral distal femoral angle (aLDFA) to the normal aLDFA of 94–98°. In most surgeons' hands the goal is 94°, although under- and overcorrection are not uncommon. Concerns with the opening wedge ostectomy primarily include osteotomy construct failure due to a relatively unstable construct and delayed healing with an appreciable bone gap present on the open aspect. Once the bone is scored, with either technique, the ostectomy is performed using a sagittal saw and a blade with enough length to traverse the patient's femoral dimensions. Great care must be taken to follow the planned cut orientation and location, avoid angulation from the transverse plane and converge the two osteotomy lines on the medial (for femoral varus correction) or lateral (for femoral valgus correction) to avoid undercorrection of the deformity. Once sectioned, control of the two femoral segments is achieved by the jig and manual manipulation at the ostectomy site.

In the case of a closing wedge it is vital that accurate, stable reduction of the wedge void is achieved. This is achieved by appropriate limb manipulation and assistance of a point-to-point bone reduction forceps placed around the jig

(b)

(a)

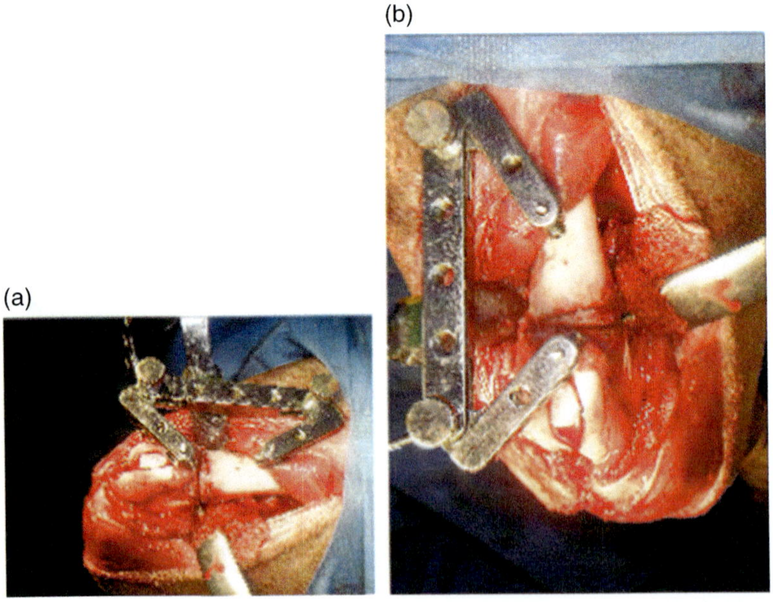

Figure 22.3 (a and b) Lateral and cranial view of the distal left femur with an attached Slocum tibial plateau leveling osteotomy (TPLO) jig in the correct location. The lateral aspect closing-wedge ostectomy is scored onto the bone surface using a sagittal saw to ensure accurate ostectomy performance.

pins under the jig. Once reduced, alteration of a perceived torsional deformity can be made in the transverse plane using the midline bone score marks made earlier to determine the degree of correction. Temporary stabilization of the osteotomy/ostectomy can be improved beyond the jig pin reduction forceps step by placing a small 1.6–2.0 mm trocar-pointed bone pin across the osteotomy site in an oblique fashion. This allows for easier plate application and helps avoid dynamic mal-reduction during the plating process. The selection of either a contoured straight plate, a custom DFO plate or a multidirectional contourable plate is one individual surgeons should make according to their training, experience, and available equipment. Recontouring to match the variations of the individual patients bone is advisable and very often necessary. The plate should be in close contact with the bone surface for a majority of its length if possible. A medial plate is theoretically not as advantageous as a lateral plate as the medial cortical wall is the compression surface whereas the lateral cortex is the tension surface; however, this concept applies to non-locking plates only. Once contoured the plate can be secured to the bone with initial cortical screws; once that process is complete, locking screws can be placed with an ideal of two locking screws per segment (Figure 22.4).

It is advisable to have three screws in the distal segment and four in the proximal segment if possible. Once the plate is secured with a minimum of two screws per segment the jig and pins can be removed (Figure 22.5).

It is also possible to remove the transosteotomy bone pin if interference with bone screws is encountered or the surgeon prefers it. Once

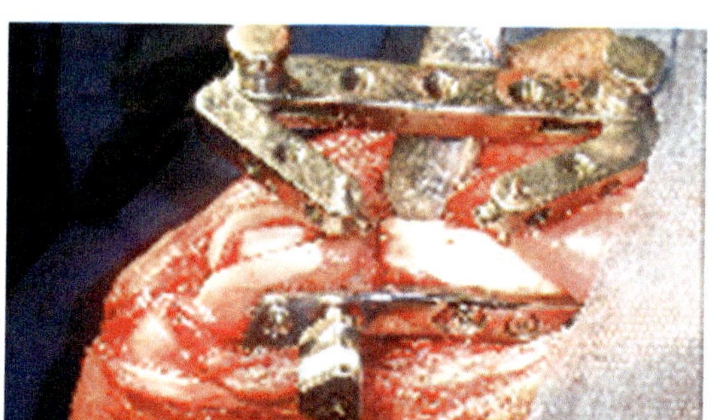

Figure 22.4 Intraoperative placement of a lateral distal femoral osteotomy (DFO) plate following ostectomy wedge reduction with temporary jig retention.

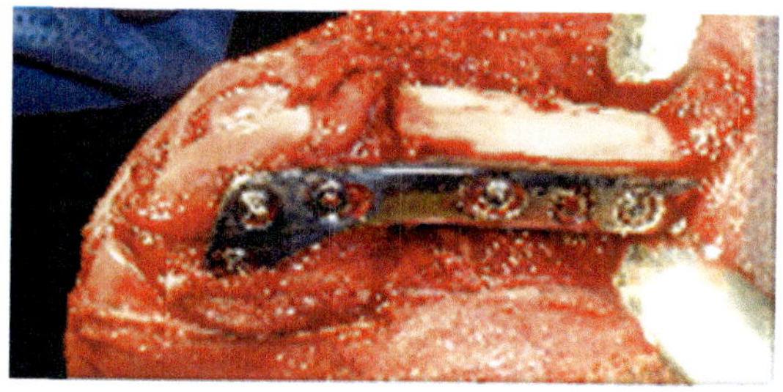

Figure 22.5 Completed placement of a lateral femoral DFO plate following jig removal.

the construct is complete, reassessment of patellar instability may be performed. If continued medial or lateral tracking is observed and significant tibial torsion is present consideration may be given to performance of a tibial crest transposition (TCT), although this is commonly not necessary. The procedure's structural alterations are completed with finalizing soft tissue release and imbrication so as to ensure a central and stable patella on the surgical table prior to closure. Closure is routine and is dictated by the initial approach. Postoperative radiographs should demonstrate correction of the excessive varus or valgus angulation with appropriate implant location (Figure 22.6a and b).

The distal femoral osteotomy, whether an opening wedge or closing wedge, must be protected postsurgery from patient overactivity and excessive loading. Failure to do so will lead to delayed healing and/or construct failure, which is disastrous in many instances and will require further surgery with a reasonable expectation of suboptimal results. Follow-up radiographic assessment must be undertaken prior to increasing patient activity to ensure that osteotomy healing is progressing satisfactorily and construct stability remains (Figure 22.7a and b).

22.4.2 Technique 2: Distal Femoral Osteotomy for Correction of Patella Luxation Using Double Plating and the Kyon ALPS System by KL Wendelburg

A novel method of DFCO uses bilateral advanced locking plate system (ALPS) plates with the smaller medially placed stabilizing plate placed prior to the osteotomy. The author believes that the bilateral plating procedure is easier to perform than some other techniques and has produced good clinical outcomes in the author's (KLW) hands.

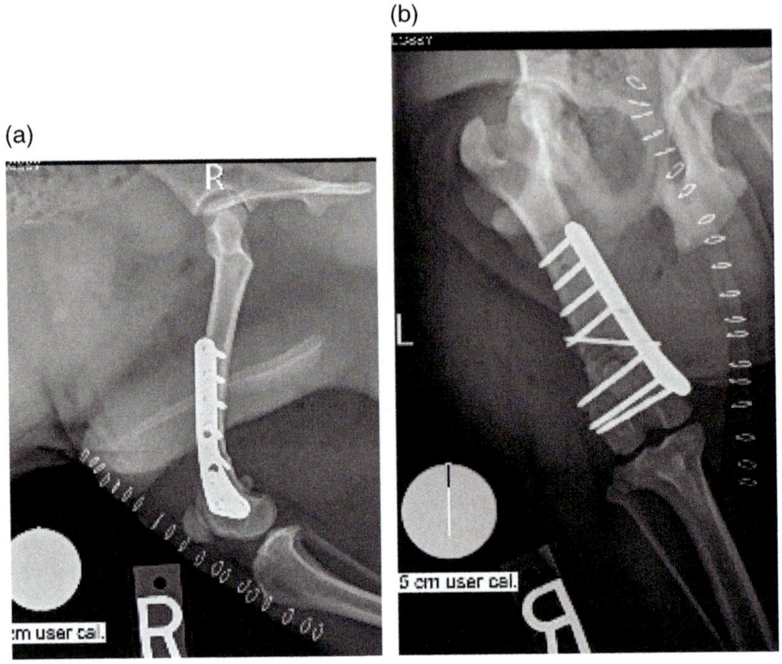

Figure 22.6 (a and b) Lateral and PA view immediately postoperatively of right femoral DFO for excessive varus correction with medial-placed locking DFO plate and trans-ostectomy stabilization pin.

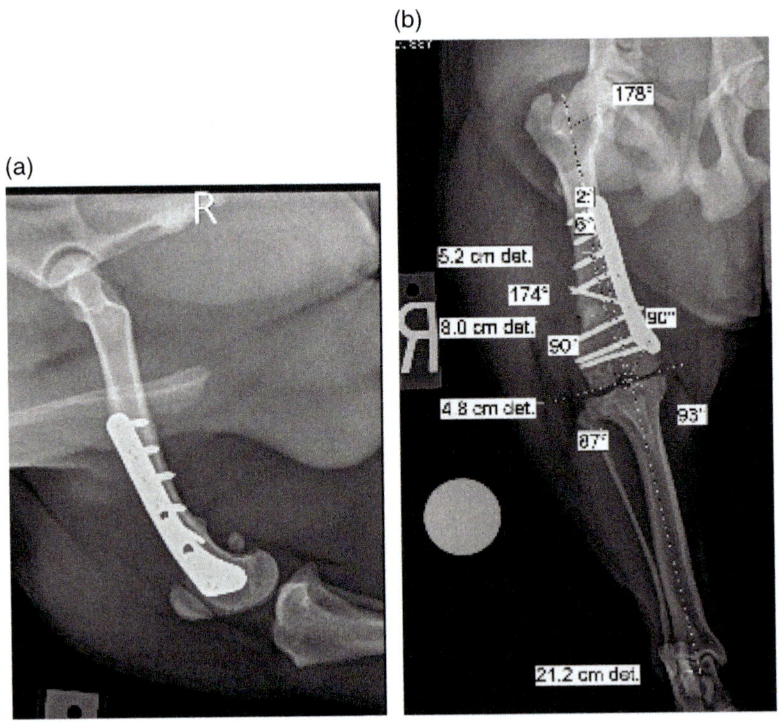

Figure 22.7 (a and b) Follow-up lateral and PA radiographs six weeks post-DFO. Ostectomy site appearance, implant location and femoral alignment appears appropriate and unchanged from post-surgery (Figure 22.6a and b). Progressive bone deposition is apparent and of an appropriate degree. Six (6) degrees of femoral varus are measured.

A medial or lateral parapatellar and distal femur skin incision is made. A routine medial approach to the distal femur is made just caudal to the quadriceps muscle group. During dissection, the majority of the geniculate vasculature and femoral periosteum is be preserved. A radiographically predetermined measurement is made from the distal aspect of the medial femoral condyle proximally and marked to indicate the CORA and osteotomy site. A combination of CT and radiographs may be necessary in some very large or giant patients to allow accurate assessment of the femur morphology (Figures 22.8 and 22.9).

A small six-hole (#5 or #6) ALPS plate is placed on the medial aspect of the femur with the center of the plate (between holes three and four) placed at the proposed osteotomy site (Figures 22.10 and 22.11). The plate is compressed to the bone with mono-cortical standard screws in the outer most holes. Mono-cortical locking screws are placed in the adjacent holes proximally and distally with the two central holes left open. The proximal and distal mono-cortical standard screws are replaced with mono-cortical locking screws.

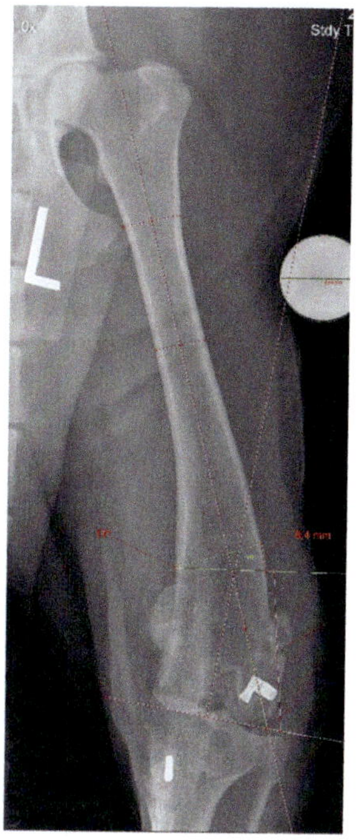

Figure 22.8 Severe distal femoral varus resulting in multiple failed attempts to correct a grade 3 MPL.

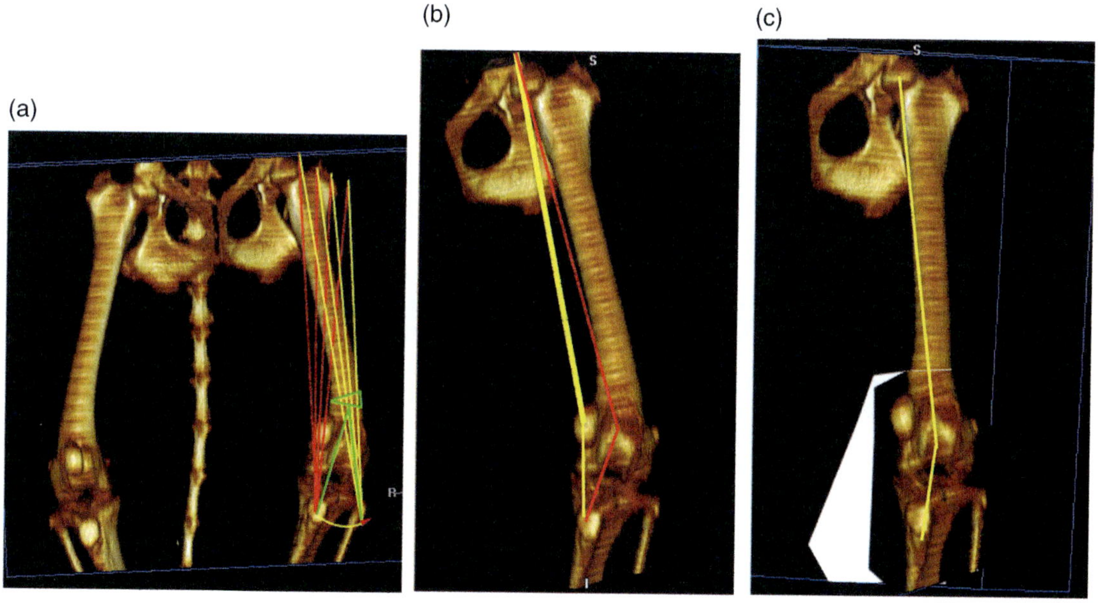

Figure 22.9 (a–c) 3D CT scan of a grade 3 MPL. Red lines show the alignment of the quadriceps mechanism. The yellow lines indicate the amount of tibial tuberosity transposition required to realign the patella into trochlear groove. The required amount of lateral translation of the tuberosity cannot be achieved, and the trochlear groove continues to be malaligned with the quadriceps mechanism. Quadriceps angle (Q angle) of the a grade 3 MPL. The yellow line represents the existing quadriceps alignment before and after a DFO. Notice how the Q angle post-osteotomy is now equal to the preexisting quadriceps alignment.

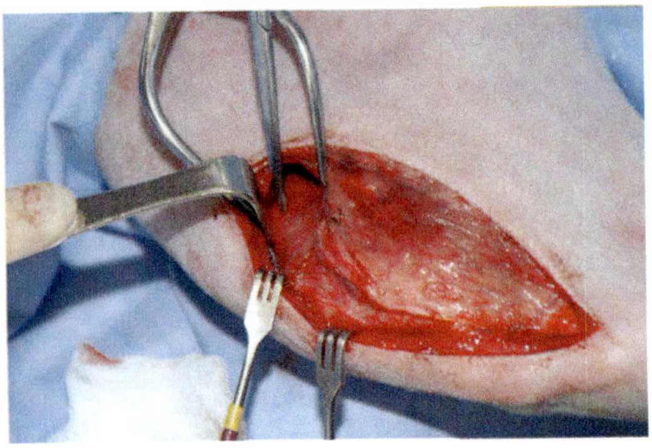

Figure 22.10 A medial approach to the distal femur. Femur is exposed with minimal dissection and the periosteum is left intact.

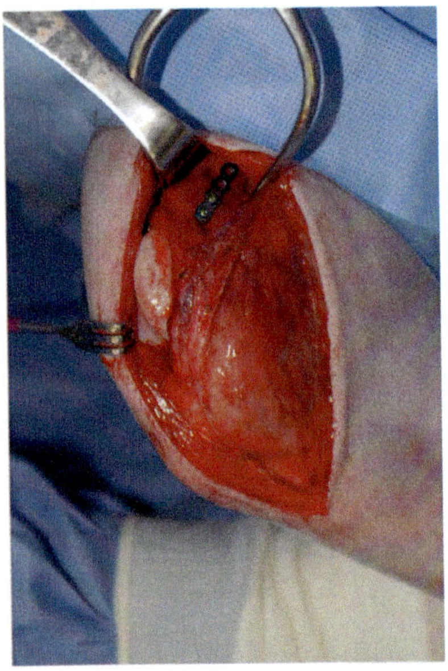

Figure 22.11 A six-hole #5 or 6 Advanced Locking Plate System (ALPS) plate is fixed to the medial femoral cortex. Notice holes three and four are left open. The CORA osteotomy location lies between those two holes. A medial or lateral approach to the stifle can be done to inspect the trochlear groove and remainder of the stifle joint.

A partial (cranial half) transverse osteotomy is then performed with a reciprocating saw over the cranial aspect of the femur, centered between middle two holes (three and four) of the medially placed ALPS plate.

A lateral approach to the distal femur, just caudal to the vastus lateralis muscle, is then made, again preserving the majority of the geniculate vasculature and the periosteum.

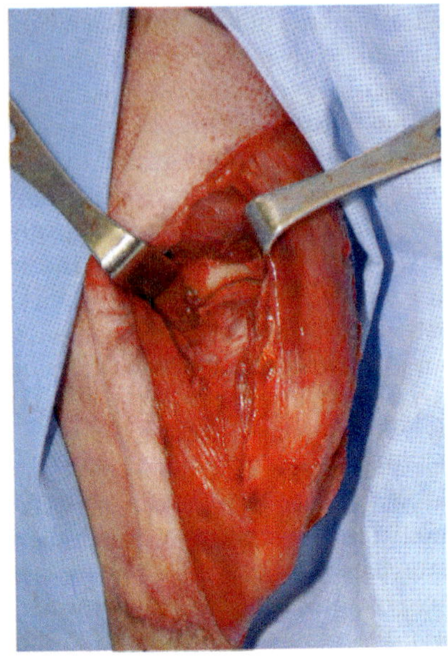

Figure 22.12 The lateral approach to the distal femur. The transverse osteotomy and the second wedge osteotomy are easily and accurately performed with the femoral alignment maintained by the previously applied medial plate.

Using the cranial partial osteotomy as a directional guide, complete the transverse osteotomy to the medial plate between screw holes three and four using a sagittal saw (Figure 22.12). If a torsion correction is planned, the proximal aspect of the medial plate should have an additional screw hole and held to the bone with one mono-cortical standard screw and a secure bone holding forceps. Following the completed transverse osteotomy, you must return to the medial plate, release the proximal bone by removing the screw, and rotate the distal segment as required. Using a Kirschner wire on each side of the osteotomy can serve as guides to achieve the correct amount of rotation. Following rotation, the proximal plate is secured as previously described using mono-cortical locking screws. For the closing wedge procedures, a lateral closing wedge ostectomy is performed to remove the premeasured section of bone proximal to the initial osteotomy. This is done by measuring the radiographically calculated distance proximally from the initial transverse osteotomy. Start the second osteotomy of the wedge directly lateral on the femur using a sagittal saw. Then, insert another sagittal saw blade into the initial transverse osteotomy to be used as a guide. While holding a radiographically predetermined angle guide against the sagittal saw blade placed in the transverse osteotomy, complete the second osteotomy from lateral to medial. The wedge of bone is created with the osteotomies coming together at the medial plate between the central holes three and four. The wedge is then removed and the lateral defect in the bone is easily collapsed and compressed manually by manipulation of the distal femur.

This will produce bending of the small medial ALPS plate between holes two and four. A larger ALPS plate is contoured in plane to the distal femur. While the distal femur is held in approximate reduction with pointed bone reduction forceps, bending and torsional contouring of the plate to the lateral surface of the femur is achieved. While being held in reduction, a standard cortical screw is placed in one of the distal two screw holes of the contoured plate. With the distal plate compressed to the distal femur, the osteotomy is collapsed and compressed, then held with a bone-holding forceps over the proximal plate and bone. After assuring alignment laterally on the femur, a proximal standard bicortical screw is placed to compress the plate to the bone. With the plate compressed to the bone both distally and proximally, mono-cortical locking screws are used to fill the remaining holes proximal and distal to the osteotomy. The distal monocortical standard screw is then replaced with a locking screw (Figure 22.13).

Alignment is then evaluated by flexing and extending along with internal and external rotation of the stifle. A trochlear groove recession is performed for patients that are assessed to have a shallow trochlear groove or worn trochlear ridge. Since the DFCO will appropriately correct the joint angle and Q angle, a tibial tuberosity transposition should not be necessary to complement this procedure. Some dogs with severe deformities having concurrent internal stifle torsion may require a lateral stabilizing suture from the lateral fabella to the tibial tuberosity to prevent or neutralize excessive internal torsion within the stifle joint. The patella should remain in the groove and appeared appropriately reduced prior to closure. A routine closure is then performed.

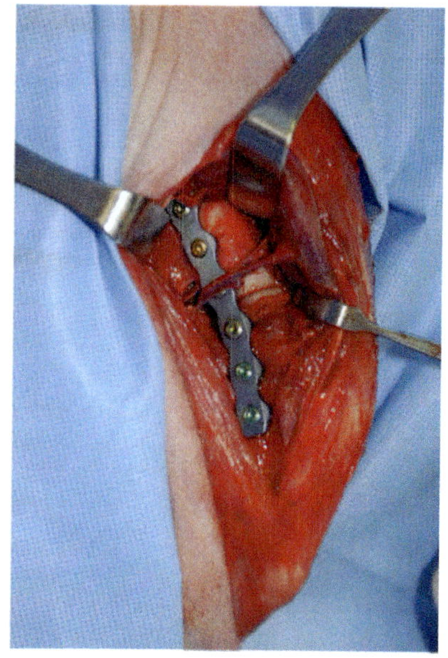

Figure 22.13 Application of the lateral ALPS plate is performed by first compressing the plate to the bone with standard cortical screws (gold color) placed proximal and distal to the osteotomy. The distal standard cortical screw has been replaced with a monocortical locking screw (green color). The smaller-diameter standard cortical screw can also be used to apply compression across the osteotomy site. Notice both in-plane and out of plane bending of the ALPS plate to allow for very distal fixation.

All stifles should be evaluated for concurrent cranial cruciate ligament rupture during surgery. If a cranial crucial ligament (CCL) rupture is diagnosed, a TPLO can be performed concurrently with the DFCO procedure. Severe cases of distal femoral varus may also have concurrent proximal tibial valgus. If the mechanical medial proximal (mMPTA) of the distal tibial in a tangential view CA-CR view radiograph is over 95°, a corrective osteotomy of the proximal tibia should also be performed to achieve a post-operative mMPTA of 90–93°.

Orthogonal femoral radiographs consisting of a mediolateral projection and either a craniocaudal or caudocranial projection are obtained postoperatively. Distal femoral angulation assessed radiographically with a goal of the aLDFA to range from 92–95° (Figures 22.14 and 22.15).

Instead of using a jig to maintain reduction, this technique uses a small ALPS plate to stabilize the site of the closing wedge osteotomy. The placement of the small ALPS plate on the

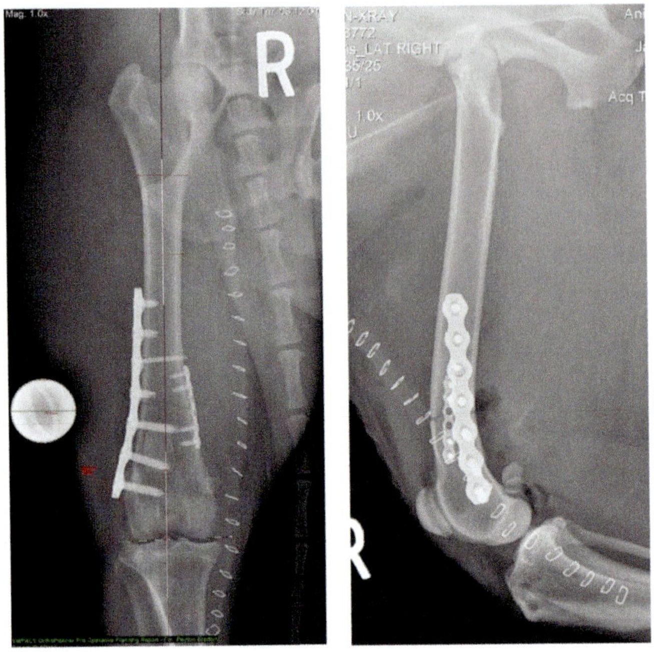

Figure 22.14 Postop distal femoral corrective osteotomy (DFCO). Note the mild amount of in-plane bending needed to keep the plate caudal to the lateral trochlear groove.

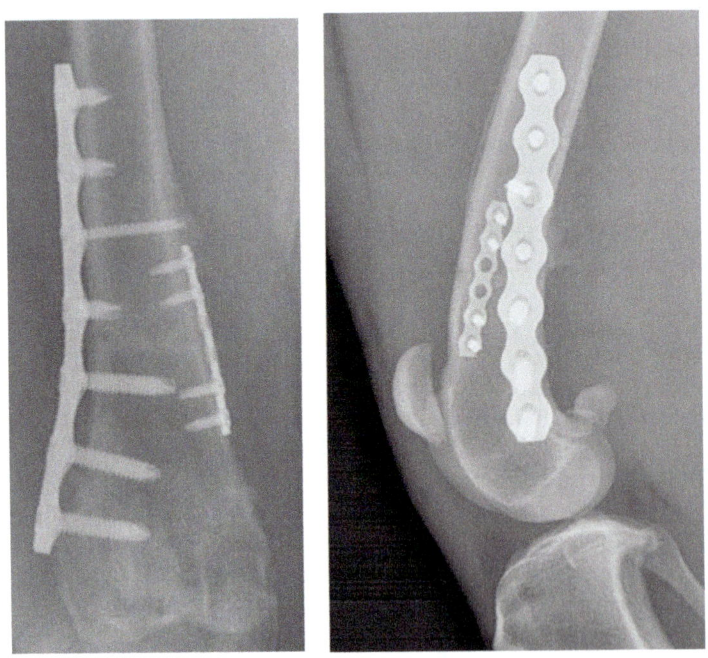

Figure 22.15 One-month postop DFCO. Nearly healed osteotomy with a return to normal function.

medial cortex prior to the osteotomies provides additional stability and reference to facilitate an accurate wedge generated with the second osteotomy. The locking plate design of the ALPS plate allows for monocortical locking screws to be used. The monocortical locking screws not only allow for both medial and lateral plates to be applied to the distal

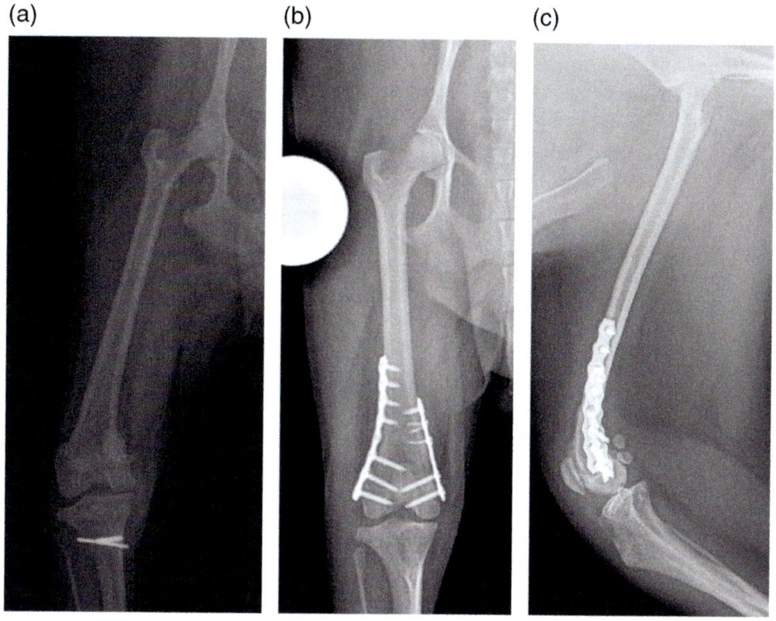

Figure 22.16 (a, b, and c) Failed traditional MPL repair in a 5 kg toy breed referred for DFCO. Two-months postop DFCO with healed osteotomy and normal function. In-plane bending allows for distal position of ALPS plate.

femur, but also make it easier to perform a lateral closing wedge osteotomy with the medial plate fixed to the bone. The in-plane bending feature gives the surgeon the ability to conform both the medial and lateral plates to distal femurs with excessive distal femoral procurvotum. Accuracy of the intended correction angle will still be maintained even if the second osteotomy exits the medial cortex proximal to the first transverse osteotomy since the plate maintains the medial cortex distance.

The author has found this method to be technically easier than other reported techniques that use TPLO jigs to assist. With just four screws placed, the small medial plate is very quickly applied, providing a guide for the osteotomy and maintaining the osteotomy in alignment for easy application of the lateral plate after the bone wedge is removed. This procedure can also be performed on toy breed dogs as small as 3–4 kg (Figure 22.16).

References

1. Tomlinson, J., Fox, D., Cook, J.L. et al. (2007). Measurement of femoral angles in four dog breeds. *Vet. Surg.* 36 (6): 593–598.
2. Olimpo, M., Piras, L.A., Peirone, B. et al. (2017). Comparison of osteotomy technique and jig type in completion of distal femoral osteotomies for correction of medial patellar luxation. An in vitro study. *Vet. Comp. Orthop. Traumatol.* 30 (1): 28–36.
3. Brower, B.E., Kowaleski, M.P., Peruski, A.M. et al. (2017). Distal femoral lateral closing wedge osteotomy as a component of comprehensive treatment of medial patellar luxation and distal femoral varus in dogs. *Vet. Comp. Orthop. Traumatol* 30 (1): 20–27.
4. Panichi, E., Cappellari, F., Olimpo, M. et al. (2016). Distal femoral osteotomy using a novel deformity reduction device. *Vet. Comp. Orthop. Traumatol.* 29 (5): 426–432.
5. Yasukawa, S., Edamura, K., Tanegashima, K. et al. (2016). Evaluation of bone deformities of the femur, tibia, and patella in Toy Poodles with medial patellar luxation using computed tomography. *Vet. Comp. Orthop. Traumatol.* 29 (1): 29–38.
6. Soparat, C., Wangdee, C., Chuthatep, S. et al. (2012). Radiographic measurement for femoral varus in Pomeranian dogs with and without medial patellar luxation. *Vet. Comp. Orthop. Traumatol.* 25 (3): 197–201.
7. Linney, W.R., Hammer, D.L., and Shott, S. (2011). Surgical treatment of medial patellar luxation without femoral trochlear groove deepening procedures in dogs: 91 cases (1998–2009). *J. Am. Vet. Med. Assoc.* 238 (9): 1168–1172.
8. Roch, S.P. and Gemmill, T.J. ((2008). Treatment of medial patellar luxation by femoral closing wedge ostectomy using a distal femoral plate in four dogs. *J. Small Anim. Pract.* 49 (3): 152–158.

9. Swiderski, J.K. and Palmer, R.H. (2007). Long-term outcome of distal femoral osteotomy for treatment of combined distal femoral varus and medial patellar luxation: 12 cases (1999–2004). *J. Am. Vet. Med. Assoc.* 231 (7): 1070–1075.

10. Dismukes, D.I., Fox, D.B., Tomlinson, J.L. et al. (2008). Determination of pelvic limb alignment in the large-breed dog: a cadaveric radiographic study in the frontal plane. *Vet. Surg.* 37 (7): 674–682.

Section V

Nontrauma Applications: Clinical Case Examples

V-B Arthrodesis

23 Arthrodesis

Fred Pike

The clinical challenges of arthrodesis in companion surgery are varied and include limited regional bone stock for fixation and the periarticular geometry that complicates the contouring of bone plates. Additionally, the postoperative period can be challenging for patients and clients due to extensive limitations on mobility and prolonged need for coaptation that is generally recommended following arthrodesis when using nonlocking plate fixation (nLPF). The author's clinical experience advocates that the use of locking plate fixation (LPF) can reduce many of the technical challenges associated with arthrodesis, reduce patient postoperative limitations, and decrease the duration of, or eliminate the need for, postoperative coaptation.

Indications for arthrodesis in companion animals are numerous and include end-stage osteoarthrosis, irreparable global ligament damage, congenital or traumatic joint luxation and loss of structural integrity of a joint. The general principals of arthrodesis, regardless of fixation method, include (i) removal of weight-bearing articular cartilage with surgical instrumentation; (ii) preservation of functional joint angle; (iii) bone grafting to expedite callus formation and promote bone union; (iv) rigid fixation with compression of the joint surfaces.

The majority of described techniques and clinical outcomes for arthrodesis in the veterinary literature are limited to the tarsus and carpus with less information available on shoulder, elbow and stifle arthrodesis outcomes. Prospective and retrospective studies directly comparing outcomes of LPF and nLPF are nonexistent. The use of LPF in human arthrodesis' (specifically tibiotalocalcaneal and metatarsocuneiform) reduces surgical time, decreases intraoperative blood loss and reduces the number of postoperative surgical visits [1, 2]). With the increasing utilization of LPF in veterinary medicine, publication of more peer-reviewed literature comparing clinical outcomes with the use LPF to nLPF is anticipated.

23.1 Shoulder Arthrodesis

Glenohumeral arthrodesis is indicated for the surgical management of congenital or traumatic luxation and end-stage osteoarthrosis. Glenohumeral arthrodesis is an alternative to glenoid or humeral excisional arthroplasty. Functional

Locking Plates in Veterinary Orthopedics, First Edition.
Edited by Matthew D. Barnhart and Karl C. Maritato.

outcomes are reported as fair to excellent [3]. The recommended angle for functional limb alignment is 110° [4].

Glenohumeral arthrodesis is technically demanding, with preservation of limb alignment a primary challenge. Limited bone stock proximal to the glenoid and the transitioning contour of the greater tubercle present major technical challenges. The use of LPF can address such concerns by limiting the need for precise plate contouring and eliminating the need for maximizing direct periosteal contact that would be required with nLPF.

The author's preference for glenohumeral arthrodesis is the use of the polyaxial (PAX) plating system for fixation, particularly for the scapula, where the ability for screw angulation with this system allows for maximum bone purchase. Fixation is applied following a craniolateral approach to the glenohumeral joint and following debridement of the articular cartilage. A tibial plateau leveling osteotomy (TPLO) saw blade of appropriate radius can facilitate removal of the articular cartilage and improve cancellous bone contact at the arthrodesis site. The curvature of the saw blade mirrors the natural contour of the articular surface in the transverse (lateromedial) plane, allowing maintenance of the shape of the glenoid and humeral head. Osteotomy of the acromion is not required. Maximizing the working length of the locking plates (LP) is critical to reduce the risk of stress concentration and plate fatigue at the level of the site of the primary arthrodesis. With the use of LPF, interfragmentary compression (lag screw or tension band fixation) is not a necessity. Intramedullary pins or Kirschner wires are helpful to provide temporary reduction prior to plate fixation (Figure 23.1).

23.2 Elbow Arthrodesis

In the author's experience, elbow arthrodesis is technically demanding with a high complication rate experienced with nLPF techniques. Fortunately, recent advances in minimally invasive orthopedic surgery, prosthetics ligaments and subcortical bone anchors have decreased the need for elbow arthrodesis to complex, non-reconstructible articular fractures of the elbow, severe end-stage osteoarthritis and failed elbow replacements may necessitate arthrodesis. The principles of arthrodesis outlined above are critical for successful elbow arthrodesis. The recommended angle for functional limb alignment is 110° [4].

Challenges for elbow arthrodesis include the triarticular nature of the joint that complicates complete debridement of the articular cartilage. Application of bone plating to the tension (caudal) surface of the elbow joint typically necessitates osteotomy of the tuber olecranon for traditional, linear nLPF application. LPF offers the advantage of limiting the need for screw purchase in the juxtaarticular region and the ability to contour the plate (dependent on LP design) to avoid periarticular bony anatomy, including the tuber olecrani and medial/lateral epicondyle. In the author's opinion, lateral application of the plate is associated with improved ability to maintain limb alignment through visualization of the entire limb in the sagittal plane. As with glenohumeral arthrodesis, maximizing the working length of the LP is critical to reduce the risk of stress concentration and resultant implant fatigue (Figure 23.2).

23.3 Carpal Arthrodesis

The literature suggests that the carpus is the most common joint necessitating arthrodesis in the canine [5]. Primary indications for pancarpal arthrodesis (PCA) include hyperextension injury and shearing injury. The recommended angle for functional limb alignment is 10–12° [4]

A technical challenge encountered when using LP for carpal arthrodesis is maximizing the working length of the bone plate. Traditionally, following cartilage debridement and bone grafting, the radiocarpal bone is engaged with a bone screw to stabilize the radiocarpal bone within the arthrodesis site and to maximize fixation across the arthrodesis. If the radiocarpal bone is engaged when using a LP, the effective working length of the plate is reduced and the construct is at risk of stress concentration and plate fatigue. With the reported high success following PCA using HDCPs or CastLess Plates (CLP), the indication for use of LP for arthrodesis of the carpus is limited [5]. An advantage of the PAX plating system for carpal arthrodesis is

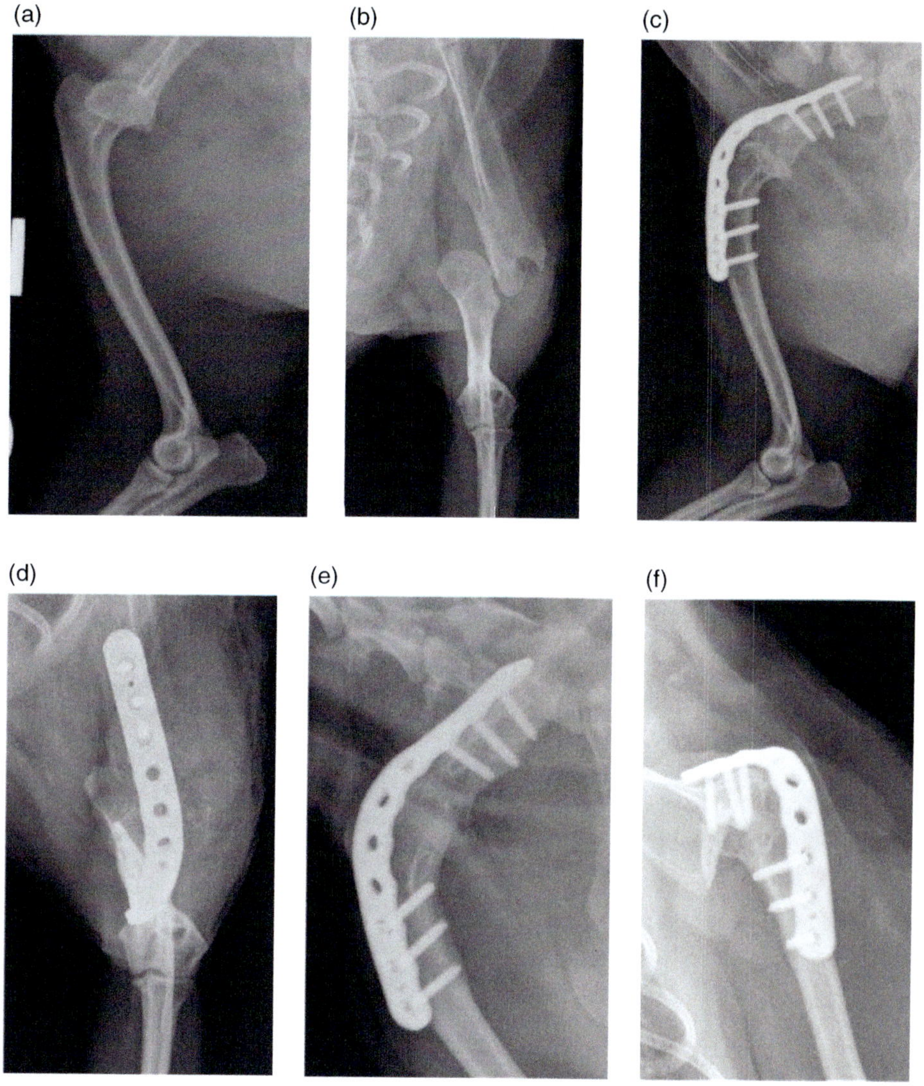

Figure 23.1 Cranial-caudal (b, d, and f) and lateral (a, c, and e) radiographs of the glenohumeral joint of a five-year-old Miniature Pincher mix with a history of a progressive left thoracic limb lameness. Preoperatively (a and d), a medial luxation of the shoulder is documented. Glenohumeral arthrodesis (b and e) was performed using a polyaxial (PAX) locking straight plate (PAX system®, Securos Surgical). Radiographic evaluation day 56 postoperative (c and f) documented stable implants and complete union of the arthrodesis.

the ability for screw angulation, which is beneficial during fixation distal to the radius. Additionally, given that the screwheads of the 2.0/2.4 and 2.7/3.5 are the same geometry, PAX plates can accommodate smaller screw diameter for use in the metacarpal bones providing an advantage similar to the hybrid dynamic compression plate (HDCP).

The author has used the PAX T-plate for partial carpal arthrodesis with excellent clinical outcomes. The T-plate is positioned distally on the dorsal surface of the radiocarpal bone and third metacarpal. The ability for screw angulation helps facilitate distal placement of the plate and decrease the risk of impingement of the radiocarpal joint. Given the limited bone stock of the radiocarpal bone, fixation is limited to two screws. In theory, LP offers an advantage of increased stiffness with two locked screws compared to two nonlocked screws (Figure 23.3).

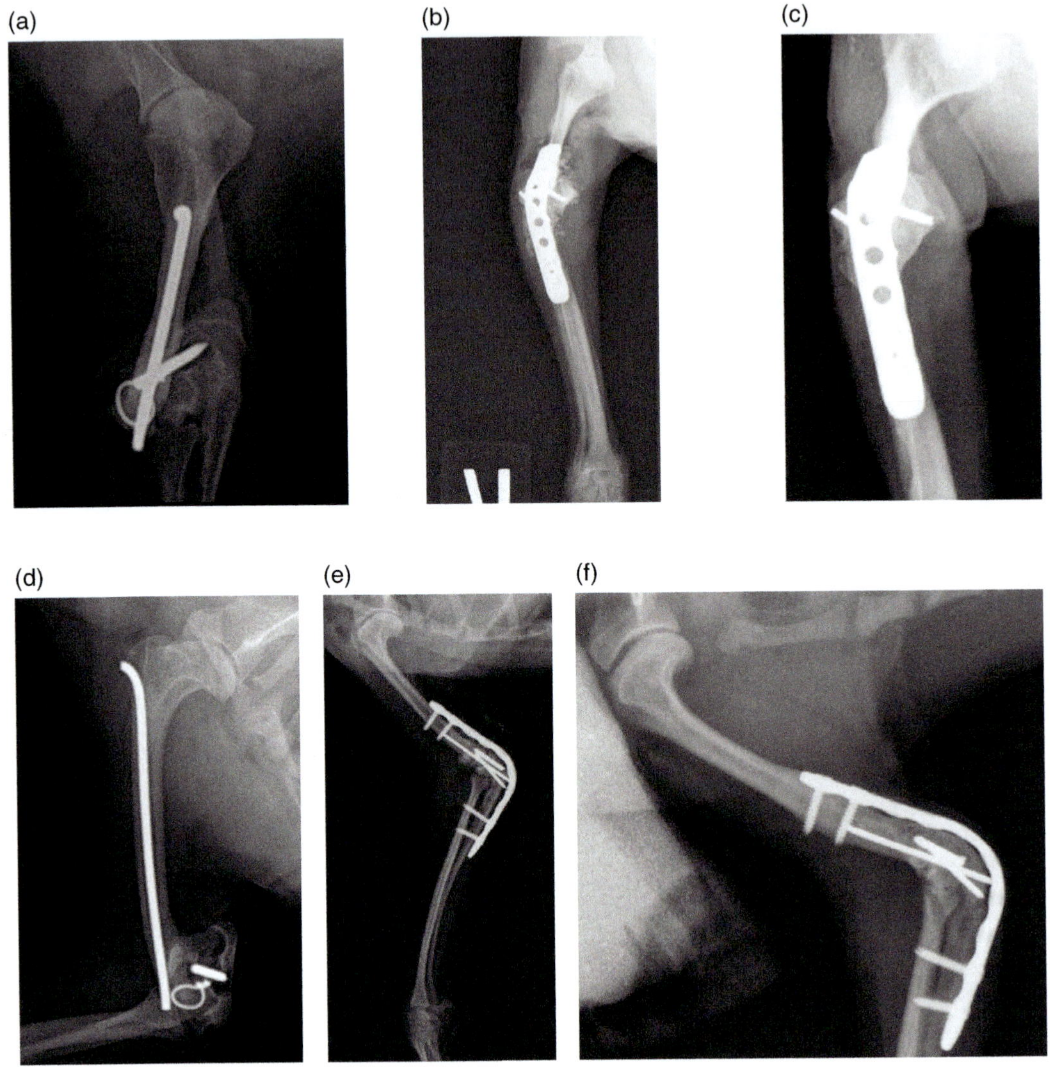

Figure 23.2 Cranial-caudal (a, b, and c) and lateral (d, e, and f) radiographs of the elbow joint of a two-year-old terrier. Preoperative radiographs (a and d) identify a chronic malunion secondary to failed repair of a type A1 distal extra-articular fracture of the humerus. Immediate postoperaitve radiographs of the elbow arthrodesis (b and e) performed using a PAX straight plate. Kirschner wires were used to achieve temporary fixation prior to plate application. Radiographic evaluation day 56 postoperative (c and f) documented stable implants and complete union of the arthrodesis.

23.4 Stifle Arthrodesis

The need for stifle arthrodesis is rare, and with the advent of the canine total knee arthroplasty (TKA) has become even more so. The main indication to perform a stifle arthrodesis is lack of the availability of TKA expertise or if conditions contraindicate a TKA. Indications for stifle arthrodesis include complex articular fractures, grade III open fractures, septic arthritis that is nonresponsive to medical management, end-stage osteoarthritis, and limb-sparing procedures that necessitate excision of significant load-bearing articular. While reasonable clinical outcomes can be achieved following stifle arthrodesis, a significant functional lameness is expected and client expectations should be established in advance of surgery. Limb circumduction is an anticipated outcome that can limit return to the functional expectations of the

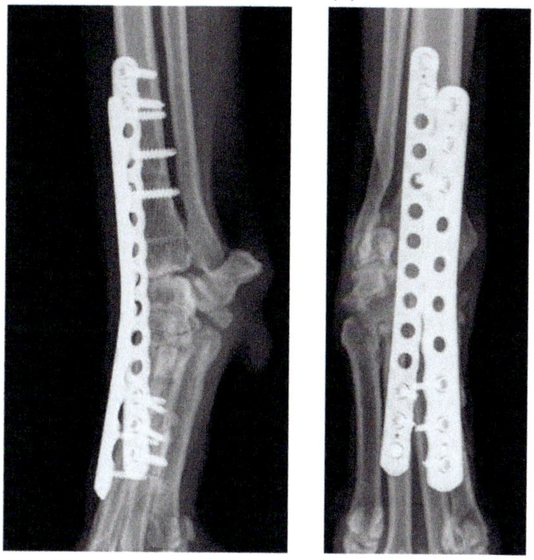

Figure 23.3 Lateral (a) and cranial-caudal (b) radiographs of the carpus of six-year-old Irish Wolfhound presented for a non-weight-bearing right thoracic limb lameness. Carpal hyperextension of 60° was documented. Patient size necessitated the use of two PAX straight plates.

owner. The recommended angle for functional limb alignment is 140° [4].

With respect to stifle arthrodesis, LPF offers the advantage of requiring a less aggressive surgical approach. Osteotomy of the tibial tuberosity is not required, as the need for sagittal placement of the bone plate is not a prerequisite to successful arthrodesis. The author's preference is to place temporary fixation following appropriate limb alignment in the sagittal and axial plane. When limb alignment is confirmed, a LP is applied to the cranial cortex of the femur and the medial aspect of the proximal tibia without the morbidity associated with tibial tuberosity osteotomy. Soft tissue dissection is minimized by medial application of the bone plate to the proximal tibia. Maximizing the working length of the LP is critical and avoids the need for excessive juxtaarticular dissection.

Linear application of LPF in the cranial plane has been described and necessitates osteotomy of the tibial tuberosity with subsequent reattachment utilizing cerclage wire or compression screw fixation following plate fixation [6].

As described for glenohumeral arthrodesis, the use of a TPLO blade of appropriate radius can facilitate stifle arthrodesis. Following a medial approach to the distal femur and proximal tibia, the saw blade is advanced in a mediolateral transverse axis, resulting in excision of the articular surface of the distal femur and proximal tibia and the associated intra-articular structures, including the menisci and cruciate ligament. The resultant concave osteotomy surfaces can be apposed with K-wires for temporary immobilization to allow evaluation of limb alignment prior to LP fixation (Figure 23.4).

23.5 Tarsal Arthrodesis

Numerous techniques for pantarsal arthrodesis have been described, including cranial, medial, and lateral application of dynamic compression plating (DCP)/ limited-contact dynamic compression plate (LC-DCP). Major and minor complication rates for tarsal arthrodesis have been reported as 32.5% and 42.5%, respectively [7] with pantarsal arthrodesis having a higher complication rate than partial tarsal arthrodesis. An advantage of LP fixation for tarsal arthrodesis is the need to engage a single metatarsal bone distally, thereby reducing the risk of trauma to the medially located dorsal pedal artery or perforating metatarsal artery. Such arterial trauma can result in plantar necrosis, which is reported to occur in 15% of clinical cases utilizing nLPF [7].

Specialty locking plates are available, with limited literature describing long-term clinical outcomes. The recommended angle for functional limb alignment is 135–145° for dogs and 115–125° for cats [4].

The challenges for pantarsal arthrodesis are similar to other joints, with the primary technical consideration being regional anatomy that complicates the surgeon's ability to contour bone plates. Without appropriate contouring, the plate-bone contact friction created by the screw tightening moment is minimized and construct fixation is compromised. In theory, the locking interface provided by LP may favor osteosynthesis by providing a more stable mechanical environment with lower strain. Given the advantages of LPs, the availability of specialty plates for arthrodesis will likely increase in the future.

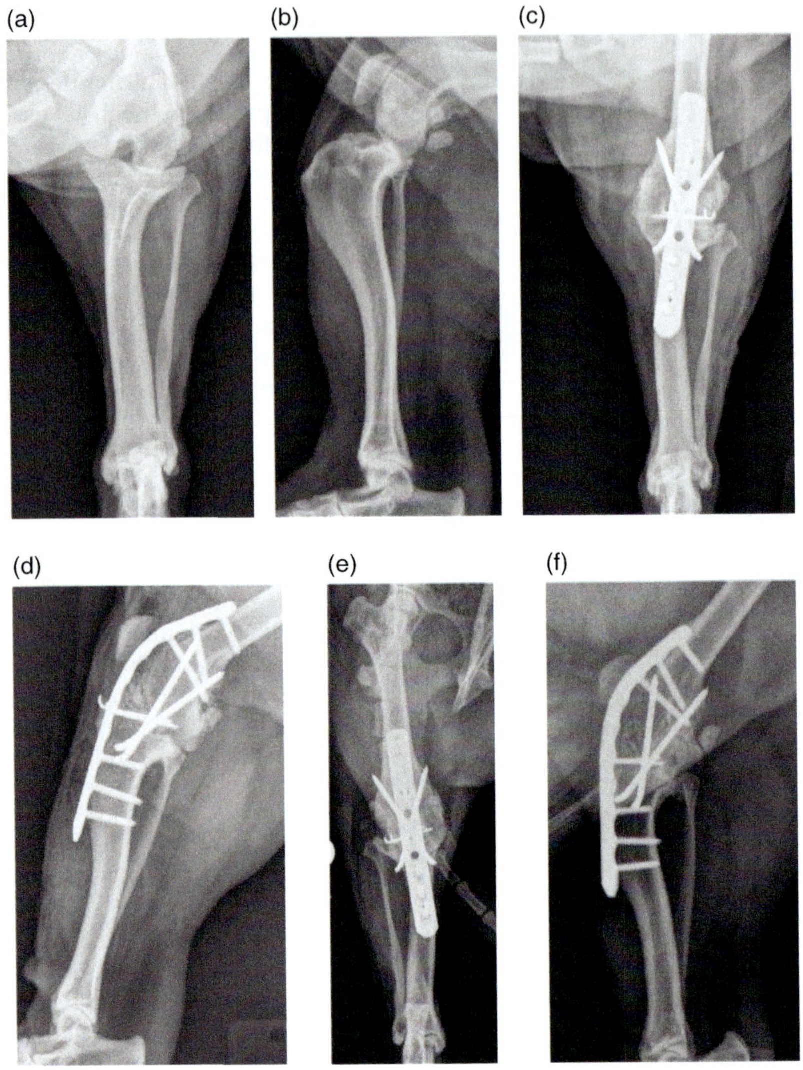

Figure 23.4 Cranial-caudal (a, b, and c) and lateral (d, e, and f) radiographs of the stifle joint of a 10-year-old Shih-Tzu with grade V outerbridge wear secondary to chronic immune mediated polyarthropathy. Immediate postoperaitve radiographs of the stifle arthrodesis (b and e) performed using a PAX straight plate and Kirschner wires. Radiographic evaluation day 60 postoperative (c and f) documented stable implants and complete union of the arthrodesis.

The author's primary clinical experience with LP for the tarsal region has been partial tarsal arthrodesis utilizing a laterally applied PAX LP. Traditional principles of arthrodesis are applied and the LP is applied proximally to the lateral aspect of the calcaneus continuing distally to the diaphysis of metatarsal V. A high-speed burr is utilized to remove the protuberance of the base of MT V at the insertion of the fibularis brevis muscle. The rigidity of the LP negates the need for interfragmentary compression. Clinical experience suggests that the duration of external coaptation can be reduced with LPF for partial tarsal arthrodesis thereby decreasing the risk of bandage related morbidity. The author typically uses external coaptation in the form of a medioplantar splint made from fiberglass casting tape. Splint coaptation is utilized for two weeks followed by one week immobilization with a soft padded bandage. Coaptation is not utilized beyond week three postoperative.

References

1. Zhang, C., Shi, Z., and Mei, C. (2015). Locking plate versus retrograde intramedullary nail fixation for tibiotalocalcaneal arthrodesis: A retrospective analysis. *Indian J. Orthop.* 49 (2): 227–232.
2. Tavakkolizadeh, A., Klinke, M., and Davies, M. (2006). Tibiotalocalcaneal arthrodesis in treatment of hindfoot pain and deformity. *Foot Ankle Surg.* 12: 59–64.
3. Pucheu, B. and Duhautois, B. (2008). Surgical treatment of shoulder instability: a retrospective study of 76 cases (1993–2007). *Vet. Comp. Orthop. Traumatol.* 21: 368.
4. Johnson, A.L., Houlton, J.E., and Vanninni, R. (2005). *AO Principles of Fracture Management in the Dog and Cat*. Switzerland: AO Publishing.
5. Bristow, P.C., Meeson, R.L., Thorne, R.M. et al. (2015). Clinical comparison of the hybrid dynamic compression plate and the castless plate for pancarpal arthrodesis in 219 dogs. *Vet. Surg.* 44 (1): 70–77.
6. Petazzoni, M. and Nicetto, T. (2015). Stifle arthrodesis using a locking plate system in six dogs. *Vet. Comp. Orthop. Traumatol.* 28 (4): 288–293.
7. Roch, S.P., Clements, D.N., Mitchell, A.S. et al. (2008). Complications following tarsal arthrodesis using bone plate fixation in dogs. *J. Small Anim. Pract.* 49 (3): 117–126.

Section V

Nontrauma Applications: Clinical Case Examples

V-C Spinal Diseases

24 Atlantoaxial Subluxation

Karl C. Maritato

24.1 Introduction

Atlantoaxial subluxation (AAS) is an uncommon disorder seen particularly in toy breeds of dogs including Chihuahuas, Yorkshire Terriers, Pomeranians, and Toy Poodles. The congenital form of the disease is most common, with abnormalities contributing to instability including dens aplasia, hypoplasia, dorsal angulation or degeneration, and failure or absence of ligamentous support. The acquired form can occur in any age or breed of dog following trauma.

Many different surgical techniques have been described for the treatment of AAS. Dorsal and ventral approaches have been advocated, with neither having been shown to be superior to the other with similar complication and success rates reported [1]. When comparing risk factors affecting outcome, similar success rates for dorsal (88.9%) and ventral (85.3%) procedures were noted; however, dogs were also noted to have a higher incidence of postoperative neurologic deficits with dorsal procedures than with ventral procedures. Acute onset of clinical signs is a known positive predictor of a success [1, 2]. In some studies, age of onset of clinical signs was predictive of outcome, whereas in others it was not [1–3]. Severity of neurologic deficits at presentation may affect outcome [1, 3]; however, most studies show even those with the most severe neurologic dysfunction can recover well [2, 4–6]. Postoperative AA reduction and radiographic positioning of the dens have not been shown to correlate with outcome [1]. This supports the suggestion that the shearing motion of the instability is the critical insult to the spinal cord, not the static position of the vertebrae (see biomechanics below). The postoperative fatality rate is 5% with ventral procedures and 8% with dorsal procedures [7].

Dorsal techniques rely on fibrosis to stabilize the AA joint, as there is no access to the joint space with these techniques. With ventral techniques, the joint space can be arthrodesed, allowing for long-term fusion of the joint to combat the instability.

Of the ventral techniques described, screws, with or without wire, and polymethylmethacrylate (PMMA) is likely the most common technique utilized. The use of PMMA has been shown to provide a strong, solid fixation. However, there are several disadvantages, including thermal damage, increased risk of infection, pressure necrosis of adjacent structures,

Locking Plates in Veterinary Orthopedics, First Edition.
Edited by Matthew D. Barnhart and Karl C. Maritato.

and inconvenience when revision surgery is required [1, 8–12]. In addition, screw placement with these techniques requires a very shallow angle of placement, which can be difficult to navigate in such small anatomic spaces.

In several studies, locking plates have been promoted over compression plates due to a loss of stabilization from screw loosening and pullout from the vertebra with compression plates [13, 14]. Additionally, monocortical screw pullout was shown in humans to be similar to bicortical screws, supporting the use of locking plates with monocortical screws [15]. Biomechanical tests have shown locking plates to be more stable than nonlocking plates in human studies [15, 16]. As early as 1995, the biomechanical advantages of locking plates were shown in experimental models comparing locking and nonlocking implants in the human cervical spine, particularly in flexion [16]. In the canine cervical spine, both biomechanical studies and clinical applications of locking plate fixation have been published for treatment of cervical spondylomyelopathy and vertebral fractures [13, 17–19]. The soft, small vertebrae in these dogs can predispose to vertebral and spinal cord damage [10]. The only evaluation of locking plate treatment of AAS published to date was in three dogs in 2011 [20], all of which recovered to near-normal neurologic function and were pain free. Two of the three dogs were grade 4 tetraparetic preoperatively, with the third being grade 2 tetraparetic. Application of the locking plate as described later in this chapter resulted in adequate arthrodesis of the C1–C2 space and improved neurologic function within two weeks of surgery in all three dogs, along with high owner satisfaction.

24.2 Anatomy

Given that AAS is most common in small-breed dogs, a solid understanding of the anatomy makes for operating in such a small area more feasible. The AA joint is differentiated from the other vertebral units due to the lack of an intervertebral disc. The vertebral canal of C1 is defined by a small vertebral body ventrally (known as the arch), the lateral masses, and the dorsal arch. Adjacent to the lateral masses are the large transverse processes (the wings). Cranially the atlas has articular processes that articulate with the occipital condyles, and caudally there are two glenoid cavities that articulate with the cranial aspect of the vertebral body of the axis.

The fovea of the dens is a depression in the ventral arch in which the dens of the axis rests. The dens arises from the cranial aspect of the body of the axis. It is retained in the fovea via the transverse ligament of the atlas, just dorsal to the dens. Three other ligaments are involved in the stability of the AA joint: the apical ligament of the dens and two alar ligaments. The apical ligament runs from the dens to the basioccipital bone and the alar ligaments bilaterally arise adjacent to the dens and attach medial to the occipital condyles. The axis has a large vertebral body for screw placement; however, the bone is thin.

24.3 Biomechanics

There is very limited information on the biomechanics of the AA joint in dogs. In 2013, a study was published that demonstrated that the alar ligaments seem to be the main stabilizing component during shear loading [21]. It is suspected that shear loading is the most important force involved in supporting the weight of the head. Disruption of the apical and alar ligaments may lead to dorsal dislocation of the dens, allowing the dens to induce concussive trauma to the spinal cord. Flexion shear force is likely the most important force to be countered when considering fixation methods. In 2015, Forterre et al, showed that ventral and lateral flexion may lead to severe spinal cord compression in these dogs, as the range of motion in a Yorkie with AAS was compared to a Coton de Tulear with a normal AA joint [22]. Figure 24.1a and b depicts an MRI of a three-year-old Chihuahua with intact dense and ruptured ligaments. This resulted in severe contusion to the spinal cord, as depicted by the hyperintensity of the spinal cord in the region of C1-2.

24.4 Materials

The author uses a 2.0 mm Polyaxial (PAX) Advanced Locking System butterfly locking plate (Securos, Fiskdale, MA, USA). These plates

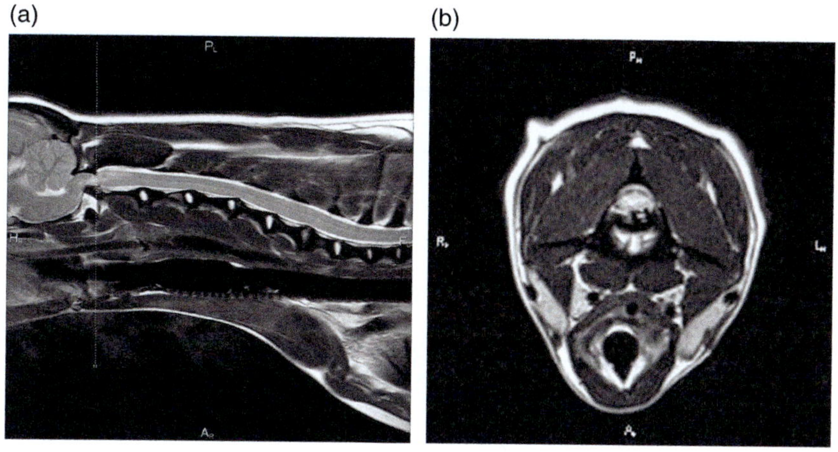

Figure 24.1 (a and b) Sagittal and axial MRI images of a dog with AA luxation. Note the dorsal tipping of the dens into the spinal canal causing ventral compression of the spinal cord.

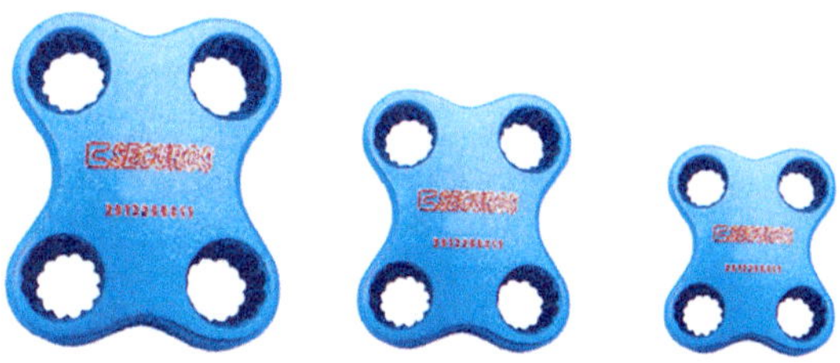

Figure 24.2 Securos butterfly atlantoaxial PAX locking plate in 12, 14, and 16 mm sizes.

are titanium, are 2 mm thick, and have lengths of 12, 14, and 16 mm. They have four holes in the "corners of the butterfly wings," which accept 2.0 mm PAX locking screws (Figure 24.2). The advantage of the PAX system is the ability to angle the screws up to 10°, allowing more freedom to place the screws where needed [23].

24.5 Surgical Approach

The patient is placed in dorsal recumbency, with a small towel under the neck to elevate gently, allowing for a more level surgical field. A ventral midline incision is made from just cranial to the palpable larynx to the mid-caudal cervical region. The subcutis is dissected and the bellies of the paired sternohyoideus muscles are separated; be cautious of the caudal thyroid vein. The trachea, larynx, thyroid gland, carotid artery, and internal jugular vein are retracted to one side. The longus colli muscle and the fibers of the ventral arch of the atlas and body of the axis are transected, which exposes the joint as well as the bodies of both the atlas and axis.

24.6 Application

The body of the axis is typically dorsally displaced upon initial observation; it is elevated into reduction via gentle traction on the remaining intact musculature. The joint surfaces of the AA joint are removed with a high-speed pneumatic drill and/or 11 blade and currette. The plate requires no contouring, and it is placed centered on the joint space with two screw holes over the atlas and two over the axis. A PAX-specific drill guide is placed into the plate hole to ensure proper angulation and prevent overangulation, which leads to poor locking mechanics [23]. A 1.3 mm drill bit is used to drill the holes into the atlas and axis. Caution must be taken to not enter the spinal canal and damage the spinal cord. The benefit of being able to angle the screws, as well as the allowance of monocortical only screws via the locking mechanism, makes this plate well suited for minimizing iatrogenic spinal cord damage. The author typically places the atlas screws first, followed by the axis screws. The screws are 2.0 mm.

Given the incredibly small size of some of these patients and the very thin bone encountered, the author has, on occasion, utilized a

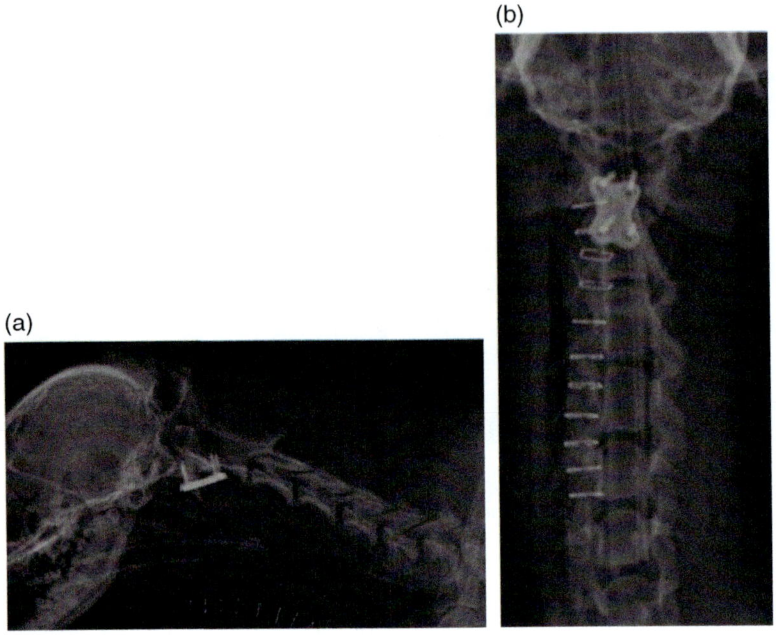

Figure 24.3 (a and b) Postoperative lateral and ventrodorsal radiographic projections showing proper plate placement and reduced AA disc space.

Jacob's chuck to complete "drilling" of the hole. This allows slower, more controlled pressure application to the thin bone, reducing iatrogenic damage. The hole is started with power drill and completed by hand.

Once completed, the area is lavaged with sterile saline, and the muscles, subcutaneous tissue, and skin are sutured with appropriately sized suture. Postoperative radiographs are made to evaluate placement and alignment (Figure 24.3a and b).

24.7 Postoperative Care

The authors make an attempt to reduce ventroflexion ability in these dogs postoperatively by placing a lightweight neck brace for approximately four to six weeks. Whether this supplemental stabilization is required is not proven; however, in the author's perspective, it is associated with minimal morbidity and may reduce complications. The brace is checked weekly to ensure that the patient is comfortable and no complications are occurring.

These dogs are allowed to recover in the intensive care unit and are monitored closely for any respiratory compromise. The intensity of the postoperative nursing care varies based on preoperative neurologic status. If the patient is nonambulatory, it is important to ensure that the patient is rotated/flipped every four hours and is not left in one recumbent state. Ideally, these dogs are kept in sternal recumbency, with hind limb side flipping, as neurologic patients are prone to aspiration pneumonia and respiratory difficulty [24]. On average, they are released within 48 hours.

Owners are instructed to confine the dog at home and encourage rest to minimize the chances of implant failure due to excessive activity. Owners are shown rehabilitation exercises they can do with their dog at home, and professional rehabilitation is instituted as soon as possible.

At week six, radiographs of the cervical spine are made to evaluate healing of the AA joint. In most cases, sufficient fusion is obtained at this point and a steady increase in activities is introduced over the following four weeks.

By week 10, patients are allowed to return to a normal lifestyle.

In summary, locking plate fixation is strongly advocated in human cervical neurosurgery and is applicable to veterinary patients. The technique and implants involved are straightforward and may reduce intraoperative iatrogenic injury, resulting in very good outcomes for these patients.

References

1. Beaver, D.P., Ellison, G.W., Lewis, D.D. et al. (2000). Risk factors affecting the outcome of surgery for atlantoaxial subluxation in dogs: 46 cases (1978–1998). *J. Am. Vet. Med. Assoc.* 216: 1104–1109.
2. Havig, M.E., Cornell, K.K., Hawthorne, J.C. et al. (2005). Evaluation of nonsurgical treatment of atlantoaxial subluxation in dogs: 19 cases (1992–2001). *J. Am. Vet. Med. Assoc.* 227: 257–262.
3. Aikawa, T., Shibata, M., and Fujita, H. (2013). Modified ventral stabilization using positively threaded profile pins and polymethylmethacrylate for atlantoaxial instability in 49 dogs. *Vet. Surg.* 42: 683–692.
4. Pujol, E., Bouvy, B., Oman˜a, M. et al. (2010). Use of the Kishigami atlantoaxial tension band in eight toy breed dogs with atlantoaxial subluxation. *Vet. Surg.* 39: 35–42.
5. Sa´nchez-Masian, D., Luja´n-Feliu-Pascual, A., Font, C. et al. (2014). Dorsal stabilization of atlantoaxial subluxation using non-absorbable sutures in toy breed dogs. *Vet. Comp. Orthop. Traumatol.* 27: 62–67.
6. Thomas, W.B., Sorjonen, D.C., and Simpson, S.T. (1991). Surgical management of atlantoaxial subluxation in 23 dogs. *Vet. Surg.* 20: 409–412.
7. Plessas, I.N. and Volk, H.A. (2014). Signalment, clinical signs and treatment of altantoaxial subluxation in dogs: a systematic review of 336 published cases from 1967 to 2013. *J. Vet. Intern. Med.* 28: 944–975.
8. Schulz, K.S., Waldron, D.R., and Fahie, M. (1997). Application of ventral pins and polymethylmethacrylate for the management of atlantoaxial instability: results in nine dogs. *Vet. Surg.* 26: 317–325.
9. Sanders, S.G., Bagley, R.S., Silver, G.M. et al. (2004). Outcomes and complications associated with ventral screws, pins and polymethylmethacrylate for atlantoaxial instability in 12 dogs. *J. Am. Anim. Hosp. Assoc.* 40: 204–210.
10. Platt, S.R., Chambers, J.N., and Cross, A. (2004). A modified ventral fixation for surgical management of atlantoaxial subluxation in 19 dogs. *Vet. Surg.* 33: 349–354.
11. Voss, K., Keller, M., and Montavon, P.M. (2004). Internal splinting of dorsal intertarsal and tarsometatarsal instabilities in dogs and cats with the ComPact Uni-lock 2.0/2.4 system. *Vet. Comp. Orthop. Traumatol.* 17: 125–230.
12. Blass, C.E., Waldron, D.R., and van Ee, T.R. (1988). Cervical stabilization in three dogs using Steinmann pins and metylmethacrylate. *J. Am. Anim. Hosp. Assoc.* 24: 61–68.
13. Trotter, E. (2009). Cervical spine locking plate fixation for treatment of cervical spondylitic myelopathy in large breed dogs. *Vet. Surg.* 38: 705–718.
14. Bergman, R.L. (2004). Cervical spondylomyelopathy in the dog: A comparison to the disease in humans. Proceedings from the Annual American College of Veterinary Internal Medicine Congress. Berlin, Germany. pg. 17–20.
15. Pitzen, T., Barbier, D., Titinger, F. et al. (2002). Screw fixation to the posterior cortical shell does not influence peak torque and pull out in anterior cervical plating. *Eur. Spine J.* 11: 494–499.
16. Smith, S.A., Lindsey, R.W., Doherty, B.J. et al. (1995). An in-vitro biomechanical comparison of the Orosco and AO locking plates for anterior cervical spine fixation. *J. Spinal Disord.* 8: 220–223.
17. Solano, M.A., Fitzpatrick, N., and Bertran, J. (2015 Jul). Cervical distraction-stabilization using an intervertebral spacer screw and string-of pearl (SOP™) plates in 16 dogs with disc-associated wobbler syndrome. *Vet. Surg.* 44 (5): 627–641.
18. Danielski, A., Vanhaesebrouck, A., and Yeadon, R. (2012). Ventral stabilization and facetectomy in a great Dane with wobbler syndrome due to cervical spinal canal stenosis. *Vet. Comp. Orthop. Traumatol.* 25 (4): 337–341.
19. Agnello, K.A., Kapatkin, A.S., Garcia, T.C. et al. (2010 Dec). Intervertebral biomechanics of locking compression plate monocortical fixation of the canine cervical spine. *Vet. Surg.* 39 (8): 991–1000.
20. Dickomeit, M., Alves, L., Pekarkova, M. et al. (2011). Use of a 1.5 mm butterfly locking plate for stabilization of atlantoaxial pathology in three toy breed dogs. *Vet. Comp. Orthop. Traumatol.* 24 (3): 246–251.
21. Reber, K., Bürki, A., Vizcaino Reves, N. et al. (2013). Biomechanical evaluation of the stabilizing function of the atlantoaxial ligaments under shear loading: a canine cadaveric study. *Vet. Surg.* 42 (8): 918–923.
22. Forterre, F., Precht, C., Riedinger, B. et al. (2015). Biomechanical properties of the atlantoaxial joint with naturally-occurring instability in a toy breed dog. A comparative descriptive cadaveric study. *Vet. Comp. Orthop. Traumatol.* 28 (5): 355–358.

23. Bufkin, B.W., Barnhart, M.D., Kazanovicz, A.J. et al. (2013). The effect of screw angulation and insertion torque on the push-out strength of polyaxial locking screws and the single cycle to failure in bending of polyaxial locking plates. *Vet. Comp. Orthop. Traumatol.* 26 (3): 186–191.

24. McMillan, M.W., Whitaker, K.E., Hughes, D. et al. (2009 Dec). Effect of body position on the arterial partial pressures of oxygen and carbon dioxide in spontaneously breathing, conscious dogs in an intensive care unit. *J. Vet. Emerg. Crit. Care* 19 (6): 564–570.

25 Caudocervical Spondylomyelopathy

Noel Fitzpatrick

25.1 Introduction

Cervical spondylomyelopathy (CSM) is a multifactorial condition affecting the cervical spine of the dog, resulting in progressive compression of the spinal cord and nerve roots [1–3]. A spectrum of distinct lesions may coexist and commonly include combinations of chronic degenerative disc disease, ligamentum flavum hypertrophy, congenital osseous vertebral malformation, articular facet hypertrophy, and vertebral column subluxation [1, 2, 4]. Large-breed dogs are generally affected, with over-representation of middle-aged Doberman Pinschers and young Great Danes [1, 2, 5–7].

25.2 Biomechanics of the Cervical Spine

The biomechanical and morphologic features of the caudal cervical spine may contribute to the high frequency of caudal cervical disc lesions. It is reported that 77% of people with neck pain have an abnormal center of motion in at least one functional spinal unit (a pair of adjacent vertebral bodies plus the intervertebral disc) [8]. Axial rotation has been suggested as a major biomechanical predicator of disc degeneration [9]. Concave-shaped articular facets allow more axial rotation [10]. A higher number of concave articular facets have been demonstrated in the cervical spine of large-breed dogs as compared to small-breed dogs and in the caudal cervical spine by comparison with the cranial cervical spine [10]. The caudal cervical spine has been recently shown by kinematics study to experience three times more axial rotation than the cranial segment [11].

25.3 Classification of CSM

Refinement of treatment protocols can be improved by accurate classification of the condition.

25.3.1 Disc-Associated Wobbler Syndrome

Disc-associated wobbler syndrome (DAWS) describes protrusion of one or more degenerative cervical discs into the spinal canal, causing

Locking Plates in Veterinary Orthopedics, First Edition.
Edited by Matthew D. Barnhart and Karl C. Maritato.

compression of the spinal cord and exacerbating any subclinical stenosis already existing at the affected cervical spinal segments due to bony abnormalities or dorsal ligamentum flavum hypertrophy [2]. Spinal cord compression typically occurs at the intervertebral disc spaces between the fifth cervical (C5) and seventh cervical (C7) vertebrae in large-breed dogs such as Dobermans [12–14].

25.3.2 Osseous-Associated Wobbler Syndrome

Osseous-associated wobbler syndrome (OAWS) is a term developed by the author to describe compression of the spinal cord by malformation and proliferation of the osseous elements of the dorsal facets and neural arch. Although giant-breed dogs such as Great Danes show a predilection for lesions of the caudal cervical spine, they also develop lesions of the vertebrae more cranial, and the osseous compression can occur concomitant with soft tissue proliferation of the facets and intervertebral disc protrusion [14, 15]. We have also observed such changes in the cranial cervical spine in chondrodystrophic breeds such as Basset Hounds [16] and sporadically in other giant- and large-breed dogs as well [17].

25.4 Decision-Making

It is the author's preference to obtain a minimum imaging database of patients with suspected CSM.

25.4.1 MRI

- MRI imaging should include T1-weighted and T2-weighted sagittal and transverse plane projections to determine localization, extension, direction, presence, and severity of spinal cord and/or nerve root compression, discogenic disease, signs of degenerative disease, and potential cysts with or without articular facet pathology [14, 15, 18]. Additionally, T2* gradient echo sequences may provide additional information on osseous margins.
- MRI parenchymal imaging is important both in terms of volume of compression for DAWS and OAWS cases and also in terms of adjudication of hyperintensity signal on T2-weighted images as a percentage of spinal cord diameter as a prognostic indicator suggestive of chronic disease (gliosis).
- For all DAWS cases at the author's facility, MRI scan sequences are obtained with the cervical spine in flexion and in extension as well as neutral to advise classification as static or dynamic (Figure 25.1). We also recommend the application of 20% of linear traction to the cervical spine to determine if compression is reduced in traction responsive cases (Figure 25.2). These factors directly influence our treatment choice of distraction-fusion or disc replacement.

25.4.2 CT

- For cases with suspected OAWS, a CT scan is routinely performed since it provides superior definition of osseous margins [19–21].
- CT scans are also mandatory for accurate manufacture of custom implants.

We believe there is a rationale to provide distraction-stabilization for multiple manifestations of CSM with the exception of DAWS where there is no osseous static compression or facet pathology. Those cases may benefit from a motion-preserving technique such as intervertebral disc replacement.

Surgical distraction provides immediate nerve root and spinal cord decompression, and mechanical stabilization with autologous graft augmentation for fusion favors osseous or fibro-osseous union, minimizing or reducing dynamic compressive forces. We no longer perform dorsal laminectomy procedures for the majority of OAWS cases and have had considerable success treating such cases with distraction-fusion alone. We have demonstrated regression of facet hypertrophy and osseous compression over time using sequential CT scans in multiple patients in association with resolution of pain and resolution or stabilization of upper motor neuron (UMN) neurologic signs.

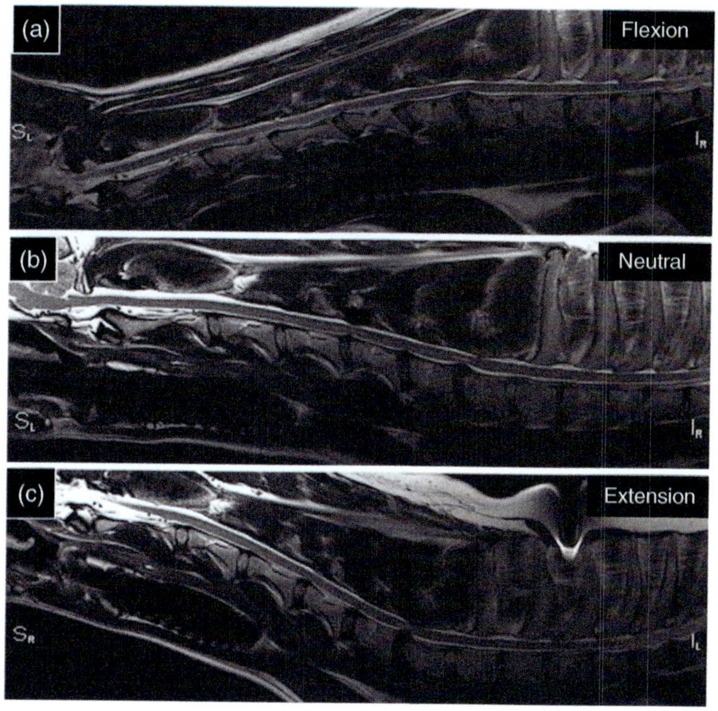

Figure 25.1 MRI investigation of dynamic and static cervical spondylomyelopathy (CSM). The variable presentation of CSM in flexion (a), in neutral positioning (b), and when extended (c) is demonstrated. Protrusion of the C6–C7 intervertebral disc is apparent, which worsens on extension and is accompanied by increased signal within the cord consistent with gliosis.

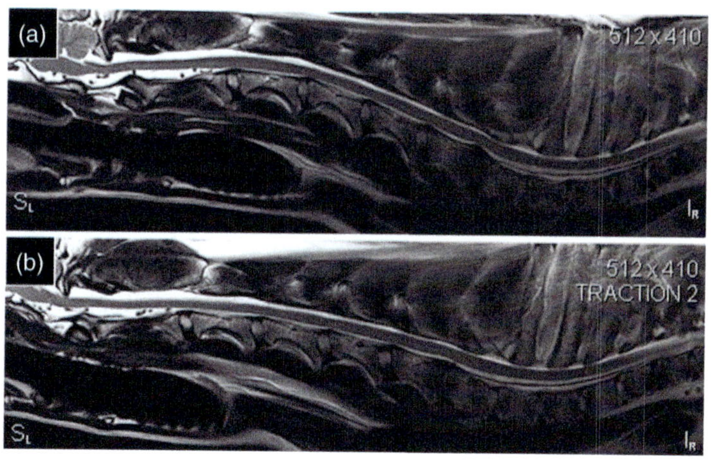

Figure 25.2 Traction application during MRI imaging. (a) Spinal cord impingement is visible at C6–C7 associated with intervertebral disc protrusion. (b) When 20% traction was applied to the same patient, the degree of impingement is reduced and continuity of CSF fluid signal is largely restored. The use of traction may help identify patients suitable for treatment using distraction-fusion and stabilization.

Cases classified as DAWS are generally dynamic and traction responsive. Dorsal annulus fibrous hypertrophy either with or without associated osseous hypertrophy can exacerbate spinal cord compression [3, 12, 13]. C5–C6 and C6–C7 are most commonly reported affected sites [22]. Disc-associated CSM is recognized in 82–96% of Dobermans with cervical myelopathy [19, 23], (Figure 25.3).

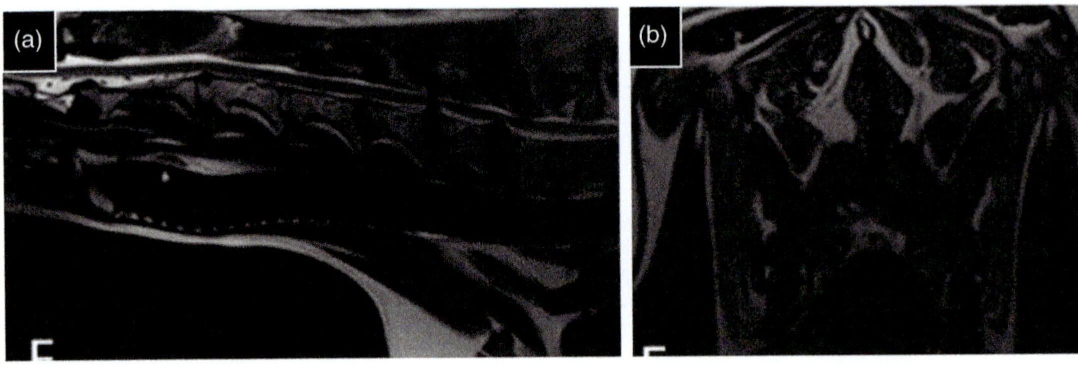

Figure 25.3 MRI presentation, DAWS. Sagittal T2-weighed MRI scan in sagittal (a) and transverse (b) planes showing multiple intervertebral sites with ventral loss of hyperintense signal (fat/csf) due to spinal cord compression at C5–C6–C7. Transverse image of the same patient at C5–C6 reveals dorsal and ventral extradural spinal cord compression due to intervertrbral disc protrusion and ligamentous hypertrophy. Hyperintensity of the spinal cord parenchyma is indicative of gliosis.

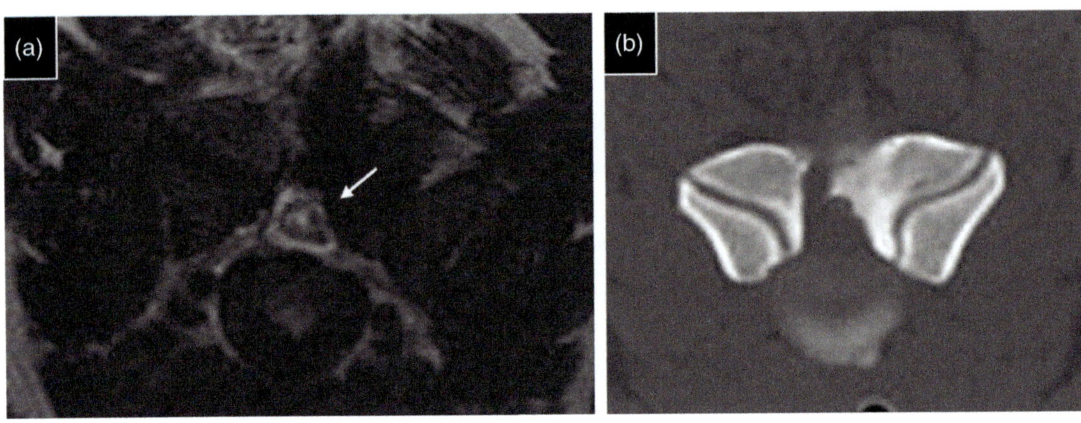

Figure 25.4 MRI and CT imaging, OAWS. (a) Transverse T2-weighed magnetic resonance image (MRI) showing dorsolateral extradural compression with central hyperintense signal in the spinal cord indicative of gliosis (white arrow). (b) Computer tomographic (CT) scan of the same patient demonstrates dorso-lateral facet hypertrophy and reduction of the spinal canal and neuroforaminal dimensions.

For OAWS patients, osseous changes account for 77% of spinal cord compression in giant breed dogs [19]. C5–C6 and C6–C7 are the most common locations for compression in large-breed dogs in 91% and 72% in giant-breed dogs, respectively [19]. The osseous compression produces an absolute stenosis of the spinal canal. Other compressive lesions are generally secondary including disc disease (Figure 25.4).

25.5 Patient Positioning and Surgical Anatomy

Dogs are placed in dorsal recumbency with padding under the trunk and caudal cervical spine. The cranial cervical spine is extended approximately 40° relative to the trunk to allow ventral access to the cervical spine. The head is secured to the operating table with tape to maintain sagittal plane alignment of the cervical spine. The thoracic limbs are crossed over the thorax and secured caudally to maximize exposure to the caudal cervical spine and to expose the proximal lateral humerus for harvesting autogenous cancellous bone graft (Figure 25.5). A ventral midline approach is performed as previously described [24].

25.6 Distraction Stabilization Techniques

The technique and results from application of ventral and dorsal decompressive techniques including laminectomy, facetectomy, and ventral

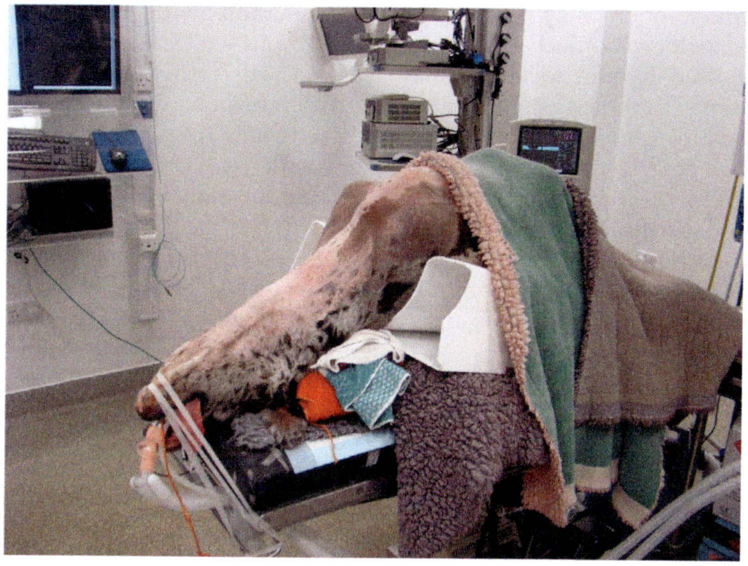

Figure 25.5 Patient positioning for surgery. Accurate positioning is required for distraction-fusion surgery in CSM cases. The patient is placed in dorsal recumbency with adequate padding supporting the caudal cervical spine and cranial thorax. Cranial cervical spine extension relative to the trunk provides ventral cervical spine exposure. The head and thoracic limbs are secured firmly and proximal humeral access is available for autograft harvest.

slot have been well documented. Recent literature suggests that distraction-stabilization may produce rapid and robust longer-term decompression for DAWS patients. Several stabilization and distraction-stabilization procedures have been reported with the use of ventral and interbody fixation with or without biological augmentation, including intervertebral spacers such as allogenic cortical bone grafts, polymethylmethacrylate (PMMA) cement plugs, washers, and other metallic spacers such as cages with or without screws [22, 25–29].

25.6.1 Unicortical Locking Systems

The application of monocortical screws provides comparable fixation to bicortical screws in the canine cervical spine [30], without the risk of vertebral canal penetration, damage of the cord, and damage of the vertebral vascular plexus. Biomechanical examination of cervical fixation identifies the use of unilateral locking systems with monocortical screws as suitable fixation in the canine cervical spine [31].

Excessive motion has been related to delayed healing or surgical failure in anterior plating of the cervical spine in humans [32]. The use of locking plates in the cervical spine has significantly improved intervertebral fusion in people [33]. The need to minimize motion to achieve union has driven the development of locking plate constructs for management of CSM in dogs.

Angular stable (locking) constructs minimize implant back out and collapse because of subsidence. Rigid fixation has gained widespread acceptance for the treatment of CSM in dogs [22, 25, 26, 34]. Locking plates provide comparable fixation to nonlocking plates and screw-PMMA systems [35, 36] while the fixed-angle interface negates the risk of screw-plate disengagement inherent in non-locking systems.

Bilateral locking plate stabilization is superior to screw-PMMA in the reduction of bending and axial rotation across a single vertebral space and may minimize the domino effect in adjacent intervertebral spaces [37]. Positive profile pin-PMMA constructs confer superior fixation in flexion and lateral bending in a lumbar spine model [38] however this stabilization modality may exert a deleterious effect on adjacent intervertebral segments and presents the risk of transverse foraminal penetration during cervical fusion [37, 39]. This risk may be minimized by using 3D printed guides to facilitate pin placement.

Veterinary specific solutions may be preferable to address CSM in dogs. Biomechanical testing of commonly used human locking plate systems demonstrated inferior stabilization and increased failure compared to screw-PMMA and cortical ring spacer fixation in a canine model [36]. By contrast, mechanical testing of veterinary-specific locking plates produced distraction stabilization comparable to screw-PMMA fixation [40]. Concomitant application of an intervertebral spacer with fixation enhanced construct stiffness [26].

Finding a reliable alternative to the application of PMMA with screw or pin fixation may be desirable from the perspective of ease of implant application and reduction in profile of fixation units, such that the possibility for neural impingement, vascular disruption, oesophagitis, and dysphagia is reduced.

25.6.2 Bone Graft and Intervertebral Spacers

Failure of the fixation construct and collapse of spacers before fusion is a common challenge for all techniques. Therefore, spacers that favor osseous union and spacers with a wide surface area over the end plates have been preferred. An integrated intervertebral fusion device for single body fusion was described with *in vitro* data demonstrating fixation comparative with locking plates alone without bone graft [41].

A variety of polymeric and metallic implants have been developed with the aim of achieving stable robust intervertebral distraction and transvertebral osseous union, and these are usually augmented with cancellous autograft.

Bone autograft is potently osteogenic, osteoconductive, and nonimmunogenic. Use of autograft should be limited to augmentation of implants in transvertebral fusion; cancellous graft is preferred over cortical and transcortical material. Application of autograft alone as an intervertebral spacer material should be avoided. Allograft and allograft-derived materials may have adequate structural strength as cortical block spacers, but lack intrinsic osteogenic capacity and demonstrate slower integration rates and lower rates of fusion by comparison with autogenous material. Locking plates applied in combination with intervertebral cancellous block and cortical ring allograft have produced satisfactory outcomes for treatment of traction responsive single site CSM [25, 26].

Activation of organic graft and synthetic graft alternatives by OP-1 (Bone Morphogenic Protein-7) and BMP-2 enhances osteogenic activity but has been associated with adverse off-target effects [42].

The use of intervertebral cement plugs for cervical distraction-fusion has yielded variable success [43–45]. Immediate decompression, symptom alleviation and limited disease progression long-term have been reported in some studies in large-breed dogs [44, 45]. However, PMMA set-curing may cause thermal injury and extrication of inaccurately placed material is challenging. Postoperative radiographs and early follow-up highlight propensity for bone cement to delocalise post application. In one study of 52 Doberman pinchers, intervertebral PMMA spacer treatment provided satisfactory initial stabilization but complications in a significant number of cases were associated with inadequate distraction, failed fusion, vertebral fracture and catastrophic cervical collapse [43].

Good outcomes were reported using a polymer cage device incorporating autologous bone graft in combination with locking plates [27]. This device was comparable to PEEK spinal cage systems described in human patients [46].

Radiographic documentation of osseous union and favorable clinical outcome has been reported in dogs affected by DAWS using an intervertebral spacer developed by the author (Fitz Intervertebral Traction Screw, FITS™) in conjunction with double ventral locking plates (SOP™, "String-of-Pearls") [22]. Short-term loosening of the plates and screws was documented but generally without clinical consequence [22].

Across all systems, long-term intervertebral fusion based on radiographic assessment has been reported with a success of 70–90% incorporating use of cancellous bone graft [22, 25–29].

25.7 New Implants and Surgical Planning

The author has developed a new intervertebral distraction-fusion system. The objectives for the system are as follows:

1. The intervertebral spacer devices should be self-distracting following preparation of the intervertebral space.
2. The intervertebral spacer devices should be applicable even in the presence of deformed end plates, including those affected by deformity and vertebral "tipping."
3. The intervertebral spacer devices should be applicable to all patient sizes.
4. The intervertebral spacer devices should have the capability of variable depth insertion and be coated for osteo-induction.
5. The intervertebral spacer devices should penetrate the end plates focally for osseous bridging but not induce end plate collapse.
6. The system should be applicable for the treatment of both OAWS and DAWS patients.
7. Intervertebral spacers should be linkable to plate fixation units to provide an integrated robust construct.
8. Plate fixation units should be as low profile as possible and be easy to centre on the mid sagittal ventral aspects of the vertebral bodies.
9. Vertebral fixation units should have fixed-angle screws that when positioned correctly result in screw divergence for maximal screw purchase without violation of the vertebral canal.
10. Vertebral fixation units should have locking screw fixation through two cortices, i.e. from ventral to dorsal lateral to the spinal cord.
11. Sequential intervertebral spacer devices linked to individual vertebral fixation units should be rigidly linkable through any number of vertebrae in the cervical spine from C2–3 caudally to C7–T1.
12. The rigid linkage system for vertebral fixation units should be amenable to contouring dorsal to ventral and left to right in order to accommodate anatomic variance and desired neck angle.
13. Each unit should be sequentially linkable so that contouring of a fixation device over a long distance is not necessary.
14. The rigid linkage system for vertebral fixation units should be resistant to intervertebral collapse, torsion and lateral, or ventro-dorsal bending.
15. The entire linkage system should facilitate easy placement of autologous cancellous graft to afford biological fusion of any number of vertebrae.

These objectives have been achieved using intervertebral spacer devices that are threaded, conical and coated in hydroxyapatite (Fitz Intervertebral Traction Screw, FITS™), linked to an integrated plate and rod system (Cervical Fitzateur). To date, the cervical spinal fixation system units have been custom made for each individual patient, but ongoing experience facilitates manufacture of standard units that can be sized based on radiographs and CT scans. At present, CT scans imported to commercially available software packages facilitate digital templating. Application of this system has allowed the author to distract and fuse from one to seven cervical intervertebral spaces.

The use of the intervertebral spacer device has previously been reported in conjunction with SOP™ plates [22]. These locking plates had monocortical screws only, were very challenging to contour over more than a single vertebral pair, and it was difficult to achieve appropriate angulation. Plates often sat too far from the ventral vertebral cortex due to contouring challenges, and because the plates were not linked to the spacers, vertebral collapse was reported before fusion. The new integrated plate and rod system has superseded all other devices in the author's practice. The implant system is part of a larger group of implants that facilitate spinal distraction-fusion at any spinal location – the Fitz Universal Spinal System (FUSS™).

The cervical Fitzateur system comprises three basic elements – an intervertebral spacer, a plate linked to the spacer and also to a saddle (Figure 25.6a) that is screwed to the vertebra and a rod linking adjacent spacers. In single site fusions, rods are not required and instead a single plate spanning the vertebrae over the spacer is employed (Figure 25.6b). The Fitz Intervertebral Traction Screw (FITS™) spacer is conical, tapered and threaded and is available in 10 sizes.

The most critical factor is to determine optimal angulation for the screws to maximize bone-purchase in the vertebral body and ventral vertebral arch and to avoid the spinal canal. Avoidance of encroachment of the venous sinus is desirable but not mandatory. Assessment

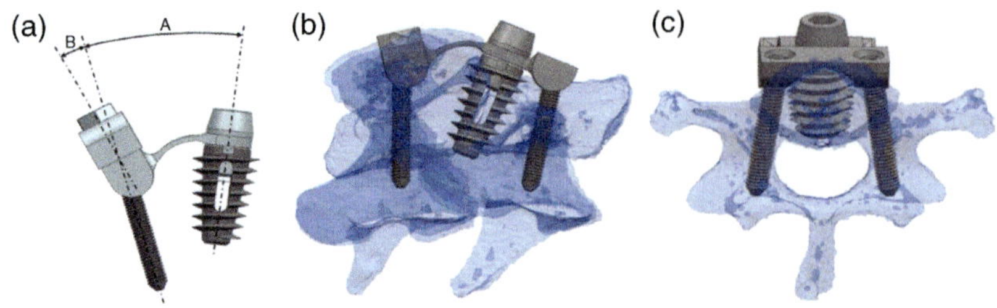

Figure 25.6 Custom fixation unit for single intervertebral fusion. Cervical Fitzateur and FITS™ (Fitz Intervertebral Traction Screw). (a) The cervical Fitzateur system comprises three elements; an intervertebral spacer (FITS device), plate and saddle. Locking screws are used to secure the saddles to adjacent vertebrae. (b) The angle of screw application is designed to maximize bone engagement, avoid incursion of the spinal canal and avoid convergence with the FITS spacer (Image a, arcs A and B). (c) Locking screws are divergent in the transverse axis and secured within the vertebral pedicle with care taken to avoid interfering with the vertebral canal and facet joints. The leading edge of the FITS device is flush but does not penetrate the ventral border of the vertebral canal (b and c).

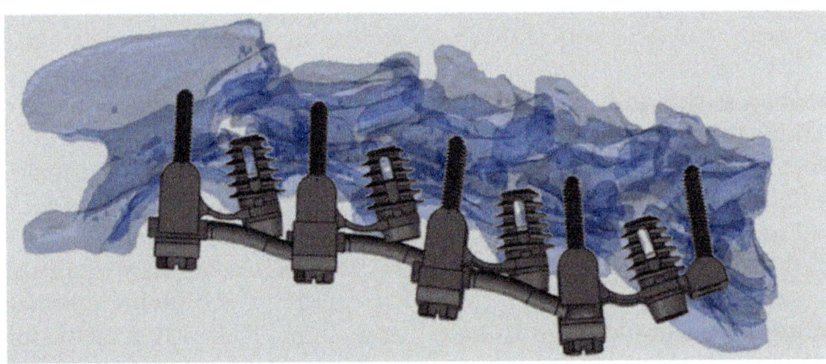

Figure 25.7 Interlinking FITS spacers and Fitzateur system. A single Fitzateur device can be linked through a rod and locking plate-saddle system and secured to adjacent FITS spacers. The modular interlinking system combines to provide immediate decompression of the spinal cord, distraction fusion and stabilization across multiple vertebrae.

of screw length is facilitated by preoperative measurement on CT scans. The goal is at least two screws per plate in each vertebral body; four in larger breed dogs.

The objective of the system is to immediately decompress the spinal cord and nerve roots caused by intervertebral disc protrusion, facet hypertrophy, or vertebral arch malformation by placing the FITS™ device. The device is coated in hydroxyapatite for fibro-osseous on-growth and fusion is augmented using cancellous bone graft harvested from the proximal humerus. The spacers are linked robustly across any number of cervical sites with custom-contoured rods and clamps (Figure 25.7).

25.8 Surgical Techniques

A standard ventral approach to the cervical spine facilitates muscular retraction, ventral annulectomy and nuclear extirpation. The end plates are debrided and a shallow groove is created perpendicular to the mid-sagittal ridge of each vertebral body to facilitate tracking of the conical FITS spacer device. The saddle and plate units are attached sequentially to the spacer devices, centred appropriately and screwed in position using 3.5 mm locking screws of appropriate length. Divergence angle is pre-determined and intrinsic to the saddle plate. Then contiguous saddles are linked using a rod and clamp system that facilitates placement of both the leading and the trailing ends of alternate rods side-by-side to form a series of units as required. One end of the rod has a ball shape and the other has a trapezoid shape, such that contouring is possible but torsion and lateral bending is prevented. The result is a rigid construct.

25.9 Outcomes

Outcomes associated with the application of this new cervical distraction-fusion fixation system has not yet been reported and patient follow-up is ongoing. An earlier version of the technique using the spacer device and more conventional locking plates (SOP™) revealed radiographic fusion in 10/16 cases at 6 weeks after surgery [22]. With the new system, we have avoided problems previously observed for plate-screw loosening. Design based on CT scan for every case avoids the possibility of screw incursion of the spinal canal when the saddles are placed appropriately and also allows purchase of greater bone stock. The rod and clamp architecture is unique and allows contouring for accurate alignment while also being torsion resistant. We have fused from one to seven intervertebral sites and complications with the most recent iteration of implants are lower than that reported for other techniques at this time, but longer-term follow-up data is not yet available for publication. Our subjective adjudication is that operative times are reduced by comparison to all other systems the author has used, patients walk quickly (within 48 hours), hospital stay is significantly reduced by comparison with both published and anecdotal experience with laminectomy, and the recovery is robust and resilient. It is important to note that spinal cord degeneration can be so severe that no distraction-fusion technique would produce improvement in some cases, with the hope merely being prevention of further deterioration for as long as possible.

We have treated all forms of disc- and osseous-associated cervical deformities including dorsal, lateral, ventral, or combination of compressive lesions on the cervical spine with this system and have documented evidence of regression of both soft tissue and osseous compressive elements over time.

25.10 Conclusion

The use of internal rigid fixation with angle stable screws in distraction-stabilization techniques for management of CSM in dogs have provided advantages and generally improved short and long term outcomes. Outcomes analysis is ongoing. Accurate decision-making to identify the particularities of each individual case affected by this complex syndrome remains paramount to achieve a successful long term outcome.

References

1. Lincoln, J.D. and G.D, P. (1985). Evaluation of fenestration for treatment of degenerative disc disease in the caudal cervical region of large dogs. *Vet. Surg.* [Internet] 14 (3): 240–246.
2. Jeffery, N.D. and W.M, M.K. (2001). Surgery for disc-associated wobbler syndrome in the dog–an examination of the controversy. *J. Small Anim. Pract.* 42 (12): 574–581.
3. Seim, H. (2002). Wobbler syndrome. In: *Small Animal Surgery*, 2 (ed. T. Fossum), 1237–1249. Mosby Inc.
4. da Costa, R.C., Echandi, R.L., and Beauchamp, D. (2012). Computed tomography myelographic findings in dogs with cervical spondylomyelopathy. *Vet. Radiol. Ultrasound* 53 (1): 64–70.
5. Rossmeisl, J.H., Lanz, O.I., Inzana, K.D. et al. (2005). A modified lateral approach to the canine cervical spine: procedural description and clinical application in 16 dogs with lateralized compressive myelopathy or radiculopathy. *Vet. Surg.* 34 (5): 436–444.
6. Voss, K., Steffen, F., and Montavon, P.M. (2006). Use of the ComPact UniLock system for ventral stabilization procedures of the cervical spine: a retrospective study. *Vet. Comp. Orthop. Traumatol.* 19 (1): 21–28.
7. Trotter, E.J., deLahunta, A., Geary, J.C. et al. (1976). Caudal cervical vertebral malformation-malarticulation in great Danes and Doberman pinschers. *J. Am. Vet. Med. Assoc.* 168 (10): 917–930.
8. Amevo, B., Worth, D., and Bogduk, N. (1991). Instantaneous axes of rotation of the typical cervical motion segments: a study in normal volunteers. *Clin. Biomech.* 6 (2): 111–117.
9. Farfan, H.F., Cossette, J.W., Robertson, G.H. et al. (1970). The effects of torsion on the lumbar intervertebral joints: the role of torsion in the production of disc degeneration. *J. Bone Joint Surg. Am* 52 (3): 468–497.
10. Breit, S. and Kunzel, W. (2001). Osteological features in pure-bred dogs predisposing to cervical spinal cord compression. *J. Anat.* 199: 527–537.
11. Johnson, J.A., da Costa, R.C., Bhattacharya, S. et al. (2011). Kinematic motion patterns of the cranial and caudal canine cervical spine. *Vet. Surg.* 40 (6): 720–727.
12. Rusbridge, C., Wheeler, S.J., Torrington, A.M. et al. (1998)). Comparison of two surgical techniques for

the management of cervical spondylomyelopathy in dobermanns. *J. Small Anim. Pract.* 39 (9): 425–431.
13. Seim, H. and Prata, R. (1982). Ventral decompression for the treatment of cervical disk disease in the dog: a review of 54 cases. *J. Am. Anim. Hosp. Assoc.* 18: 233–240.
14. Lipsitz, D., Levitski, R.E., Chauvet, A.E. et al. (2001). Magnetic resonance imaging features of cervical stenotic myelopathy in 21 dogs. *Vet. Radiol. Ultrasound* 42 (1): 20–27.
15. da Costa, R.C., Parent, J.M., Partlow, G. et al. (2006). Morphologic and morphometric magnetic resonance imaging features of Doberman pinschers with and without clinical signs of cervical spondylomyelopathy. *Am. J. Vet. Res.* 67 (9): 1601–1602.
16. Palmer, A.C. and Wallace, M.E. (1967). Deformation of cervical vertebrae in basset hounds. *Vet. Rec* 80 (14): 430–433.
17. Murthy, V.D., Gaitero, L., and Monteith, G. (2014). Clinical and magnetic resonance imaging (MRI) findings in 26 dogs with canine osseous-associated cervical spondylomyelopathy. *Can. Vet. J.* 55 (2): 169–174.
18. Guillem Gallach, R., Suran, J., Cáceres, A.V. et al. (2011). Reliability of t2-weighted sagittal magnetic resonance images for determining the location of compressive disK herniation in dogs. *Vet. Radiol. Ultrasound* 52 (5): 479–486.
19. da Costa, R.C. and Johnson, J.A. (2012). Intervertebral and intravertebral ratios in doberman pinscher dogs with cervical spondylomyelopathy. *Vet. Radiol. Ultrasound* 53 (5): 518–523.
20. Newcomb, B., Arble, J., Rochat, M. et al. (2012). Comparison of computed tomography and myelography to a reference standard of computed tomographic myelography for evaluation of dogs with intervertebral disc disease. *Vet. Surg.* 41 (2): 207–217.
21. Penderis, J. and Dennis, R. (2004). Use of traction during magnetic resonance imaging of caudal cervical spondylomyelopathy ("wobbler syndrome") in the dog. *Vet. Radiol. Ultrasound* 45 (3): 216–219.
22. Solano, M.A., Fitzpatrick, N., and Bertran, J. (2015). Cervical distraction-stabilization using an intervertebral spacer screw and string-of pearl (SOPTM) plates in 16 dogs with disc-associated wobbler syndrome. *Vet. Surg.* 44 (5): 627–641.
23. McKee, W.M., Butterworth, S.J., and Scott, H.W. (1999). Management of cervical spondylopathy-associated intervertebral, disc protrusions using metal washers in 78 dogs. *J. Small Anim. Pract.* 40 (10): 465–472.
24. Johnson, K.A. (2014). *Piermattei's Atlas of Surgical Approaches to the Bones and Joints of the Dog and Cat*, 5, 33–45. Elsevier Health Sciences.
25. E.J, T. (2009). Cervical spine locking plate fixation for treatment of cervical Spondylotic myelopathy in large breed dogs. *Vet. Surg.* 38 (6): 705–718.
26. Bergman, R.L., Levine, J.M., Coates, J.R. et al. (2008). Cervical spinal locking plate in combination with cortical ring allograft for a one level fusion in dogs with cervical spondylotic myelopathy. *Vet. Surg.* 37 (6): 530–536.
27. Steffen, F., Voss, K., and Morgan, J.P. (2011). Distraction-fusion for caudal cervical Spondylomyelopathy using an intervertebral cage and locking plates in 14 dogs. *Vet. Surg.* 40 (6): 743–752.
28. Shamir, M.H., Chai, O., and Loeb, E. (2008). A method for intervertebral space distraction before stabilization combined with complete ventral slot for treatment of disc-associated wobbler syndrome in dogs. *Vet. Surg.* 37 (2): 186–192.
29. De Decker, S., Caemaert, J., Tshamala, M.C. et al. (2011). Surgical treatment of disk-associated wobbler syndrome by a distractable vertebral titanium cage in seven dogs. *Vet. Surg.* 40 (5): 544–554.
30. Hettlich, B.F., Allen, M.J., Pascetta, D. et al. (2013). Biomechanical comparison between bicortical pin and monocortical screw/polymethylmethacrylate constructs in the cadaveric canine cervical vertebral column. *Vet. Surg.* 42 (6): 693–700.
31. Agnello, K.A., Kapatkin, A.S., Garcia, T.C. et al. (2010). Intervertebral biomechanics of locking compression plate Monocortical fixation of the canine cervical spine. *Vet. Surg.* 39 (8): 991–1000.
32. Spivak, J.M., Chen, D., and Kummer, F.J. (1999). The effect of locking fixation screws on the stability of anterior cervical plating. *Spine* (Phila Pa 1976) [Internet] 24 (4): 334–338.
33. Kaiser, M.G., Haid, R.W., Subach, B.R. et al. (2002). Anterior cervical plating enhances arthrodesis after discectomy and fusion with cortical allograft. *Neurosurgery* 50 (2): 229–236.
34. Pfeil, I. (2012). Treatment of 65 dogs with wobbler syndrome by distraction and fusion with TTA cages. Proceedings 16th ESVOT congress. Bologna.
35. Lehmann, W., Briem, D., Blauth, M. et al. (2005). Biomechanical comparison of anterior cervical spine locked and unlocked plate-fixation systems. *Eur. Spine J.* 14 (3): 243–249.
36. Morrison, E.J., Litsky, A.S., Allen, M.J. et al. (2016). Evaluation of three human cervical fusion implants for use in the canine cervical vertebral column. *Vet. Surg.* [Internet] 45 (7): 901–908.
37. Hakozaki, T., Ichinohe, T., Kanno, N. et al. (2016). Biomechanical assessment of the effects of vertebral distraction-fusion techniques on the adjacent segment of canine cervical vertebrae. *Am. J. Vet. Res.* 77 (11): 1194–1199.

38. Sturges, B.K., Kapatkin, A.S., Garcia, T.C. et al. (2016). Biomechanical comparison of locking compression plate versus positive profile pins and polymethylmethacrylate for stabilization of the canine lumbar vertebrae. *Vet. Surg* 45 (3): 309–318.
39. Koehler, C.L., Stover, S.M., LeCouteur, R.A. et al. (2005). Effect of a ventral slot procedure and of smooth or positive-profile threaded pins with polymethylmethacrylate fixation on intervertebral biomechanics at treated and adjacent canine cervical vertebral motion units. *Am. J. Vet. Res* 66 (4): 678–687.
40. Hettlich, B.F., Fosgate, G.T., and Litsky, A.S. (2017). Biomechanical comparison of 2 veterinary locking plates to monocortical screw/polymethylmethacrylate fixation in canine cadaveric cervical vertebral column. *Vet. Surg* 46 (1): 95–102.
41. Schöllhorn, B., Bürki, A., Stahl, C. et al. (2013). Comparison of the biomechanical properties of a ventral cervical intervertebral anchored fusion device with locking plate fixation applied to cadaveric canine cervical spines. *Vet. Surg* 42 (7): 825–831.
42. James, A.W., LaChaud, G., Shen, J. et al. (2016). A review of the clinical side effects of bone morphogenetic protein-2. *Tissue Eng. Part B Rev.* 22 (4): 284–297.
43. McKee, W.M., Pink, J.J., and Gemmill, T.J. (2016). Cement plug technique for the management of disc-associated cervical spondylopathy in 52 Dobermann Pinscher dogs. *Vet. Comp. Orthop. Traumatol.* 29 (3): 195–201.
44. Sterna, J. (2007). Distraction with bone cement plug as a treatment of caudal cervical spondylomyelopathy–report of three cases. *Pol. J. Vet. Sci.* 10 (3): 179–182.
45. Dixon, B.C., Tomlinson, J.L., and Kraus, K.H. (1996). Modified distraction-stabilization technique using an interbody polymethyl methacrylate plug in dogs with caudal cervical spondylomyelopathy. *J. Am. Vet. Med. Assoc.* [Internet] 208 (1): 61–68.
46. Chou, Y.-C., Chen, D.-C., Hsieh, W.A. et al. (2008). Efficacy of anterior cervical fusion: comparison of titanium cages, polyetheretherketone (PEEK) cages and autogenous bone grafts. *J. Clin. Neurosci* 15 (11): 1240–1245.

26 Lumbosacral Stabilization

Noel Fitzpatrick

26.1 Introduction

Degenerative lumbosacral stenosis (DLSS) is a common cause of caudal spinal pain in medium- and large-breed dogs. It is seen less commonly in small dogs and cats. DLSS results in a narrowing of the vertebral canal and intervertebral foramina at the level of the lumbosacral junction. The narrowing results in compressive radiculopathy of the L7 nerve roots and the nerve roots of the cauda equina. Compression of the nerve roots is a multifactorial process. Direct compression of the nerve roots can be caused by prolapse of the annulus fibrosus, hypertrophy of the joint capsule of the L7-S1 (LS) articular facets and hypertrophy of the interarcuate ligament. Osteophytosis / spondylosis at the level of the intervertebral foramena may also cause direct compression of the L7 nerve roots abaxially. The compressive process may also have a dynamic component whereby compression of the nerve roots is exacerbated or relieved depending on degree of flexion or extension at the LS junction. This is the result of further disc protrusion, motion of the spondylotic new bone on the caudal aspect of L7 and the cranial aspect of S1, ventral migration of the dorsal lamina of the sacrum relative to L7 and relative motion of the inflamed articular facets. It is well established that the intervertebral foramen undergoes narrowing when the LS junction is placed into extension [1, 2].

26.2 Clinical Examination

Though direct consequences of compression of the L7 and cauda equina nerve roots can be observed with neurogenic deficits producing paresis, muscle weakness and urinary issues, the most commonly encountered clinical signs are related to pain, both acute and chronic, and lameness, both profound and subtle. In the author's experience, pain only or pain and lameness are often the only signs manifested. Because muscle spasms can be associated with persistent or intermittent claudication of the L7 nerve roots, the condition is commonly confused with other scenarios such as iliopsoas muscle strain-sprain or sacroiliac pain.

In dogs affected by DLSS, pain may often be elicited during physical examination by application of direct pressure over the lumbo-sacral junction dorsally, but one must be careful to

Locking Plates in Veterinary Orthopedics, First Edition.
Edited by Matthew D. Barnhart and Karl C. Maritato.

neutralize the coxofemoral joints so as not to confuse hip pain. Simultaneous hyperextension of the LS spine may also produce a painful response. Along the sciatic nerve pathway, pain may be evoked on deep digital pressure application, either externally by placing the thumb in the caudal thigh recess between the biceps femoris and the semitendinosus-membranosus (Holsworth Test) or per rectum using a gloved index finger where the sciatic nerve can be palpated on the axial aspect of the lesser ischiatic notch (Fitzpatrick Test). Clinical signs are caused by direct compression of the cauda equina and impingement of the ganglia of the spinal nerve roots as they exit through the intervertebral foramena [3].

26.3 Decision-Making

26.3.1 Radiography

- Plain and dynamic radiography has been evaluated in the diagnosis of LS disease. However, the author never undertakes surgery in cases affected by DLSS without advanced imaging [4].
- The effect of intervertebral disc protrusion, spondylosis, and facet inflammation on the cauda equina and L7 nerve roots cannot be determined without cross-sectional imaging.

26.3.2 CT Scan

- The author prefers CT scan over MRI scan for evaluation of the osseous compressive elements of DLSS, especially in the neuroforamina on transverse planar imaging and evaluation of positional alignment of the dorsal lamina of the sacrum relative to L7 in neutral and hyperextended positions. CT scan can demonstrate a reduction in the volume of the intervertebral foramena of dogs abaxially (by bone and soft tissue) but unlike MRI, cannot evaluate the neuronal structures traveling through the intervertebral foramena [5].
- CT scan is also a very important tool for patients undergoing instrumented surgical management of DLSS so that implant sizes can be estimated presurgically, thus facilitating operative planning.

26.3.3 MRI

- MRI is the gold standard modality for evaluating the anatomic and dynamic features of DLSS. This modality allows accurate assessment of the neuronal structures and the soft tissue components of compression while also demonstrating osseous compressive elements.
- Dynamic imaging sequences, whereby the dog is scanned in different degrees of extension of the LS junction, are very useful to fully understand how neural impingement changes as the dog moves. This is pertinent to the L7 nerve roots abaxially and the cauda equina when affected by protrusion, spondylosis, facet inflammation and ventral migration of the dorsal lamina of the sacrum relative to L7 (Figure 26.1a).
- Traditional parasagittal imaging of the neuroforamena has been shown to underestimate neuroforaminal volume. Angled cross-section imaging of the L7-S1 neuroforamena using parasagittal oblique sequences allow a more clinically relevant understanding of the compression of the nerve root at the entry, middle, and exit zones, (Figure 26.1b). This imaging is a key tool in the decision-making process of the author regarding stabilization of the L7-S1 junction, and we have published this data recently [6].

26.4 Surgical Planning: Patient Positioning and Surgical Approach

The patient is positioned in ventral recumbency and supported in the midline with positioning aids to maintain patient stability. The hind limbs are drawn forward with the metatarsal bones parallel to the top of the surgical table to flex the lumbosacral spine and open the L7-S1 space. A standard dorsal approach to the L7-S1 junction is adopted [7] with dorsal laminectomy involving approximately one-third of the cranial to caudal width of the L7 lamina and two-thirds of the cranial extent of the sacral lamina. Meticulous hemostasis is important to maintain a clear surgical field during implant positioning, but this can be very challenging because frequently in chronic cases there is

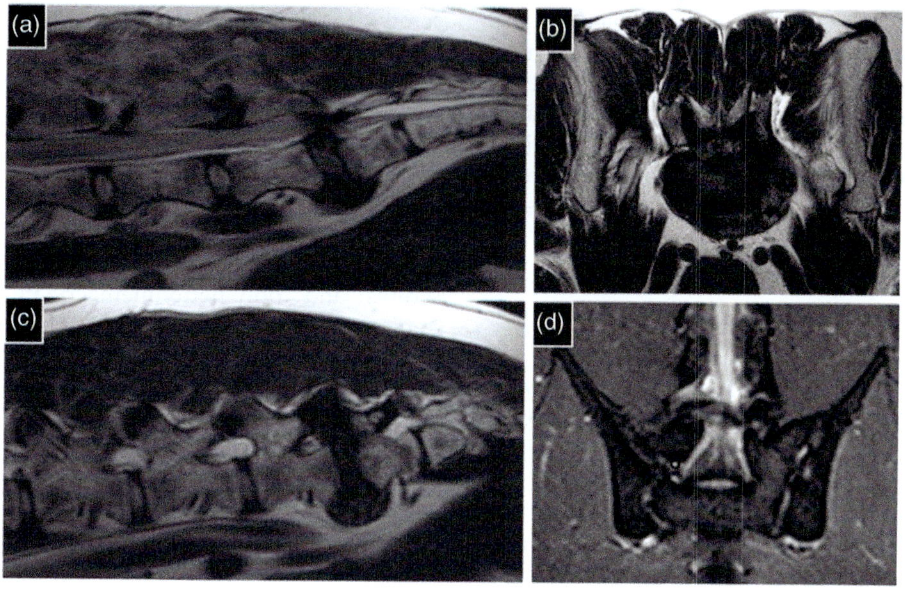

Figure 26.1 Typical MRI findings in DLSS. T2 weighted (a–c) and STIR (d) MRI scans of a typical presentation of degenerative lumbosacral stenosis (DLSS). (a) Sagittal plane demonstrating marked compression of the cauda equina dorsal to L7-S1 intervertebral space. Nucleus pulposus signal is reduced and irregular. (b) Transverse plane through L7-S1 disc with dramatically reduced nucleus pulposus signal and obliteration of both the spinal canal and the L7 neuroforamina, which normally manifest nerve roots within fat signal. (c) Parasagittal plane manifesting hypointensity of lateralized disc protrusion within the neuroforamen when compared with more cranial segments. (d) Dorsal plane demonstrating near-complete discontinuation of nerve root and fat signal at junction of conus medullaris and cauda equina.

significant bleeding associated with chronic inflammation, and bleeding from the ventral venous sinuses can be considerable. Muscular dissection is extended cranially to allow access for screw placement on either side of the L7 vertebral body.

26.5 Surgical Techniques

26.5.1 Decompression Alone – Dorsal Laminectomy and Foraminotomy

Surgical management of LS disease involves either decompression alone, stabilization alone, or distraction-stabilization, with dorsal facet and /or ventral vertebral body fusion being preferable for any stabilization technique. Decompression without surgical stabilization may provide immediate symptomatic relief for some patients, and this may be maintained indefinitely, although analysis of long-term outcomes is required to validate this approach [8]. However, laminectomy alone can only be successful for central protrusion or extrusion, and this accounts for a very small proportion of clinical cases of DLSS in the author's practice. Decompression via dorsal laminectomy alone does not address lateralized neuroforaminal impingement and it can be difficult to achieve adequate decompression of all of the entry, middle, and exit zones by foraminotomy techniques alone. The possibility for iatrogenic damage of the L7 nerve roots must also be considered and impairment of visibility produced by hemorrhage potentially compromises optimal removal of osseous and soft tissue compressive elements.

Dorsal laminectomy and dorsal disc annulectomy destabilize the L7-S1 spinal segment and increase the range of motion in flexion and extension [9–11]. Extension of the mobile L7-S1 junction that ensues may decrease the foraminal aperture and exacerbate the effect of foraminal stenosis on nerve root impingement [12], even when foraminotomy has been performed. Foraminotomy may be a successful intervention for lateralized L7 compression but fails to address the dynamic compressive effect of spinal motion on foraminal occlusion. Ongoing lumbosacral instability can accelerate the progression of lumbosacral disease and may exacerbate clinical signs associated with nerve root occlusion [1, 12]. Additionally, even if satisfactory decompression is achieved at the time of foraminotomy, bone and scar tissue may grow back such that longer-term success of decompression might not be maintained.

26.5.2 Decompression + Dorsal Fixation

26.5.2.1 Dorsal Fixation with Facet Screws

Transarticular fixation of the facet joints with screws following decompression seeks to preserve relative vertebral position and to maintain foraminal aperture (Figure 26.2a), but it has been observed that such stabilization may not significantly alter long-term outcomes versus decompression alone [13, 14]. Furthermore, the author has observed fracture of the L7-S1 facets following screw stabilization after both dorsal laminectomy and foraminotomy, separately or combined. Additionally, facet screws do not result in distraction and therefore may not adequately resolve clinical signs because of residual static impingement.

26.5.2.2 Dorsal Fixation with Screws + Plates or Screws /Pins + Cement

Stabilization of the L7-S1 junction has been achieved using a variety of methods. Pins or screws and polymethylmethacrylate cement deployed either in neutral or flexed lumbo-sacral positions have been deployed most commonly (Figure 26.2d). Custom locking plates have purportedly been employed but not yet reported. The string-of-pearls (SOP™, Orthomed, Huddersfield, UK) locking plate applied dorsally has been reported (Figure 26.2c) but found to have no biomechanical benefit over pins and PMMA cement [15]. It is challenging to effectively deploy fixed-angle locking systems in the lumbosacral area as the anatomy makes it difficult to obtain sufficient bone stock and plates can be challenging to contour. Variable angle locking systems may be more suitable for use, however

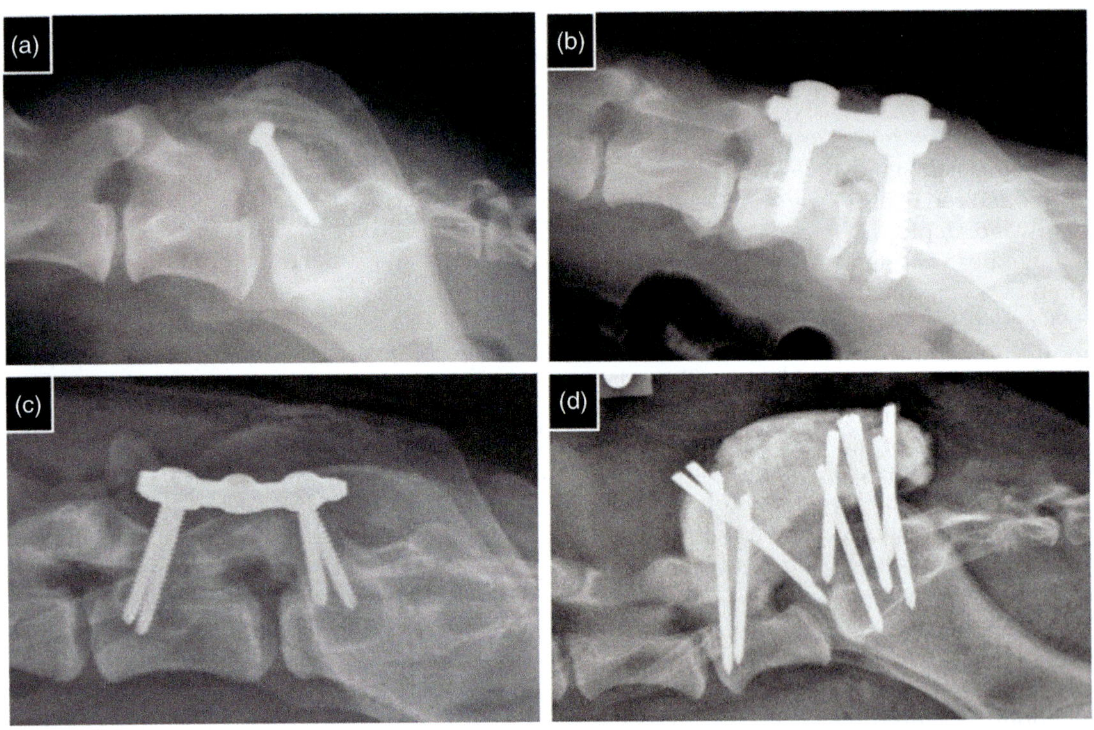

Figure 26.2 Fixation modalities in lumbosacral fusion. (a) Facet screw fixation. (b) Noncustomized pedicle screw with fixed-angle connecting rod and clamp. (c) Contoured SOP plate with fixed-angle pedicle screws. (d) Multi-angled pins secured with PMMA.

these systems often lack the angular freedom needed for successful deployment.

Some authors have advocated fusion in mild flexion with dorsal fixation, but this results in abnormal loading of the lumbosacral spine and may contribute to fixation failure with implant breakage over time. The author has observed this with all screws up to 3.5 mm in diameter linked with either polymethylmethacrylate cement or SOP locking plates and also with pins up to 3 mm in diameter. There is considerable load exerted and failure in such circumstances is largely dependent on core diameter of the screw or pin. In the opinion of the author, the core diameter of 3.5 mm screws and even solid 3 mm pins may be too weak to sustain such loading, especially with the lumbosacral spine fixed in permanent flexion, and sometimes patient size prohibits deployment of screws of larger diameter such as 4.5 mm standard screws or 4 mm pins.

26.5.2.3 Dorsal Fixation with Pedicle Screws

Pedicle screw and rod fixation following dorsal laminectomy stabilizes the lumbosacral joint (Figure 26.2b), maintaining the intervertebral space and foraminal dimensions and may slow the progression of degenerative changes [9, 10, 16, 17]. Clinical data reporting the use of a pedicle screw and rod fixation system developed for humans and deployed to treat 12 dogs with severe lumbosacral stenosis demonstrated alleviation of symptoms in 8/12 animals and improvement in 4/12 as measured by hind limb function and force plate analysis with no implant failure [18]. The screws were placed vertically into the arches of L7 vertebrae and the lateral aspects of the sacrum but available screw sizes limit patient applicability, and there is a risk of iatrogenic trauma to the L7 nerve roots in the lateral recesses of the caudal aspect of the L7 vertebra. Purportedly, some distraction in the pedicle screw-rod construct is imbued by dorsal tension across the device. However, the absence of an implant between adjacent end-plates fails to contribute ventral distraction and does not provide vertebral segments with an osteoconductive scaffold necessary to promote interbody bone union. This is evidenced by the lack of intervertebral bone growth in pedicle screw-rod fixation systems.

The goal of decompression combined with dorsal fixation of the L7-S1 vertebrae is to remove the static elements of compression of osseous or soft tissue origin and permanently stabilize relative motion of the L7-S1 functional spinal unit. This aims to prohibit dynamic impingement of the L7 nerve roots and cauda equina and render ongoing degenerative changes less clinically relevant to the patient. The fundamental challenge is that even if a locking plate or screws / pins and cement or rods are used, fixation is persistently vulnerable to failure if the dorsal facets do not fuse and become adequately robust independent of the mechanical fixation employed. The surface area of the facet joints is very small and even when all cartilage is debrided and bone graft is applied, this surface area available for biological fusion is intrinsically small. Therefore, fusion ventrally between the L7 vertebral body and the sacrum would be desirable. Apart from the formation of further ventral and abaxial spondylosis, which in and of itself can cause further L7 nerve root compression, there is no mechanism by which dorsal fixation alone can achieve this. With all decompression and dorsal stabilization systems there remains an inherent risk of implant failure and sudden intervertebral and foraminal collapse.

26.5.2.4 Decompression + Ventral Distraction + Dorsal Fixation

In contrast to decompression and placement of screws across the facets or decompression and placement of screws / plates or screws / pins / cement or screws/ rods dorsally with the lumbosacral spine in mild flexion, ventral distraction plus dorsal fixation aims to linearly distract the L7 vertebra relative to the sacrum before stabilization and also aims for inter-body vertebral fusion. The goal of distraction-stabilization-fusion is to distract the L7-S1 vertebral end-plates and neuroforaminae in an anatomically favorable position prior to stabilization such that the volume of the intervertebral foramena is enlarged and thus nerve root pain and dysfunction may be alleviated immediately and indefinitely. This may also result in relative realignment of the L7 vertebral body and the sacrum, which is superior rather than inferior to the preoperative position in that hyperextension may be reduced and the functional spinal unit is not being placed in forced flexion (Figures 26.3, 26.4, and 26.5).

The use of a titanium intervertebral cage as a stand-alone device or in combination dorsal fixation was recently investigated in vitro [19]. Application of the intervertebral device

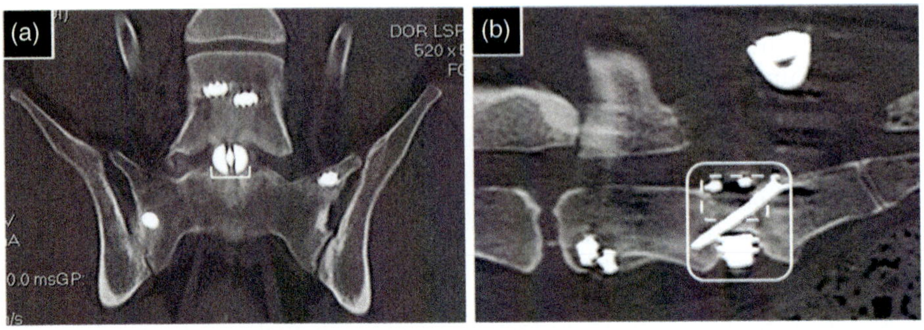

Figure 26.3 Measurement of L7-S1 endplate distraction on CT scan. (a) Dorsal plane measurements across the FITS™ spacer demonstrated over 80% increase from pre-operative values. (b) Sagittal plane measurements of entire intervertebral space (solid white) and dorsal segment (dashed) on sagittal view was up to twice that of the pre-operative distance and persistent at six months.

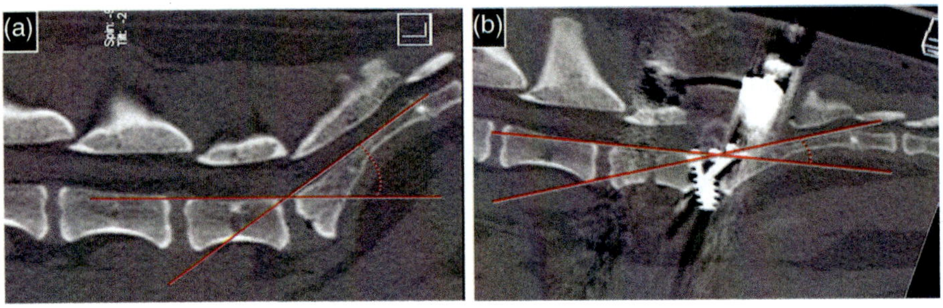

Figure 26.4 CT scan in the sagittal plane. Demonstration of the reduction in lumbosacral angle following application of the FITS-Fitzateur™ system. (a) Lumbosacral angle measured comparing the intersection of two lines projected across the dorsal aspect of the lumbar and sacral vertebral segments. (b) Angle postoperatively. Angle reduction is sustained through six-month follow up.

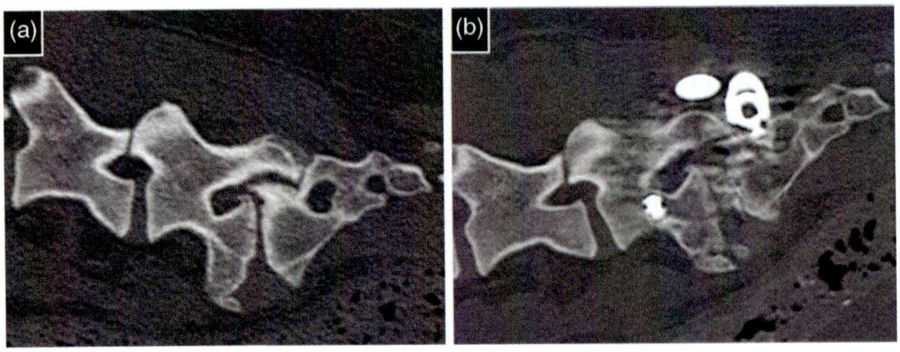

Figure 26.5 CT scan Parasagittal view. (a) Lateralized stenosis of the neuroforaminal aperture obscuring nerve root outflow at L7. (b) Application of FITS spacer between L7-S1 vertebral bodies generates ventral distraction of the impinged functional spinal unit. Realignment of vertebral bodies into greater flexion enhances neuroforaminal dimensions measured in the cranial-caudal and dorso-ventral plane. Significant opening of the neuroforaminal aperture was sustained at six months following surgery.

(a) (b)

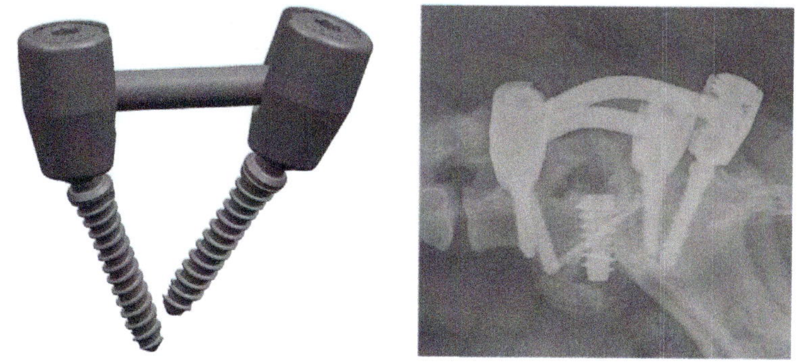

Figure 26.6 The Fitzateur™ dorsal fixation construct and the Fitz Intervertebral Traction Screw (FITS) spacer. (a) Schematic of the variable angle pedicle screw and locking system. Customization of the locking angle enables the surgeon to adapt the angle of pedicle screw placement. (b) Radiograph of dorsal fixation using the Fitzateur system. Dorsal fixation is achieved by careful pedicle screw placement into the vertebral bodies of L7 and the sacrum and linkage by the rod and locking clamp assembly. Screw size and angle are patient specific and derived from CT scan assessment to maximize bone purchase and avoid violation of any neural structures. Bilateral screws are linked by a unique "dumbbell" rod and clamp system dorsally between adjacent vertebral segments.

without supplementary fixation recapitulated a normal range of motion and resistance to bending and axial forces in spinal samples. Concurrent application of the spacer with dorsal fixation further enhanced lumbosacral segment stabilization. To date no system incorporating an intervertebral distraction device in combination dorsal fixation has yet been published for clinical patients clinically affected by DLSS.

The author has reported in abstract form the application of a novel titanium intervertebral spacer device in association with a dorsal screw and rod stabilization system using a multidirectional clamp system [20] (Figure 26.6). The distraction device is a conical screw of various sizes (Fitz Intervertebral Traction Screw, FITS™) that can be placed via dorsal laminectomy following dorsal annulectomy and nuclear extirpation. The nerves of the cauda equina are retracted laterally to permit intervertebralL7-S1 FITS placement (Figure 26.7). The device alleviates compression across the neuroforamina by distracting the end-plates of L7 and S1. An adjunctive dorsal fixation rod–clamp–screw system (Fitzateur, Figures 26.8 and 26.9) uses pedicle screws placed bilaterally in the body of L7 and in the alar wings of the sacrum and dorsally linked using clamps and rods to achieve rigid stabilization (Figure 26.3).

26.5.2.4.1 Objectives of the FITS–Fitzateur System

1. The FITS device is conical to facilitate passage past the nerve roots of the cauda equina, and also to be self-distracting – i.e. as it is driven, the end-plates are distracted.
2. The FITS device is manufactured in five diameters, with two lengths in each diameter, yielding 10 devices capable of deployment in patients of any size over 10 kg bodyweight.
3. The FITS device is coated in hydroxyapatite to encourage osseous on-growth and through-growth to facilitate interbody fusion (Figure 26.3b).
4. Back-out of the FITS device is prevented by application of a 2.4 mm screw through a slot in the device (Figures 26.3b and 26.6b).
5. Large-diameter 5 mm screws are employed for the dorsal Fitzateur system, which taper from their apex to base such that the hub of the screw subjacent to the head is largest at the maximum point of loading at the cis-cortex. The profile is designed to minimize possibility of screw breakage (Figure 26.8b).
6. The screws penetrate the L7 vertebral body abaxially at an angle that reduces the possibility for inadvertent penetration of

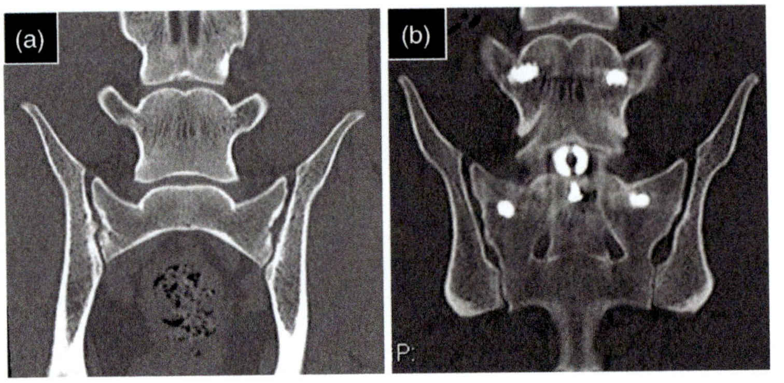

Figure 26.7 CT scan, dorsal plane, pre- (a) and post- (b) operatively. (b) Axial placement of FITS spacer between L7-S1 end plates with concurrent placement of a cross-locking screw directed caudoproximal to distocranial through the central aperture of the FITS™ device preventing screw backout. Accurate vertebral body screw placement is demonstrated within the cortices of L7 and S1 vertebral bodies.

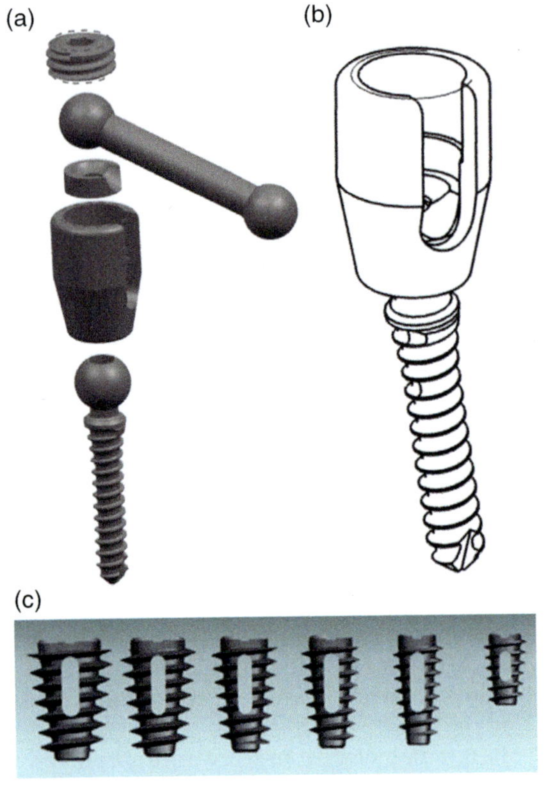

Figure 26.8 Multidirectional clamp-rod lumbosacral fixation system with tapered self-distracting screw spacer device. This constitutes a unique adjustable rod and locking system enabling variability in screw angle placement. (a) Demonstrates the individual components of the pedicle screw, rod, and locking system. (Fitzateur™) (b) Schematic of the screw-washer-clamp assembly. (c) Some examples of the various distraction devices available (Fitz Intervertebral Traction Screw, FITS).

the lateral recess of the L7 nerve roots (Figures 26.7 and 26.9).

7. The screws are bicortical in the L7 vertebral body, with the aim of increasing pullout strength (Figure 26.9).
8. The clamps, washers, and screwheads are specifically designed to allow multidirectional capability (Figure 26.8a). The angle between the rod and the screw connected via the clamp can vary from 37–124° (Figures 26.10b and c).
9. The clamp-rod connector system of the Fitzateur is designed such that the base of the clamp tapers so as to fit flush with the vertebral arch of L7 in the narrow angle between the lateral aspects of the L7 vertebral bodies and the wings of the ilii (Figure 26.8b).
10. The rods have ball-shaped enlargements on either end to fit inside C-shaped clamps such that collapse between clamps is prohibited (Figure 26.8).
11. Specific washers within each clamp allow compression of the ball-end of the rod with a locknut within the clamp to prevent loosening (Figure 26.8).
12. The rods can be bent in any direction and can be contoured over and flush with the articular facets to provide added rigidity by three-point contact – each end in clamps and the midpoint flush dorsal to the facet on either side (Figure 26.6b).

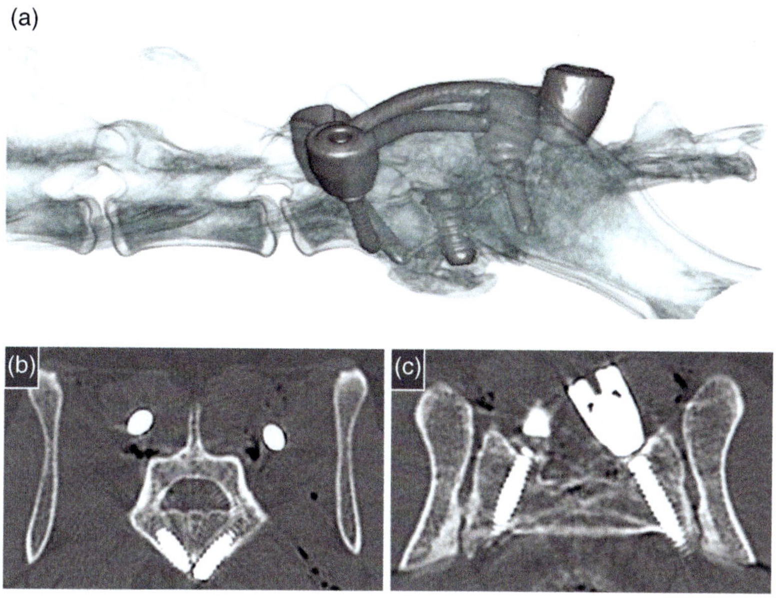

Figure 26.9 Lumbosacral distraction fusion using Fitz Intervertebral Traction Screw (FITS™) and Fitzateur assembly. (a) CT reconstruction following successful lumbosacral distraction fusion. FITS device in situ following dorsal annulectomy of L7-S1 with 2.4 mm locking screw applied to prevent device migration. Bilateral screws placed within vertebral bodies are linked with the angle-variable rod and clamp system designed to permit appropriate rod contouring. (b) Transverse plane CT scan of 7th lumbar vertebra demonstrating convergent screw placement within vertebral body. (c) Screws placed into the alar wings of S1 are divergent in the transverse axis. Bicortical screw placement is achieved in both L7 and S1 enhancing pullout strength and construct integrity (note that in larger dogs, bicortical fixation is not always achieved in the sacrum but should always be achieved in the L7 vertebral body).

26.6 Outcomes

There is a lack of standardization when it comes to classifying DLSS and this makes it difficult to compare outcomes between surgical approaches and even the outcomes between patients within a treatment group. An analysis of the published data suggests that around 80% of dogs will improve with surgical intervention and clinical signs will resolve for about 50% in the medium-to-long term with stabilization [21].

The FITS–Fitzateur distraction-stabilization technique allows immediate and indirect decompression of the neuroforaminae (Figure 26.10) without the potential for iatrogenic trauma to the L7 nerve roots, which could be associated with foraminotomy, and follow-up CT scan supports that foraminal decompression is sustained to at least six months postoperatively [3]. In a recent analysis of 21 clinical cases measured by CT scan, the dorsal to ventral neuroforaminal dimension mean across all zones (entry, middle, and exit) postoperatively was 107% greater than the preoperative measurement and sustained to 91% greater at six months. The sagittal distraction postoperative mean across the dorsal aspect of the LS intervertebral space was 99%, with 98% being maintained at six months post-operatively (Figure 26.3). Pre to postoperative reduction in LS angle was 41% with maintenance at 35% at six months postoperatively [3] (Figure 26.4).

We have performed mechanical testing of the FITS–Fitzateur system in vitro wherein instrumented lumbo-sacral spinal units were subjected to nondestructive four-point bending under compressive loading [6]. Angular displacement at L6-L7 and L7-S1 in flexion at 150 N was compared between three constructs (intact – laminectomy – instrumented). Dorsal laminectomy/discectomy resulted in a modest increase in the range of motion at L6-L7 and L7-S1 as compared with the intact spine when subjected to compressive loading. Application of

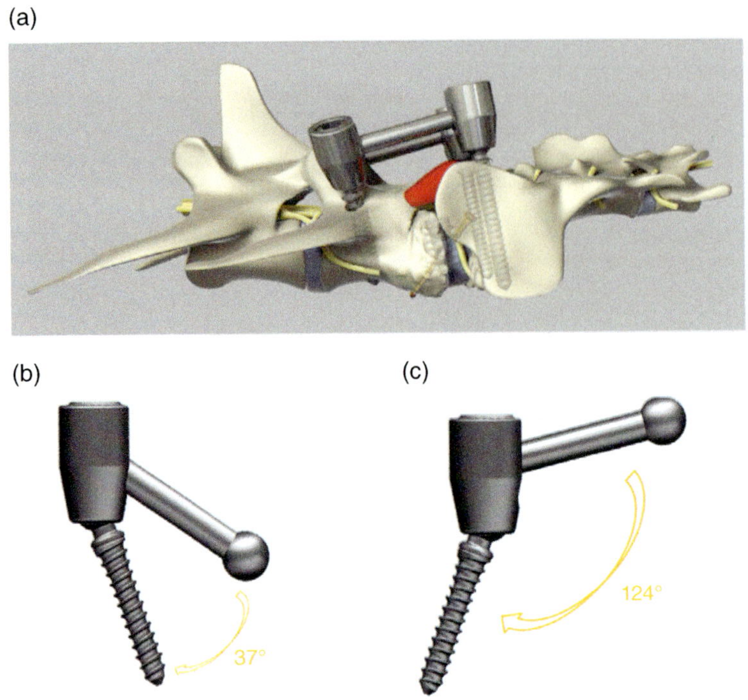

Figure 26.10 Multidirectional functionality of FITS – Fitzateur™ pedicle screws relative to clamp-rod fixation. (a) Schematic of Fitzateur™ and FITS assembly in-situ. Variable angulation of pedicle screws in L7 is independent of screw angulation in sacral body. (b) and (c) The angles between the rod, screw, and clamp construct allow for a screw-rod angle variation 37–124°. This linear angularity combines with a rotational freedom afforded by the spherical screw-clamp integration and dumbbell style connecting rod providing multiple degrees of freedom in construct morphology and screw placement.

the spinal instrumentation at L7-S1 resulted in a significant reduction in flexion, extension, and lateral bending at L7-S1 as compared with laminectomy alone but no significant change in motion at the L6-L7 junction. Therefore, the system should reliably stabilize the L7-S1 junction and, hopefully, in clinical cases longer term would not result in increased propensity for disease further cranially.

In a clinical study presented recently as an abstract pre-publication by the author, 73 dogs affected by DLSS where cauda equina and neuroforaminal stenosis was identified were operated using FITS-Fitzateur constructs [3]. According to owner and veterinary assessment at an average of 290 days, clinical signs improved for 72 dogs with one euthanized due to lack of response. Veterinary examination included musculature score, pain score, and lameness examination. Owner questionnaire included assessment of walking, sitting, rising, running, climbing stairs, getting into car and exercise more than 10 minutes in addition to perceived pain. Major complications included three surgical site infections and screw breakage in three cases where a 3.5 mm screw was employed, which we no longer deploy in clinical cases over 15 kg bodyweight. Minor complications included tail flaccidity in approximately 60% of cases, 90% of which resolved by 12 weeks postoperatively. Also, 4% were affected by transient urinary incontinence, all of which was resolved.

26.7 Conclusion

DLSS is a complex multifactorial disease for which treatment is challenging. Decompression by dorsal laminectomy has limited success where abaxial impingement of the L7 nerve roots is present. Foraminotomy may be successful, but longer-term instability or reocclusion can be problematic. Facet screw fixation following decompression may be fraught with failure because of facet breakage and paucity of surface area for attainment of fusion, plus residual static compression may persist. Locking plate systems have been deployed with limited success to achieve stabilization of the L7-S1 spinal segment but screw failure is common. Screws and pins with cement may be used to stabilize the LS junction in mild flexion, but implants may fail in this nonphysiologic position. Human pedicle screws provide rigidity of the LS functional spinal unit but static compression may remain. Deployment of a cage plus dorsal fixation has been explored in cadaver patients only and application *in vivo* has not yet been reported.

The application of a new conical intervertebral spacer device (FITS) that can be placed via a dorsal approach, in conjunction with a specifically designed vertebral body screw-clamp-rod construct (Fitzateur) has yielded favorable medium to long term clinical results. The author submits that distraction of the L7-S1 end-plates and neuroforamina plays a key role in the short and long-term success of this treatment. Further research is warranted into the categorization of lumbosacral disease and comparisons of the various modalities for surgical management of this challenging condition.

References

1. da Costa, R.C. and Johnson, J.A. (2012). Intervertebral and intravertebral ratios in Doberman pinscher dogs with cervical spondylomyelopathy. *Vet. Radiol. Ultrasound* 53 (5): 518–523.
2. Zindl, C., Fitzpatrick, N. (2014). Variations in lumbosacral intervertebral foraminal dimensions comparing parasagittal standard and oblique magnetic resonance imaging measurements in dogs with hyper- extended and neutral positioning. In: WVOC & VOS Abstracts. p. 12.
3. Fitzpatrick, N. (2017). Lumbosacral spine as a cause of lameness in dogs. In: American College of Veterinary Surgeons, 412–415.
4. Mattoon, J.S. and Koblik, P.D. (1993). Quantitative survey radiographic evaluation of the lumbosacral spine of normal dogs and dogs with degenerative lumbosacral stenosis. *Vet. Radiol. Ultrasound* 34: 194–206.
5. Worth, A.J., Hartman, A., Bridges, J.P. et al. (2017). Computed tomographic evaluation of dynamic alteration of the canine lumbosacral intervertebral neurovascular foramina. *Vet. Surg.* 46: 255–264.
6. Zindl, C., Tucker, R.L., Jov, J. et al. (2017). Effects of image plane, patient positioning, and foraminal zone on magnetic resonance imaging measurements of canine lumbosacral intervertebral foramina. *Vet. Radiol. Ultrasound* 58: 206–215.
7. Gomes, S.A., Lowrie, M., and Targett, M. (2017). Lateral foraminotomy as treatment for lumbosacral foraminal stenosis in forty-five dogs with degenerative lumbosacral stenosis. In: European College of Veterinary Neurology, 59.
8. Johnson, K. (2014). *Piermattei's Atlas of Surgical Approaches to the Bones and Joints of the Dog and Cat*, 33–45. Elsevier Health Sciences.
9. Smith, M.E.H., Bebchuk, T.N., Shmon, C.L. et al. (2004). An in vitro biomechanical study of the effects of surgical modification upon the canine lumbosacral spine. *VCOT Arch.* 17 (1): 17.
10. Meij, B.P., Suwankong, N., VenDerDeen, A.J. et al. (2007). Biomechanical flexion–extension forces in normal canine lumbosacral cadaver specimens before and after dorsal laminectomy_ discectomy and pedicle screw–rod fixation. *Vet. Surg.* 36 (8): 742–751.
11. Smolders, L.A., Kingma, I., Bergknut, N. et al. (2012). Biomechanical assessment of the effects of decompressive surgery in non-chondrodystrophic and chondrodystrophic canine multisegmented lumbar spines. *Eur. Spine J.* 21 (9): 1692–1699.
12. Jones, J.C., Davies, S.E., Werre, S.R. et al. (2008). Effects of body position and clinical signs on L7-S1 intervertebral foraminal area and lumbosacral angle in dogs with lumbosacral disease as measured via computed tomography. *Am. J. Vet. Res.* 69 (11): 1446–1454.
13. Hankin, E.J., Jerram, R.M., Walker, A.M. et al. (2012). Transarticular facet screw stabilization and dorsal laminectomy in 26 dogs with degenerative lumbosacral stenosis with instability. *Vet. Surg.* 41 (5): 611–619.
14. Golini, L., Kircher, P.R., Lewis, F.I. et al. (2014). Transarticular fixation with cortical screws combined with dorsal laminectomy and partial discectomy as surgical treatment of degenerative lumbosacral stenosis in 17 dogs: clinical and computed tomography follow-up. *Vet. Surg.* 43 (4): 405–413.
15. Nel, J.J., Kat, C.-J., Coetzee, G.L. et al. (2017). Biomechanical comparison between pins and polymethylmethacrylate and the SOP locking plate system to stabilize canine lumbosacral fracture-luxation in flexion and extension. *Vet. Surg.* 46 (6): 789–796.
16. Fitzpatrick, N., Egan, P., Murphy, S. et al. (2014). Lumbosacral distraction-fusion using an

intervertebral spacer and screw-rod fixation system for treatment of degenerative lumbosacral stenosis. In: 4th World Veterinary Orthopaedic Congress & 41st Veterinary Orthopedic Society Conference Abstracts. p. 8.

17. Zindl, C., Litsky, A.S., Fitzpatrick, N. et al. (2018). Kinematic behavior of a novel pedicle screw-rod fixation system for the canine lumbosacral joint. *Vet. Surg.* 47 (1): 114–124.
18. Tellegen, A.R., Willems, N., Tryfonidou, M.A. et al. (2015). Pedicle screw-rod fixation: a feasible treatment for dogs with severe degenerative lumbosacral stenosis. *BMC Vet. Res.* 11: 299.
19. Teunissen, M., van der Veen, A.J., Smit, T.H. et al. (2017). Effect of a titanium cage as a stand-alone device on biomechanical stability in the lumbosacral spine of canine cadavers. *Vet. J.* 220: 17–223.
20. Fitzpatrick, N. and Danielski, A. (2012). Lumbosacral distraction-fusion using a novel intervertebral distraction spacer and dorsally applied screw-rod fixation system for treatment of degenerative lumbosacral stenosis in 12 dogs [abstract]. 21st Annual scientific meeting Proceedings – small animals. 243.
21. Meij, B.P. and Bergknut, N. (2010). Degenerative lumbosacral stenosis in dogs. *Vet. Clin. North Am. Small Anim. Pract.* 40 (5): 983–1009.

Index

Page locators in **bold** indicate tables. Page locators in *italics* indicate figures.

Locking Plates in Veterinary Orthopedics, First Edition.
Edited by Matthew D. Barnhart and Karl C. Maritato.

Printed and bound by CPI Group (UK) Ltd, Croydon, CR0 4YY

21/09/2026

14965829-0001